Surgical Management of Inflammatory Eye Disease

Matthias D. Becker · Janet L. Davis (Eds.)

Surgical Management of Inflammatory Eye Disease

With 104 Figures and 26 Tables

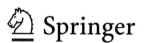

Matthias D. Becker, MD PhD FEBO MSc
Professor of Ophthalmology
Interdisciplinary Uveitis Center
Dept. of Ophthalmology
University of Heidelberg
Im Neuenheimer Feld 400
D-69120 Heidelberg
Germany

Current Address:
Department of Ophthalmology
Triemli Hospital Zürich
Co-chairman
Head of Posterior Segment & Uveitis Division
Birmensdorfer Str. 497
CH-8063 Zürich
Switzerland
Matthias.Becker@triemli.stzh.ch

Janet L. Davis, M.D.
Ophthalmology
University of Miami Bascom Palmer
900 NW 17th Street
33136 Miami, Florida, USA
Jdavis@med.miami.edu

ISBN 978-3-540-33861-1

e-ISBN 978-3-540-33862-8

DOI 10.1007/978-3-540-33862-8

Library of Congress Control Number: 2008925095

© 2008 Springer-Verlag Berlin Heidelberg

This work is subject to copyright. All rights are reserved, whether the whole or part of the material is concerned, specifically the rights of translation, reprinting, reuse of illustrations, recitation, broadcasting, reproduction on microfilm or in any other way, and storage in data banks. Duplication of this publication or parts thereof is permitted only under the provisions of the German Copyright Law of September 9, 1965, in its current version, and permission for use must always be obtained from Springer Verlag. Violations are liable to prosecution under the German Copyright Law.

The use of general descriptive names, registered names, trademarks, etc. in this publication does not imply, even in the absence of a specific statement, that such names are exempt from the relevant protective laws and regulations and therefore free for general use.

Cover design: Frido Steinen-Broo, eStudio Calamar, Spain
Production: le-tex publishing services oHG, Leipzig, Germany

Printed on acid-free paper

9 8 7 6 5 4 3 2 1

springer.com

Some copies of this book previously printed are missing chapter 7. If you are aware of such a copy, please return it to Springer for replacement.

The publisher and the authors accept no legal responsibility for any damage caused by improper use of the instructions and programs contained in this book and the DVD. Although the software has been tested with extreme care, errors in the software cannot be excluded.

Product liability: The publishers cannot guarantee the accuracy of any information about dosage and application contained in this book. In every individual case the user must check such information by consulting the relevant literature.

Foreword

If the number of jokes is any indication, surgeons and internists have a natural antipathy. Every first-year medical student should know the answer to: "How does a surgeon stop an elevator door from closing?" Only slightly fewer students are taught: "What do you call two ophthalmologists reading an electrocardiogram?" The answer is: a double blind study.

As an internist whose stomach becomes queasy at the sight of a suture, who better to comment on Matthias Becker's and Janet Davis' edited volume, *Surgical Treatment of Ocular Inflammation*? It is my pleasure to have this privilege.

While surgeons and internists do in general have different personalities and differing approaches to disease (internists halt the elevator doors with their hands; surgeons use their heads), their roles are ultimately complementary and the whole that results is truly greater than the sum of the parts. The morbidity of an operation can be avoided often by proper medical management, while the direction and ultimate success of medical therapy may need the assistance of a skillful surgeon.

In this internationally represented collection, Becker and Davis have approached a critical topic that has never been the subject of a single volume before. Their effort is richly illustrated, logically organized, and eminently practical. The accompanying 44 videos will prove a resource to many practitioners and to every training program.

Education, of course, prepares us for the future. One could argue that the rapidly expanding understanding of the immune response will markedly diminish the role of the surgeon in the care of patients with uveitis. I would argue the opposite. Although local therapy with intraocular corticosteroids is fraught with complications, mainly due to the medication's effect on the lens and trabecular meshwork, future, more targeted intraocular therapies have the potential for greater efficacy and less toxicity. And while biopsy now yields a specific diagnosis in the minority of instances, evolving molecular and surgical techniques could eventually make this approach routine.

I am sure that readers will find this volume to be timely and practical. I will read it wishing that my hand could be extricated from the elevator door, but grateful that my surgical colleagues are nearby to rescue me.

James T. Rosenbaum
Oregon Health & Science University

Preface

Intraocular inflammation comprises a wide variety of clinical entities. Its relative rarity makes diagnosis and therapy difficult. However, great progress has been made in the management of ocular inflammatory disorders as our knowledge has increased over the past decade, especially in the analysis of ocular specimens and in the use of immunosuppressive medication. We hope and expect that this is a prelude to even greater progress in this field.

Despite adequate medical therapy, ocular inflammatory diseases often cause secondary complications that require surgical intervention. The indications for surgical treatment, preoperative medical therapy, and intraoperative management require experience both as a surgeon and as a doctor managing ocular inflammatory disease in order to obtain successful outcomes with the best prognosis for the control of postoperative inflammation. We aim to improve the understanding of nonmedical therapy of ocular inflammatory disease so as to help the clinician who is faced with performing surgery on a patient with uveitis.

This book will provide the practitioner with practical information on planning surgical intervention in these difficult cases. It is designed to bridge the gap between primary research literature and daily practice. Although current and practical information is stressed, new research and trends are also highlighted. The book is designed to be user-friendly with numerous tables and illustrations. The "Core Messages" help the reader focus on the most important themes in each chapter. Finally, all procedures are explained in detail to facilitate their use by ophthalmologists in practice and in training.

In the first section, current thinking on the surgical treatment of uveitis is discussed in relation to invasive drug delivery and to surgery to modify uveitic activity. The emphasis is on drugs and devices used to influence inflammatory activity by local therapy.

The second section includes a wide variety of topics concerning the surgical treatment of uveitic complications, including general treatment strategies for uveitis. Diagnosis is discussed in relation to clinical decision making. Surgical procedures are comprehensively described.

The third section describes surgical biopsies for the diagnosis of ocular inflammatory disease and masquerades.

To our knowledge, this is the first book dealing with this topic. The book is accompanied by a DVD illustrating the various surgical procedures, making the book a "hands-on" experience. We hope to engage the reader's interest and look forward to feedback that will enhance the next edition.

The editors gratefully acknowledge the effort of the contributing authors who, despite intensive clinical and research work, found time to assist in the completion of this project. More than 30 internationally recognized leaders in ophthalmology have made a significant contribution through these pages to state-of-the-art surgery for uveitis.

We are indebted to the editorial and production staff at Springer for their commitment to timely publication. We thank Marion Philipp and Martina Himberger, who helped design this book's unique presentation.

We believe that the topics and authors that we have selected will improve understanding of the many facets of uveitis surgery and will contribute to better care for our patients. Our hope is that *Surgical Management of Inflammatory Eye Disease* will ultimately inspire clinicians to make further advances in this field.

Heidelberg, Miami
February 2008
Matthias D. Becker
Janet L. Davis

Contents

Part A
A Surgical Treatment of Uveitis

I Invasive Drug Delivery

1 Injectable Intraocular Corticosteroids . . 5
Paul A. Kurz, Eric B. Suhler,
Christina J. Flaxel, James T. Rosenbaum

2 Intraocular Corticosteroid Implants . . . 17
David Callanan

**3 Noncorticosteroid Intraocular Drug
Therapy** 23
Francine Behar-Cohen, Jean-Louis Bourges

II Surgery to Modify Uveitic Activity

**4 Therapeutic Vitrectomy for Noninfectious
Uveitis** 35
Kathrin Greiner, Andrew D. Dick

**5 Cryotherapy and Laser for Intermediate
Uveitis** 47
Javier A. Montero, Jose M. Ruiz-Moreno

Part B
**Surgical Treatment
of Uveitic Complications**

I Anterior Segment

Cornea

6 Surgery for Band Keratopathy 63
Ruth Lapid-Gortzak,
Jan Willem van der Linden,
Ivanka J. E. van der Meulen,
Carla P. Nieuwendaal

**7 Surgical Management of Diffuse
Corneal Opacities** 67
Thomas John

Lens

**8 Selection of Surgical Technique
for Complicated Cataract in Uveitis** . . . 85
Mauricio Miranda, Jorge L. Alió

9 Perioperative Medical Management . . . 99
Manfred Zierhut, Peter Szurman

10 Pars Plana Lensectomy 103
Emilio Dodds

**11 Extracapsular Extraction
by Phacoemulsification** 111
Antoine P. Brézin, Dominique Monnet

**12 Selection of Intraocular Lenses: Materials,
Contraindications, Secondary Implants** 121
Gerd U. Auffarth

**13 Management of Posterior Synechiae,
Peripheral Anterior Synechiae,
Iridocorneal Adhesions, and Iridectomy** 131
Yosuf El-Shabrawi

**14 Complications Post Cataract Surgery
in the Uveitic Eye** 137
Marie-José Tassignon, Dimitrios Sakellaris

15 Cataract Surgery in Childhood Uveitis . . 145
Arnd Heiligenhaus, Carsten Heinz,
Bahram Bodaghi

Glaucoma

**16 Surgical Management of Uveitis-Induced
Angle-Closure Glaucoma** 167
Kaweh Mansouri, Tarek Shaarawy

17 Surgical Management of Open-Angle Glaucoma Associated with Uveitis 173
Herbert P. Fechter, Richard K. Parrish II

18 Cyclodestructive Procedures 193
Torsten Schlote

II Posterior Segment

19 Macular Surgery for Posterior Segment Complications of Uveitis 203
Janet L. Davis

20 Surgical Treatment of Retinal Vasculitis with Occlusion, Neovascularization or Traction 209
Jose M. Ruiz-Moreno, Javier A. Montero

21 Surgical Treatment of Uveitic Complications: Retinal Detachment ... 219
Heinrich Heimann

22 Surgical Management of Ocular Hypotony 231
Mark Hammer, W. Sanderson Grizzard

Part C
Surgery for Diagnosis of Uveitis

23 Anterior Chamber Tap and Aqueous Humor Analysis 239
Uwe Pleyer, Justus G. Garweg

24 Surgery for the Diagnosis of Uveitis – Anterior Segment Biopsy 245
Bahram Bodaghi

25 Diagnostic Vitrectomy 255
Christoph M.E. Deuter, Sabine Biester, Karl Ulrich Bartz-Schmidt

26 Choroidal Biopsy 267
Christoph M.E. Deuter, Sabine Biester, Karl Ulrich Bartz-Schmidt

27 Retinal Biopsy 271
Janet L. Davis

Subject Index 277

Contributors

Jorge L. Alió, M.D. Ph.D., Prof.
Miguel Hernández University
Instituto oftalmologico de Alicante
Avda. de Denia, 111
03015 Alicante, Spain
jlalio@vissum.com

Gerd U. Auffarth, Prof. Dr.
University of Heidelberg
International Vision Correction Research Centre
(IVCRC)
Department of Ophthalmology
69120 Heidelberg, Germany
gerd_auffarth@med.uni-heidelberg.de

Karl Ulrich Bartz-Schmidt, Prof. Dr.
University of Tübingen
Department of Ophthalmology
Schleichstraße 12
72076 Tübingen, Germany
bartz-schmidt@med.uni-tuebingen.de

Francine Behar-Cohen, M.D.
INSERM, U598, Hôtel-Dieu
Department of Ophthalmology
15 rue de l'Ecole de Médecine
74006 Paris, France
behar@idf.inserm.fr

Sabine Biester, Dr.
University of Tübingen
Department of Ophthalmology
Schleichstraße 12
72076 Tübingen, Germany
sabine.biester@med.uni-tuebingen.de

Bahram Bodaghi, M.D.
Pierre and Marie Curie University
Pitié-Salpêtrière Hospital
Department of Ophthalmology
47–83 boulevard de l'Hopital
75651 Paris, Cedex 13, France
bahram.bodaghi@psl.aphp.fr

Jean-Louis Bourges, M.D.
INSERM U598, Hôtel-Dieu
Department of Ophthalmology
Paris, France

Antoine P. Brézin, M.D., Ph.D.
Université Paris 5, Faculté de Médecine
Service d'Ophtalmologie, Hôpital Cochin
27 rue du Faubourg Saint-Jacques
75679 Paris, Cedex 14, France
antoine.brezin@cch.aphp.fr

David Callanan, M.D.
Texas Retina Associates
Arlington, TX 76012 USA
dcallanan@texasretina.com

Janet L. Davis, M.D., M.A. Prof.
University of Miami, Bascom Palmer
Ophthalmology
900 NW 17th Street
33136 Miami, Florida, USA
jdavis@med.miami.edu

Christoph M.E. Deuter, Dr.
University of Tübingen
Department of Ophthalmology
Schleichstraße 12
72076 Tübingen, Germany
christoph.deuter@med.uni-tuebingen.de

**Andrew D. Dick, M.D., FRCOopth,
FRDS, FRCS, FRCP, Prof.**
Bristol Eye Hospital
Department of Ophthalmology
Lower Maudlin Street
Bristol, BS1 2LX, UK

Emilio Dodds, M.D.
Consultores Oftalmologicos
Buenos Aires, Argentina
emdodds@consultoresoftalmologicos.com

Yosuf El-Shabrawi, Prof. Dr.
University of Graz
Department of Ophthalmology
Auenbruggerplatz 4
8036 Graz, Austria
yosuf.elshabrawi@meduni-graz.at

Herbert P. Fechter, Dr. M.D.
Ophthalmology Service
Walter Reed Army Medical Center
Washington, DC, USA

Christina J. Flaxel, M.D., Ass. Prof.
Casey Eye Institute
3375 SW Terwilliger Blvd.
Portland, Oregon 97239-4197
USA

Justus G. Garweg, Prof. Dr.
Swiss Eye Institute
Bern, Switzerland

Kathrin Greiner, M.D., Ph.D.
St. Johns Eye Hospital
PO Box 19960
Sheikh Jarrah
Jerusalem 97200, Israel
greiner@doctors.org.uk

W. Sanderson Grizzard, M.D.
Retina Associates of Florida
Tampa, Florida, USA

Mark Hammer, M.D.
Retina Associates of Florida
Tampa, Florida, USA
drhammer@retinaassociatesflorida.com

Arnd Heiligenhaus, Prof. Dr.
Department of Ophthalmology
St. Franziskus Hospital
Hohenzollernring 74
48145 Muenster, Germany
arnd.heiligenhaus@uveitis-Zentrum.de

Heinrich Heimann, Prof. Dr.
Consultant Ophthalmic Surgeon
St. Paul's Eye Unit
Royal Liverpool University Hospital
Liverpool, UK
heinrichheimann@yahoo.de

Carsten Heinz, Dr.
St. Franziskus Hospital
Department of Ophthalmology
Hohenzollernring 74
48145 Muenster
Germany

Thomas John, MD
Loyola University at Chicago
Thomas John Vision Institute
10315 South Cicero Avenue
Oak Lawn, Illinous 60453
USA
tjcornea@gmail.com

Paul A. Kurz, M.D.
Casey Eye Institute
3375 SW Terwilliger Blvd.
Portland, Oregon 97239-4197
USA

Ruth Lapid-Gortzak, M.D.
Academic Medical Centre, University of Amsterdam
Amsterdam, the Netherlands
Cornea, External Diseases, and Cataract Service
Department of Ophthalmology
Retina Total Eye Care—Refractive Surgery Clinic
Driebergen, The Netherlands
r.lapid@amc.uva.nl

Jan Willem van der Linden, B.Optom.
Retina Total Eye Care – Refractive Surgery Clinic
Traay 42
3971 GP Driebergen
The Netherlands

Kaweh Mansouri, M.D., M.P.H.
University of Geneva
Glaucoma Sector
Ophthalmology Service
Department of Clinical Neurosciences
Geneva, Switzerland
kaweh.mansouri@ophtal.vd.ch

Ivanka J.E. van der Meulen, M.D.
Academic Medical Centre, University of Amsterdam
Cornea, External Diseases, and Cataract Service
Department of Ophthalmology
Amsterdam, The Netherlands

Mauricio Miranda, M.D., M.Sc.
Instituto de Ojos Oftalmosalud
Avenida Javier Prado Este 1142
Lima 27 San Isidro, Peru
mauricio_mvfmd@hotmail.com

Dominique Monnet, M.D.
Université Paris 5, Faculté de Médecine
Service d'Ophtalmologie, Hôpital Cochin
Paris, France

Javier A. Montero, M.D.
Pio del Rio Hortega University Hospital
Instituto Oftalmológico de Alicante, VISSUM
Valladolid, Spain
msm02va@wanadoo.es

Carla P. Nieuwendaal, M.D.
Academic Medical Centre, University of Amsterdam
Cornea, External Diseases, and Cataract Service
Department of Ophthalmology
Amsterdam, The Netherlands

Richard K. Parrish, II, M.D.
Bascom Palmer Eye Institute
University of Miami Miller School of Medicine
Miami, Florida, USA
rparrish@med.miami.eu

Uwe Pleyer, Prof. Dr.
Charité, Universitätsmedizin Berlin
Campus Virchow-Klinikum
Department of Ophthalmology
Augustenburger Platz 1
13353 Berlin, Germany
uwe.pleyer@charite.de

James T. Rosenbaum, M.D., Prof.
Casey Eye Institute
3375 SW Terwilliger Blvd.
Portland, Oregon 97239-4197
USA

Jose M. Ruiz-Moreno, M.D.
Castilla La Mancha University School of Medicine
Department of Ophthalmology
Albacete, Spain
Instituto Oftalmológico de Alicante, VISSUM
Alicante, Spain
josemaria.ruiz@uclm.es

Dimitrios Sakellaris, M.D.
Antwerp University Hospital
City Campus
Gratiekapelstraat 10
2000 Antwerp
Belgium

Torsten Schlote, Prof. Dr.
Clinic Ambimed
Klingenstrasse 9
4057 Basel
Switzerland
basel@ambimed.ch

Tarek Shaarawy, MD, PhD
University of Geneva
Department of Clinical Neurosciences
Ophthalmology Service
Geneva, Switzerland
tarek.shaarawy@hcuge.ch

Marc D. de Smet, MDCM, PhD, FRCSC, Prof.
University of Amsterdam
Department of Ophthalmology
ZNA Middelheim Campus
Antwerp, Belgium
mddesmet1@mac.com

Eric B. Suhler, M.D., M.P.H., Ass. Prof.
Casey Eye Institute
3375 SW Terwilliger Blvd.
Portland, Oregon 97239-4197
USA
and Department of Ophthalmology
Portland Veterans Administration Medical Center
Portland, Oregon, USA

Peter Szurman, P.D., Dr.
University of Tübingen
Department of Ophthalmology
Schleichstraße 12
72076 Tübingen
Germany

Marie-José Tassignon, M.D., Ph.D., F.E.B.O.
Antwerp University Hospital
Department of Ophthalmology
Antwerp, Belgium
marie-jose.tassignon@uza.be

Manfred Zierhut, Prof. Dr.
University of Tübingen
Department of Ophthalmology
Schleichstraße 12
72076 Tübingen, Germany
manfred.zierhut@med.uni-tuebingen.de

Part A

A Surgical Treatment of Uveitis

I Invasive Drug Delivery

Chapter 1

Injectable Intraocular Corticosteroids

Paul A. Kurz, Eric B. Suhler, Christina J. Flaxel, James T. Rosenbaum

Core Messages

- Although risks are present, intravitreal corticosteroid injection is a relatively safe and effective treatment in a variety of conditions.
- Risks of intravitreal steroid injection include, but are not limited to, elevation of intraocular pressure, infection, cataract, retinal detachment, and central retinal artery occlusion.
- Although most observations regarding intravitreal corticosteroid injection derive from treating diabetic macular edema and age-related macular degeneration, this approach is beneficial in a number of uveitic conditions.

Contents

1.1	Introduction	5
1.2	Types and Formulations	6
1.3	Doses	6
1.4	Distribution After Injection	6
1.5	Duration of Effect and Frequency of Injections	6
1.6	Mechanism of Action	7
1.7	Risks	7
1.7.1	Elevation of Intraocular Pressure	7
1.7.2	Infectious Endophthalmitis	8
1.7.3	Sterile Inflammatory Reaction	8
1.7.4	Pseudoendophthalmitis	8
1.7.5	Cataract	9
1.7.6	Retinal Detachment and Vitreous Hemorrhage	9
1.7.7	Central Retinal Artery Occlusion	9
1.7.8	Central Serous Chorioretinopathy	9
1.7.9	Toxic Effects	9
1.8	Steps of Administration	9
1.9	Uses	10
1.9.1	Retinal Disease and Surgery	10
1.9.2	Uveitis and Ocular Inflammation	10
1.9.2.1	Cystoid Macular Edema	10
1.9.2.2	Sarcoidosis	12
1.9.2.3	Behçet's Disease	12
1.9.2.4	Eales Disease	12
1.9.2.5	Vogt-Koyanagi-Harada Syndrome	12
1.9.2.6	Sympathetic Ophthalmia	12
1.9.2.7	Choroidal Neovascularization	12
1.9.2.8	Toxoplasmic Retinochoroiditis	12
1.9.2.9	Hypotony	13
1.9.2.10	Endophthalmitis	13
1.10	Future	13
References		14

This chapter contains the following video clip on DVD: Video 1 shows Injection of intraocular Corticosteroids (Surgeon: Christina J. Flaxel).

1.1 Introduction

Corticosteroids have been used to treat ocular inflammation since the 1950s [1]. Use of systemic corticosteroids subjects the patient to numerous side effects. Local therapy with drops or injections can minimize side effects. Periocular or intravitreal injections can be particularly useful, if tolerated, in patients with unilateral disease that is not amenable to topical therapy alone. If systemic manifestations of the disease exist, or if ocular disease is bilateral and repeat injection, particularly frequently repeated intravitreal injection, is necessary, use of a systemic steroid-sparing immunosuppressive agent may be a better option.

Prednisolone acetate drops are often effective in cases in which the inflammation is restricted to the anterior chamber. However, adequate levels are not achieved in the vitreous cavity and retina. Periocular corticosteroid injection can be useful in many cases of inflammation involving the posterior segment, but most experts find that intraocular delivery is more potent.

In the late 1970s, Machemer and McCuen established the safety of intravitreal triamcinolone acetonide (TA) and studied its effect on intraocular proliferation [2, 3]. Intravitreal injection has the advantage of delivering the drug more directly to the target tissue. However, a trade-off is increased risk of complications that arise from injection directly into the eye.

By the late 1990s, there was increased clinical study of intravitreal TA as a treatment for conditions including refractory macular edema and choroidal neovascularization [4–6]. Although the United States Food and Drug Administration has not approved this indication, intravitreal injection of TA became commonplace after 2002. With the advent of various intravitreal anti-vascular endothelial growth factor (anti-VEGF) injections, the use of TA has declined for treatment of neovascular age-related macular degeneration. However, it still remains a useful option in a number of conditions, many of which are uveitic.

1.2 Types and Formulations

While a number of forms of corticosteroids exist, in most cases triamcinolone acetonide is the preferred formulation for injection into the eye. It is a minimally water-soluble suspension and acts essentially as a depot of sustained-release crystals when injected into the vitreous cavity. This leads to a longer half-life compared to more water-soluble forms such as dexamethasone. In cases in which intraocular pressure (IOP) rise is a significant concern, a corticosteroid with a shorter half-life is sometimes used. This, in theory, may decrease the risk of prolonged IOP rise, but may also decrease the duration of effect.

Triamcinolone acetonide has been commonly purchased in single-dose vials at a concentration of 40 mg/ml. Some patients may have a sterile inflammatory reaction to the injection. This is thought to be due to an additive in the formulation rather than the triamcinolone itself. Various methods exist for purifying the drug for injection, and preservative-free formulations are now available. Centrifugation removes most benzyl alcohol and thus reduces potential toxic effects [7]. One retrospective study of 310 eyes that received intravitreal TA suggested that sterile inflammatory reactions may be more common in uveitic eyes than in eyes without an underlying inflammatory predilection. In this study, 4 of 20 uveitic eyes experienced a sterile inflammatory reaction. By contrast, only 2 of 290 eyes treated for non-inflammatory posterior segment disease developed this complication [8]. This finding has not been validated by other investigators to date.

1.3 Doses

The typical dose injected in the United States is currently 4 mg. At the time of this writing, the SCORE (Standard of Care versus Corticosteroids for Retinal Vein Occlusion) Study is investigating the use of 1-mg versus 4-mg injections, versus placebo. In Europe, 25-mg injections have been used [9].

1.4 Distribution After Injection

In a study of 20 patients, following injection of a high dose (20–25 mg) of TA into the vitreous cavity, TA was not detectable in serum samples of 90% of the patients. Two patients showed marginally detectable amounts of serum TA, one at 5 days after injection and the other at 7 days after injection [1, 10].

Studies comparing the intravitreal concentration of TA after periocular injection to those after intravitreal injection have been performed. One study of vitreous samples from 12 patients, six of whom had intravitreal injection and six of whom had periocular injection, showed higher concentrations of TA after intravitreal injection [11]. A study by Thomas compared the intravitreal concentrations of TA after sub-Tenon injection in 20 patients versus that after intravitreal injection in 5 patients previously reported by Beer et al. The findings showed that, in some cases, intravitreal concentrations after sub-Tenon injection were comparable to those after intravitreal injection [1, 12].

1.5 Duration of Effect and Frequency of Injections

The duration of effect of intravitreal TA appears to be dose-dependent and is considerably shorter in vitrectomized patients. In the absence of vitrectomy, doses of 20 mg give a duration of effect of 6–9 months while the more typical dose of 4 mg shows a duration of effect of 4–6 months, although a longer duration can be seen [11]. Jonas showed that up to 8 months after injection of 25 mg of TA into eyes that had previous pars plana vitrectomy with silicone oil endotamponade, detectable levels of TA were present in extracted silicone oil samples [13].

Beer showed that after a single 4-mg injection, the mean elimination half-life was 18.6 days. In eyes that had undergone vitrectomy, the mean elimination half-life was 3.2 days. However, considerable variation of peak concentration and half-life occurred among subjects. The range of measurable concentration of intravitreal triamcinolone in humans was 71–132 days. This is longer than the 42 days of measurable dexamethasone concentration >1 μg/ml in rabbits after receiving a dexamethasone sustained delivery device (DEX-BDD, Posurdex™) [1].

Reinjection can be considered if necessary after the effect from the prior injection is likely to have faded. If clinical signs suggest worsening of a condition that had improved after the first injection, reinjection would ideally occur before more pronounced worsening. Obviously, the risk–benefit ratio of reinjection must be considered. Retreatment has been performed as often as every month to every 3–6 months [14].

1.6 Mechanism of Action

The exact mechanism(s) by which intravitreal TA has its effects is not fully known. Glucocorticoids appear to have a variety of actions, including inhibition of expression of genes contributing to inflammation and thus decreased production of cytokines, enzymes, receptors, and adhesion molecules [15]. They have been shown to interfere with fibroblast and endothelial cell function and reduce fluid transudation. In animal studies, they have been shown to inhibit neovascularization. Studies have also documented reduction of endothelial cell permeability and down-regulation of inflammatory markers [16–18].

A common use of intravitreal triamcinolone is for treatment of macular edema. It is thought that in most cases, macular edema develops following breakdown of the inner blood–retinal barrier. The breakdown of the outer blood–retinal barrier with disruption of the tight junctions between RPE cells may also play a role. TA stabilizes the blood–retinal barrier. It may also down-regulate the production of VEGF, which has been shown to be a vascular permeability factor that may be released by ischemic retina in diabetes mellitus. Inhibition of prostaglandins, which are known vascular permeability factors, may be an additional mechanism for reduction of macular edema [19, 20].

1.7 Risks

There are a number of risks associated with intravitreal TA injection. Explanation of these risks to the patient should be documented with a written informed consent. The patient should be aware that further intervention may be needed, the problem may not be rectified, and that vision or even the eye could conceivably be lost as a result of the procedure. The patient should be warned to contact the ophthalmologist with any concerns and definitely for symptoms of worsening pain, worsening vision, increasing redness, flashes, and symptoms of retinal detachment.

1.7.1 Elevation of Intraocular Pressure

Corticosteroids taken by any route can increase intraocular pressure (IOP). Obviously, the most direct way for corticosteroids to produce ocular effects, both good and bad, is application directly into the eye. While in some cases of hypotony, the IOP-raising effect can be beneficial, in most cases it is an unwanted side effect. Elevated IOP can occur immediately after injection or develop up to 7 months after injection [21].

A study by Rhee et al. of 570 consecutive eyes of 536 patients who underwent intravitreal TA (4 mg/0.1 cc) revealed that a baseline IOP of greater than 16 was a risk factor for developing IOP elevation after intravitreal injection. In addition, receiving a second injection of TA increased the risk of IOP elevation. Of eyes receiving a single injection, 53.2% had IOP elevation. This included 50.6% experiencing an elevation of at least 30% of baseline, 45.8% experiencing an elevation of 5 mmHg or more, and 14.2% experiencing an elevation of 10 mmHg or more. Of eyes receiving a second injection, 65.1% experienced IOP elevation of at least 30% [22].

Cardillo et al. studied 12 patients with bilateral diabetic macular edema and randomly assigned one eye of each patient to receive 4 mg of TA intravitreally and the fellow eye to receive 40 mg of TA by posterior sub-Tenon's injection. Interestingly, IOP did not show any statistically significant difference between the two delivery routes at 1, 3, and 6 months. While a controlled IOP elevation was noted in a number of the treated eyes, no eyes in that study had an increase in IOP above 25 mmHg [23]. Another small study of 28 eyes in 28 patients showed a significant increase in the mean IOP at 4 and 8 weeks after sub-Tenon's TA injection, while there was a smaller but significant IOP increase in the intravitreal TA group at 8 weeks only [24]. Other larger studies have shown IOP rise in 27% [25] and 36% [26] after sub-Tenon's injection of TA. Hayashi's study of 60 patients showed the incidence of IOP rise to be less when 40 mg of TA was injected by retrobulbar route than when 4 mg was injected intravitreally [27].

A study of patients with uveitic CME suggested that younger patients are more likely to have IOP rise in response to intravitreal TA injection. In this study, an IOP rise greater than 10 mmHg was more likely in patients younger than 40 years of age (61%) than in those older than 40 years of age (30%) [28].

Obviously patients who have had increased IOP in response to corticosteroids administered by another route in the past are more likely to have increased IOP in response to intravitreal corticosteroids. Depending upon the amount of IOP elevation and the ability to control the IOP in the past, intravitreal injection may still be a reasonable option.

Some advocate a trial with topical corticosteroid drops for several weeks prior to intravitreal injection to determine if patients are "steroid responders." This may be beneficial in filtering out the patients likely to have the worst IOP responses but is certainly not foolproof. In addition, it would essentially delay the time to effective posterior segment treatment and, particularly in cases of macular edema (ME), earlier treatment may lead to better visual outcome. In one study, despite exclusion of patients who had a rise of IOP greater than 15 mmHg after 1 month of treatment with 0.1% dexamethasone drops, 50% of patients who received intravitreal TA had an IOP rise [29].

It is generally thought that patients with chronic open-angle glaucoma (COAG) are more likely to be steroid responders, although one study did not show any difference in postinjection IOP in patients with or without COAG. This may have been related to a small sample size of COAG patients [30].

In many cases of steroid responders, the IOP returns to normal as the duration of steroid effect is exceeded. However, IOP can remain persistently elevated. Some suggest that intractable glaucoma is more common after intravitreal TA in cases of macular edema due to central retinal vein occlusion (CRVO) than in other indications for intravitreal TA injection [18].

1.7.2 Infectious Endophthalmitis

Recent studies have reported the incidence of infectious endophthalmitis following intravitreal injection of TA to range from 0% (0/700) to 0.87% (8/992) [31]. Sterile technique can help reduce the risk of endophthalmitis. Particularly important is instillation of povidone-iodine drops (either 5% or 10%; the 5% solution is less irritating to the cornea and conjunctiva) directly onto the injection site prior to injection. Some also advocate use of an antibiotic drop (commonly a fluoroquinolone) just before the injection and 4 times a day for 3–5 days following the injection. Use of a single-injection vial of TA, or at least a brand new bottle, for each injection is also recommended. Based on animal studies, some have suggested that intravitreal methotrexate injection may reduce the risk of development of infectious endophthalmitis and may be a safer alternative to corticosteroid injection in the treatment of noninfectious uveitis [32].

Signs and symptoms of infectious endophthalmitis can develop at any time following intravitreal TA injection, but will typically appear by postinjection day 5. In one retrospective study of eight patients who developed postinjection endophthalmitis, the median time to presentation was 7.5 days. Characteristic symptoms were pain, redness, blurry vision secondary to iritis, vitritis, and/or hypopyon [33]. However, one must keep in mind that patients with infectious endophthalmitis following intravitreal corticosteroid injection may not experience the level of pain typically experienced in eyes without intraocular steroids [31]. Despite aggressive and early treatment, visual outcomes may be poor.

There is one report of de novo development of cytomegalovirus (CMV) retinitis in an immunocompetent patient who received intravitreal TA [34]. Thankfully this appears to be quite rare. There is also a report of CMV retinitis developing in a patient after a fluocinolone acetonide (Retisert™) implant. This patient had numerous periocular and intravitreal corticosteroid injections in the contralateral eye but only developed CMV retinitis in the eye with the fluocinolone acetonide implant [35].

1.7.3 Sterile Inflammatory Reaction

If a sterile inflammatory reaction develops, it typically does so within 2 days following intravitreal TA injection. This inflammatory reaction is thought to be a response to a chemical used in the formulation of TA. Typically, patients can present with symptoms similar to that of infectious endophthalmitis. However, visual outcomes are generally good [36]. Since preservative-free formulations of TA are used in the SCORE study, additional data on the incidence of infectious and noninfectious endophthalmitis plus data on the effectiveness and potential benefits of preservative-free formulations may soon be available [18].

1.7.4 Pseudoendophthalmitis

Pseudoendophthalmitis occurs when TA crystals move into the anterior chamber and form a "pseudohypopyon." This occurs most often in pseudophakic and aphakic patients, although it has been described in phakic patients. The patients typically do not experience any pain and the pseudohypopyon resolves. The eye is frequently otherwise quiet.

1.7.5 Cataract

Corticosteroids are a well-known cause of cataract, particularly posterior subcapsular cataract (PSC). Thus, although increased visual acuity is often noticed relatively soon after intravitreal corticosteroid injection, over time, visually significant cataracts may form and may require cataract surgery.

A recent retrospective study of 93 eyes that received a 4-mg TA injection showed visually significant PSC formation in almost 50% by 1 year after injection. Patients younger than 50 years of age had about half the rate of progression compared to patients over 50. There were slight increases in the formation of nuclear sclerotic and cortical cataracts as well [21].

Another study of 33 eyes found that 2 years after injection, nuclear sclerosis increased in 9.1% of eyes, cortical cataracts increased in 12.1%, while PSC increased in 24.2% over that same time period. This study also found that PSC progression was much more frequent in eyes with at least a 5-mmHg rise in IOP [37, 38].

1.7.6 Retinal Detachment and Vitreous Hemorrhage

Retinal detachment and vitreous hemorrhage have been reported following intravitreal injection [39]. Conceivably, with introduction of triamcinolone into the vitreous, disruption of the vitreous could take place. This could lead to traction on the retina, retinal tears, and subsequent retinal detachment. In addition, if during the process of injection, traumatic damage occurs to the retina, retinal holes, retinal detachment, or vitreous hemorrhage may occur. These complications are rare, and in a recent study of 348 eyes by Jonas, none developed rhegmatogenous retinal detachment [30].

1.7.7 Central Retinal Artery Occlusion

Central retinal artery occlusion (CRAO) may occur immediately following an intravitreal injection if the postinjection IOP is high enough to stop retinal artery perfusion. Careful examination to ensure retinal vessel perfusion should be done immediately following the procedure. If postinjection IOP is sufficiently high to prevent adequate retinal vessel perfusion, an immediate anterior chamber paracentesis should be performed to lower the IOP and allow reperfusion of the retinal vessels before permanent retinal damage and cell death from ischemia can occur. Intraocular pressure should be documented soon after the injection and checked again in approximately 30 minutes to make sure the pressure is not rising and is at a safe level prior to discharging the patient home.

1.7.8 Central Serous Chorioretinopathy

Corticosteroids are known to exacerbate central serous chorioretinopathy (CSCR). Development of CSCR has been reported following vitrectomy with intravitreal TA [40]. It is unclear whether this represented a true cause-and-effect relationship. CSCR has also been reported with periocular corticosteroid injection treatment for HLA-B27-associated iritis [41].

1.7.9 Toxic Effects

Although the lack of toxicity of intravitreal TA has been documented in rabbits and widespread clinical use has proven beneficial in many cases, in vitro evidence for toxicity to human retinal pigment epithelium (ARPE-19) cells exists. At in vitro concentrations of 1 mg/ml, ARPE-19 cell viability was reduced to the greatest extent by the commercially available TA (including the vehicle preserved with benzyl alcohol), to a lesser extent by the vehicle alone, and least by preservative-free TA. While 1 mg/ml vitreous concentrations are theoretically achieved with clinical injection, it is thought that this probably does not indicate the actual exposure to cells in their biologic environment [42].

1.8 Steps of Administration

The following steps go along with the technique used in the video accompanying this chapter. There are multiple variations to this technique which are acceptable. Of note, many experts skip the subconjunctival injection of lidocaine described in step 4, and simply use a cotton swab pledgitt soaked in tetracaine or proparacaine for anesthesia. In addition, 30-gauge needles are quite prone to clogging with the preserved formulation of triamcinolone; this can complicate the injection. The clogging of the needle can lead to the needle actually rocketing off the syringe prior to or during the injection process. Many experts advocate the use of 27-gauge needles for triamcinolone injection to decrease the likelihood of these complications. Of note, some formulations of preservative-free triamcinolone are more easily able to make it through a 30-gauge needle. It seems that the preservative-free preparations may be cleared from the vitreous faster. The increased particle surface area is thought to account for this.

Acceptable sterile techniques vary as well. The crucial point is that the triamcinolone being injected and the needle remain sterile. It is important that the antiseptic, betadine, be used to prepare the injection site. This can be accomplished without sterile gloves and drapes. The use of topical antibiotics is less important and not essential, although in practice they are frequently used. Some argue that the eyelid speculum is unnecessary. Many do not wear the indirect headpiece for viewing while injecting. The needle tip is simply aimed towards the optic nerve head and the injection performed.

1. Place 2 drops of topical anesthetic in the eye to be treated.
2. Prep the eye to be treated with a prepackaged povidone-iodine swab × 2.
3. Place a drop of 5% povidone-iodine in the cul-de-sac.
4. After scrubbing and donning sterile gloves, in a sterile fashion, draw up the subconjunctival injection of 2% lidocaine with epinephrine 0.5 cc (from a fresh vial daily) and the triamcinolone 0.2 ml from a freshly opened vial. A sterile cotton tip is soaked in tetracaine solution. A 30-gauge needle is placed on both the anesthetic syringe and the triamcinolone syringe, but the solution is not pushed through.
5. Place a sterile lid speculum between the eyelids.
6. Place the topical-anesthetic soaked cotton tip on the conjunctiva for approximately 1 minute, then inject the local anesthetic to balloon the conjunctiva, using the cotton tip to disperse the anesthetic.
7. Using a sterile caliper, measure 4 mm from the limbus (in a phakic eye) or 3 mm from the limbus in a pseudophakic or aphakic eye.
8. Push the triamcinolone through to the tip of the needle to 0.1 cc total, and using a sterile cotton tip to stabilize the eye, inject 0.1 cc of triamcinolone into the vitreous cavity while observing the needle tip. Remove the needle and place a sterile cotton tip over the needle entry site for several seconds.
9. Immediately place a drop of topical broad-spectrum antibiotic solution over the injection site.
10. Observe the retina for perfusion of the central retinal artery.
11. Clean the eye, especially irrigating profusely with sterile water to remove all povidone-iodine solution.
12. Check the intraocular pressure 30 minutes post procedure and discharge if at a safe level.

1.9 Uses

Given that uveitis is relatively rare compared to macular degeneration and retinal vascular causes of macular edema, much of the data we have regarding the use of intravitreal TA is from the retinal literature. Nonetheless, intravitreal TA has been used numerous times for treatment in uveitis as well.

1.9.1 Retinal Disease and Surgery

Common retinal uses for intravitreal TA include treatment of macular edema in various diseases (including diabetes, central retinal vein occlusion, branch retinal vein occlusion, juxtafoveal telangiectasia, retinitis pigmentosa), neovascular age-related macular degeneration, Coats' disease, proliferative vitreoretinopathy (PVR), proliferative diabetic retinopathy, neovascularization of the iris (rubeosis iridis), as a visual aid in vitrectomy surgery, and as an adjunct in cataract surgery. Detailed discussion of the use in these conditions is beyond the scope of this text.

1.9.2 Uveitis and Ocular Inflammation

By definition, uveitis involves ocular inflammation. Macular edema can be a complication of many forms of uveitis. Thus, it is not surprising that intravitreal TA can be of significant benefit as a local therapy for uveitis. Local therapy to control inflammation and treat macular edema could allow the patient to avoid or reduce systemic immunosuppression.

1.9.2.1 Cystoid Macular Edema

Cystoid macular edema (CME) is a significant cause of vision loss in patients with uveitis. Inflammatory "pseudophakic" CME can also cause vision loss following cataract surgery. Dramatic improvement in uveitic CME can occur with intravitreal TA injection (Figs. 1.1 and 1.2). As with other causes of CME, eradication of uveitic CME can, but does not always, correlate with improved visual acuity.

Kok et al. studied the effect of intravitreal injection of 4 mg of TA in 65 eyes of 54 patients with uveitis-related CME. Mean follow-up time was 8 months, and the best visual acuity occurred at a mean of 4 weeks following injection. They reported that 83% had a detectable improvement in visual acuity, of which 51% had at least either two Snellen lines or three Early Treatment Diabetic Retinopathy Study (ETDRS) lines of improvement. One third of those that initially improved had subsequent worsening of their visual acuity that correlated with worsening of CME in all cases. Mean follow-up time for this group was 12.1 months. Two thirds maintained visual improvement for the follow-up period, but the mean follow-up period for this group was shorter (mean 6.7 months, range 3–13 months). Visual acuity in eyes with CME for greater than 24 months improved least while those with CME less than or equal to 12 months improved most. The mean improvement in visual acuity was only statistically significant in patients less than or equal to 60 years of age [28].

Intravitreal TA may improve CME secondary to birdshot retinochoroidopathy, immune recovery uveitis, chronic idiopathic uveitis, panretinal photocoagulation, multifocal choroiditis, refractory pseudophakic CME, and for treatment of CME and simultaneous reduction of graft rejection in patients who have undergone penetrating keratoplasty [30, 43–47]. In addition, patients with known uveitis at high risk for developing CME fol-

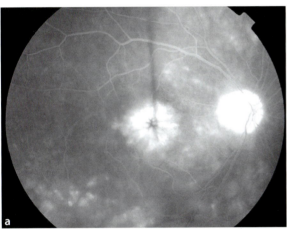
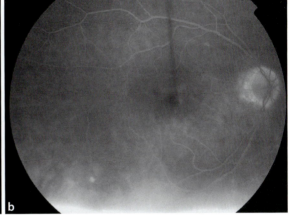

Fig. 1.1 A patient with a history of multifocal choroiditis, retinal vasculitis, and CME. **a** Late-phase fluorescein angiogram showing significant leakage consistent with CME. Visual acuity measured 20/70−1. **b** Late-phase fluorescein angiogram of the same eye 3 months following treatment with 4 mg of TAAC by intravitreal injection. The leakage has improved significantly, but the visual acuity only improved to 20/60

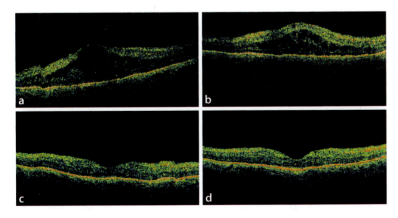

Fig. 1.2 OCT was used to document the response of CME in a 37-year-old female with bilateral panuveitis. She was treated with 4 mg of TAAC injected intravitreally. Baseline (**a**, **b**) OCT showing resolution of CME at 1 month (**c**) and 3 months (**d**) after injection. At baseline, visual acuity was counting fingers at 2 feet. At 1 month, it had improved to 20/200. At 3 months, postinjection visual acuity was recorded as 20/400+1

lowing cataract surgery can be given intravitreal or periocular TA at the time of cataract surgery to help prevent formation of CME and control inflammation. Patients with CME and pars planitis may benefit from intravitreal corticosteroid injection, although inflammation of the pars plana may complicate injection of the corticosteroid.

1.9.2.2 Sarcoidosis

Sarcoidosis is typically quite responsive to corticosteroid treatment. It is not surprising that intravitreal TA injection may have a role in some cases of sarcoid uveitis. Case reports have shown benefit in treatment of CME in patients with sarcoidosis [48]. In addition, regression of choroidal granuloma in sarcoidosis following three injections of TA at 2-month intervals has been reported [49].

1.9.2.3 Behçet's Disease

Reports have shown the benefit of intravitreal TA for treatment of CME and vitritis secondary to Behçet's disease. Duration of effect lasted 2–6 months [47, 50]. The TNF-α antagonist infliximab has proven to be very effective for the treatment of Behçet's. Since Behçet's is a systemic disease, it will frequently be preferable to treat systemically with infliximab, rather than locally with TA.

1.9.2.4 Eales Disease

Eales disease often presents with retinal periphlebitis and may progress to retinal ischemia, neovascularization, and vision loss. A case report has shown resolution of periphlebitis in a patient treated with intravitreal TA [51].

1.9.2.5 Vogt-Koyanagi-Harada Syndrome

Oral prednisone is the mainstay of treatment for Vogt-Koyanagi-Harada (VKH) Syndrome. Currently, it is generally well-accepted that long-term therapy (6–12 months) with oral prednisone following the diagnosis will reduce the risk of recurrence of inflammation. Commonly, high doses of oral prednisone are required in the acute phase, but clinical response will usually allow them to be tapered to lower doses within weeks. With this knowledge, it is not surprising that the serous detachments in the acute phase of VKH have responded to intravitreal TA injection [52]. However, since long-term systemic prednisone therapy is generally recommended for this systemic disease, the additional risks posed by intravitreal injection in combination with its ability to only have a local effect, make it less desirable in cases of VKH. However, for patients who cannot tolerate the initial high doses of systemic corticosteroid that are often necessary, intravitreal injection may be a viable option. In the presence of serous retinal detachments, special precautions may need to be taken to avoid mechanical damage to the retina from the needle.

1.9.2.6 Sympathetic Ophthalmia

In contrast to VKH, inflammation in sympathetic ophthalmia is clinically localized to the ocular tissues. It is usually chronic, often requires long-term systemic immunosuppression, and may be difficult to control. Studies have shown short-term benefit of intravitreal TA injection in eyes with inflammation due to sympathetic ophthalmia. Long-term corticosteroid delivery devices may alleviate the need for repeat intraocular injection and may be a reasonable option in patients with sympathetic ophthalmia [53, 54]. Of course, the risk of devastating complications, such as endophthalmitis, must be given special consideration in patients who are functionally monocular.

1.9.2.7 Choroidal Neovascularization

Choroidal neovascularization (CNV) can be a complication of any disease in which there is a break in Bruch's membrane. In presumed ocular histoplasmosis syndrome (POHS), CNV can develop at sites of chorioretinal scars and, especially in the macula, can lead to significant vision loss. Oral and periocular corticosteroids have been reported to have a stabilizing effect on CNV due to POHS [55]. Intravitreal triamcinolone has also been reported to have a beneficial effect on CNV in POHS [56].

Other uveitic diseases such as multifocal choroiditis and serpiginous choroiditis can lead to development of CNV. Corticosteroids can be useful for inflammatory CNV, and use of intravitreal TA for treatment of CNV secondary to serpiginous choroiditis has been reported [57].

1.9.2.8 Toxoplasmic Retinochoroiditis

Use of intravitreal dexamethasone in combination with intravitreal clindamycin has shown some benefit in toxoplasmic retinochoroiditis. One study of four eyes in four patients showed a favorable response within

2 weeks after intravitreal injection of 1.0 mg/0.1 ml clindamycin and 1.0 mg/0.1 ml of dexamethasone. Two to four injections were required to achieve control of the retinochoroiditis. In addition, three of the patients continued on one systemic drug for treatment as well [58]. It should be emphasized that corticosteroid therapy, whether intraocular, periocular, or oral should not be initiated in toxoplasmic retinochoroiditis without sufficient antibiotic coverage. Corticosteroid therapy alone can promote recurrence or worsening of toxoplasmic retinochoroiditis. For similar reasons, longer acting depot steroids such as TA should be avoided as the corticosteroid effect may outlast the antibiotic effect, leading to unopposed steroid effect.

1.9.2.9 Hypotony

Chronic inflammation of the ciliary body can lead to decreased aqueous production, chronic hypotony, and hypotony maculopathy with visual loss. The IOP-raising side effect of intravitreal corticosteroid injection can be beneficial in these cases. In addition, reduction of ciliary body inflammation may also contribute to increased aqueous production, increased IOP, and resolution of hypotony maculopathy. Figure 1.3 shows the response to intravitreal TA injection as documented by OCT in a patient with hypotony maculopathy secondary to chronic uveitis associated with juvenile idiopathic arthritis (JIA).

1.9.2.10 Endophthalmitis

The role of systemic or intravitreal corticosteroids in the treatment of infectious endophthalmitis is a controversial topic. Some think that after adequate antimicrobial therapy is initiated, corticosteroid therapy can decrease inflammation and ocular tissue damage and therefore improve outcome. Studies in rabbits have shown that in conjunction with intravitreal vancomycin, intravitreal dexamethasone can decrease inflammation and tissue destruction. Studies in rabbits with *Streptococcus pneumoniae* endophthalmitis have shown that vancomycin is eliminated less readily from eyes which are concurrently treated with intravitreal dexamethasone. One hypothesis for this is that the corticosteroid decreases breakdown of the blood–ocular barrier, reducing this route of elimination. It is not known whether the dexamethasone alters the bactericidal activity of the vancomycin [59]. Further study is needed before any definitive conclusions can be drawn regarding the use of corticosteroids in the treatment of endophthalmitis.

1.10 Future

Intravitreal corticosteroid injections have become part of the therapeutic armamentarium of physicians who treat intraocular inflammatory diseases. Further advances are needed to limit the toxicity of intravitreal

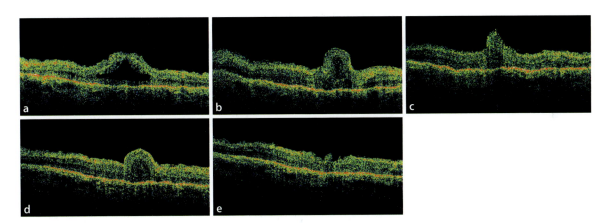

Fig. 1.3 Response as documented by OCT following injection of 4 mg of intravitreal TAAC in a patient with hypotony maculopathy secondary to chronic uveitis associated with JIA. **a** Baseline OCT showing hypotony maculopathy. Baseline visual acuity was 20/60. One week following the injection, the hypotony maculopathy had decreased, IOP was 4 mmHg, and visual acuity had decreased to 20/150. On biomicroscopy, the retina appeared to have folded upon itself, forming a cylindrical cone with the apex at the fovea. **b** Line scan slightly nasal to the fovea where the retinal fold is broader. **c** Line scan through the fovea showing the apex of the cone where the retinal fold is sharper. By 2 weeks after injection, IOP increased to 6 mmHg, and the extent of retinal folding decreased. **d** Line scan nasal to the fovea at this time. **e** Line scan through the fovea at the same visit, documenting the decreased extent of folding at the fovea. Visual acuity improved to 20/60+1

therapy while maximizing the benefits. Injectable, longer-lasting steroid depots, such as the sustained-release dexamethasone implant (Posurdex™, Allergan) offer the potential of increased duration of action and have been postulated to have a lower likelihood of pressure elevation than standard intravitreal injection. The results of ongoing clinical trials in the treatment of anterior and intermediate uveitis may demonstrate whether these hypothesized benefits are significant. The implantable fluocinolone acetonide depot (Retisert™; Bausch and Lomb) is the subject of another chapter in this book. It is associated with significant benefit in some cases, although the rate of adverse effects such as cataract formation and glaucoma that requires trabeculectomy surgery is high. Other steroid delivery devices or molecules may someday provide different safety and toxicity profiles. Lastly, exploration in the use of other immunosuppressives, including the biologics, will surely be an area of interest in the future.

Take Home Pearls

- When performed by an experienced retina or uveitis specialist, intravitreal corticosteroid injection can be a safe and effective treatment for many conditions.
- Reports of benefit support the use of intravitreal corticosteroid for various types of uveitis that lead to CME, hypotony, inflammatory CNV, Behcet's Disease, VKH, and sympathetic ophthalmia.
- Numerous risks are present with injection. The most common are elevation of intraocular pressure, which may be transient or permanent, and cataract formation. The most severe is endophthalmitis.
- Intraocular delivery of medication has become more common in recent years. While other medications with fewer known side effects than corticosteroids may be preferred in some situations, intravitreal corticosteroid injection will likely play a role for years to come.

References

1. Beer, P. M., Bakri, S. J., Singh, R. J., Liu, W., Peters, G. B., 3rd and Miller, M., Intraocular concentration and pharmacokinetics of triamcinolone acetonide after a single intravitreal injection. Ophthalmology 2003. 110: 681–686
2. Machemer, R., Sugita, G. and Tano, Y., Treatment of intraocular proliferations with intravitreal steroids. Trans Am Ophthalmol Soc 1979. 77: 171–180
3. McCuen, B. W., 2nd, Bessler, M., Tano, Y., Chandler, D. and Machemer, R., The lack of toxicity of intravitreally administered triamcinolone acetonide. Am J Ophthalmol 1981. 91: 785–788
4. Danis, R. P., Ciulla, T. A., Pratt, L. M. and Anliker, W., Intravitreal triamcinolone acetonide in exudative age-related macular degeneration. Retina 2000. 20: 244–250
5. Challa, J. K., Gillies, M. C., Penfold, P. L., Gyory, J. F., Hunyor, A. B. and Billson, F. A., Exudative macular degeneration and intravitreal triamcinolone: 18 month follow up. Aust N Z J Ophthalmol 1998. 26: 277–281
6. Martidis, A., Duker, J. S., Greenberg, P. B., Rogers, A. H., Puliafito, C. A., Reichel, E. and Baumal, C., Intravitreal triamcinolone for refractory diabetic macular edema. Ophthalmology 2002. 109: 920–927
7. Hernaez-Ortega, M. C. and Soto-Pedre, E., Removal of benzyl alcohol from a commercially available triamcinolone acetonide suspension for intravitreal use. Ophthalmic Surg Lasers Imaging 2006. 37: 162–164
8. Taban, M., Singh, R., Chung, J., Lowder, C., Perez, V. and Kaiser, P., Sterile endophthalmitis after intravitreal triamcinolone: a possible association with uveitis. Am J Ophthalmol 2007. In press
9. Jonas, J. B., Kreissig, I. and Degenring, R., Intraocular pressure after intravitreal injection of triamcinolone acetonide. Br J Ophthalmol 2003. 87: 24–27
10. Degenring, R. F. and Jonas, J. B., Serum levels of triamcinolone acetonide after intravitreal injection. Am J Ophthalmol 2004. 137: 1142–1143
11. Jonas, J. B., Intravitreal triamcinolone acetonide for treatment of intraocular oedematous and neovascular diseases. Acta Ophthalmol Scand 2005. 83: 645–663
12. Thomas, E. R., Wang, J., Ege, E., Madsen, R. and Hainsworth, D. P., Intravitreal triamcinolone acetonide concentration after subtenon injection. Am J Ophthalmol 2006. 142: 860–861
13. Jonas, J. B., Concentration of intravitreally injected triamcinolone acetonide in intraocular silicone oil. Br J Ophthalmol 2002. 86: 1450–1451
14. Peyman, G. A. and Moshfeghi, D. M., Intravitreal triamcinolone acetonide. Retina 2004. 24: 488–490
15. Barnes, P. J., Anti-inflammatory actions of glucocorticoids: molecular mechanisms. Clin Sci (Lond) 1998. 94: 557–572
16. Penfold, P. L., Wen, L., Madigan, M. C., Gillies, M. C., King, N. J. and Provis, J. M., Triamcinolone acetonide modulates permeability and intercellular adhesion molecule-1 (ICAM-1) expression of the ECV304 cell line: implications for macular degeneration. Clin Exp Immunol 2000. 121: 458–465
17. Penfold, P. L., Wong, J. G., Gyory, J. and Billson, F. A., Effects of triamcinolone acetonide on microglial morphol-

ogy and quantitative expression of MHC-II in exudative age-related macular degeneration. Clin Experiment Ophthalmol 2001. 29: 188–192
18. Sobrin, L. and D'Amico, D. J., Controversies in intravitreal triamcinolone acetonide use. Int Ophthalmol Clin 2005. 45: 133–141
19. Regillo, C. D., Brown, G. C. and Flynn, H. W., Vitreoretinal disease: the essentials. Thieme, New York: 1999
20. Nauck, M., Karakiulakis, G., Perruchoud, A. P., Papakonstantinou, E. and Roth, M., Corticosteroids inhibit the expression of the vascular endothelial growth factor gene in human vascular smooth muscle cells. Eur J Pharmacol 1998. 341: 309–315
21. Thompson, J. T., Cataract formation and other complications of intravitreal triamcinolone for macular edema. Am J Ophthalmol 2006. 141: 629–637
22. Rhee, D. J., Peck, R. E., Belmont, J., Martidis, A., Liu, M., Chang, J., Fontanarosa, J. and Moster, M. R., Intraocular pressure alterations following intravitreal triamcinolone acetonide. Br J Ophthalmol 2006. 90: 999–1003
23. Cardillo, J. A., Melo, L. A., Jr., Costa, R. A., Skaf, M., Belfort, R., Jr., Souza-Filho, A. A., Farah, M. E. and Kuppermann, B. D., Comparison of intravitreal versus posterior sub-Tenon's capsule injection of triamcinolone acetonide for diffuse diabetic macular edema. Ophthalmology 2005. 112: 1557–1563
24. Bonini-Filho, M. A., Jorge, R., Barbosa, J. C., Calucci, D., Cardillo, J. A. and Costa, R. A., Intravitreal injection versus sub-Tenon's infusion of triamcinolone acetonide for refractory diabetic macular edema: a randomized clinical trial. Invest Ophthalmol Vis Sci 2005. 46: 3845–3849
25. Okada, A. A., Wakabayashi, T., Morimura, Y., Kawahara, S., Kojima, E., Asano, Y. and Hida, T., Trans-Tenon's retrobulbar triamcinolone infusion for the treatment of uveitis. Br J Ophthalmol 2003. 87: 968–971
26. Lafranco Dafflon, M., Tran, V. T., Guex-Crosier, Y. and Herbort, C. P., Posterior sub-Tenon's steroid injections for the treatment of posterior ocular inflammation: indications, efficacy and side effects. Graefes Arch Clin Exp Ophthalmol 1999. 237: 289–295
27. Hayashi, K. and Hayashi, H., Intravitreal versus retrobulbar injections of triamcinolone for macular edema associated with branch retinal vein occlusion. Am J Ophthalmol 2005. 139: 972–982
28. Kok, H., Lau, C., Maycock, N., McCluskey, P. and Lightman, S., Outcome of intravitreal triamcinolone in uveitis. Ophthalmology 2005. 112: 1916
29. Massin, P., Audren, F., Haouchine, B., Erginay, A., Bergmann, J. F., Benosman, R., Caulin, C. and Gaudric, A., Intravitreal triamcinolone acetonide for diabetic diffuse macular edema: preliminary results of a prospective controlled trial. Ophthalmology 2004. 111: 218–224; discussion 224–215
30. Jonas, J. B., Kreissig, I. and Degenring, R., Intravitreal triamcinolone acetonide for treatment of intraocular proliferative, exudative, and neovascular diseases. Prog Retin Eye Res 2005. 24: 587–611
31. Jonas, J. B., Intravitreal triamcinolone acetonide: a change in a paradigm. Ophthalmic Res 2006. 38: 218–245
32. Deng, S. X., Penland, S., Gupta, S., Fiscella, R., Edward, D. P., Tessler, H. H. and Goldstein, D. A., Methotrexate reduces the complications of endophthalmitis resulting from intravitreal injection compared with dexamethasone in a rabbit model. Invest Ophthalmol Vis Sci 2006. 47: 1516–1521
33. Moshfeghi, D. M., Kaiser, P. K., Scott, I. U., Sears, J. E., Benz, M., Sinesterra, J. P., Kaiser, R. S., Bakri, S. J., Maturi, R. K., Belmont, J., Beer, P. M., Murray, T. G., Quiroz-Mercado, H. and Mieler, W. F., Acute endophthalmitis following intravitreal triamcinolone acetonide injection. Am J Ophthalmol 2003. 136: 791–796
34. Saidel, M. A., Berreen, J. and Margolis, T. P., Cytomegalovirus retinitis after intravitreous triamcinolone in an immunocompetent patient. Am J Ophthalmol 2005. 140: 1141–1143
35. Ufret-Vincenty, R. L., Singh, R. P., Lowder, C. Y. and Kaiser, P. K., Cytomegalovirus retinitis after fluocinolone acetonide (Retisert) implant. Am J Ophthalmol 2007. 143: 334–335
36. Moshfeghi, D. M., Kaiser, P. K., Bakri, S. J., Kaiser, R. S., Maturi, R. K., Sears, J. E., Scott, I. U., Belmont, J., Beer, P. M., Quiroz-Mercado, H. and Mieler, W. F., Presumed sterile endophthalmitis following intravitreal triamcinolone acetonide injection. Ophthalmic Surg Lasers Imaging 2005. 36: 24–29
37. Gillies, M. C., Kuzniarz, M., Craig, J., Ball, M., Luo, W. and Simpson, J. M., Intravitreal triamcinolone-induced elevated intraocular pressure is associated with the development of posterior subcapsular cataract. Ophthalmology 2005. 112: 139–143
38. Gillies, M. C., Simpson, J. M., Billson, F. A., Luo, W., Penfold, P., Chua, W., Mitchell, P., Zhu, M. and Hunyor, A. B., Safety of an intravitreal injection of triamcinolone: results from a randomized clinical trial. Arch Ophthalmol 2004. 122: 336–340
39. Ozkiris, A. and Erkilic, K., Complications of intravitreal injection of triamcinolone acetonide. Can J Ophthalmol 2005. 40: 63–68
40. Imasawa, M., Ohshiro, T., Gotoh, T., Imai, M. and Iijima, H., Central serous chorioretinopathy following vitrectomy with intravitreal triamcinolone acetonide for diabetic macular oedema. Acta Ophthalmol Scand 2005. 83: 132–133
41. Baumal, C. R., Martidis, A. and Truong, S. N., Central serous chorioretinopathy associated with periocular corticosteroid injection treatment for HLA-B27-associated iritis. Arch Ophthalmol 2004. 122: 926–928
42. Shaikh, S., Ho, S., Engelmann, L. A. and Klemann, S. W., Cell viability effects of triamcinolone acetonide and preservative vehicle formulations. Br J Ophthalmol 2006. 90: 233–236

43. Nelson, M. L. and Martidis, A., Managing cystoid macular edema after cataract surgery. Curr Opin Ophthalmol 2003. 14: 39–43
44. Martidis, A., Duker, J. S. and Puliafito, C. A., Intravitreal triamcinolone for refractory cystoid macular edema secondary to birdshot retinochoroidopathy. Arch Ophthalmol 2001. 119: 1380–1383
45. Morrison, V. L., Kozak, I., LaBree, L. D., Azen, S. P., Kayicioglu, O. O. and Freeman, W. R., Intravitreal triamcinolone acetonide for the treatment of immune recovery uveitis macular edema. Ophthalmology 2007. 114: 334–339
46. Degenring, R. F. and Jonas, J. B., Intravitreal injection of triamcinolone acetonide as treatment for chronic uveitis. Br J Ophthalmol 2003. 87: 361
47. Kramer, M., Ehrlich, R., Snir, M., Friling, R., Mukamel, M., Weinberger, D. and Axer-Siegel, R., Intravitreal injections of triamcinolone acetonide for severe vitritis in patients with incomplete Behçet's disease. Am J Ophthalmol 2004. 138: 666–667
48. Larsson, J., Hvarfner, C. and Skarin, A., Intravitreal triamcinolone in two patients with refractory macular oedema in sarcoid uveitis. Acta Ophthalmol Scand 2005. 83: 618–619
49. Chan, W. M., Lim, E., Liu, D. T., Law, R. W. and Lam, D. S., Intravitreal triamcinolone acetonide for choroidal granuloma in sarcoidosis. Am J Ophthalmol 2005. 139: 1116–1118
50. Karacorlu, M., Mudun, B., Ozdemir, H., Karacorlu, S. A. and Burumcek, E., Intravitreal triamcinolone acetonide for the treatment of cystoid macular edema secondary to Behçet disease. Am J Ophthalmol 2004. 138: 289–291
51. Pathengay, A., Pilli, S. and Das, T., Intravitreal triamcinolone acetonide in Eales' disease: a case report. Eye 2005. 19: 711–713
52. Andrade, R. E., Muccioli, C., Farah, M. E., Nussenblatt, R. B. and Belfort, R., Jr., Intravitreal triamcinolone in the treatment of serous retinal detachment in Vogt-Koyanagi-Harada syndrome. Am J Ophthalmol 2004. 137: 572–574
53. Ozdemir, H., Karacorlu, M. and Karacorlu, S., Intravitreal triamcinolone acetonide in sympathetic ophthalmia. Graefes Arch Clin Exp Ophthalmol 2005. 243: 734–736
54. Jonas, J. B., Intravitreal triamcinolone acetonide for treatment of sympathetic ophthalmia. Am J Ophthalmol 2004. 137: 367–368
55. Martidis, A., Miller, D. G., Ciulla, T. A., Danis, R. P. and Moorthy, R. S., Corticosteroids as an antiangiogenic agent for histoplasmosis-related subfoveal choroidal neovascularization. J Ocul Pharmacol Ther 1999. 15: 425–428
56. Rechtman, E., Allen, V. D., Danis, R. P., Pratt, L. M., Harris, A. and Speicher, M. A., Intravitreal triamcinolone for choroidal neovascularization in ocular histoplasmosis syndrome. Am J Ophthalmol 2003. 136: 739–741
57. Navajas, E. V., Costa, R. A., Farah, M. E., Cardillo, J. A. and Bonomo, P. P., Indocyanine green-mediated photothrombosis combined with intravitreal triamcinolone for the treatment of choroidal neovascularization in serpiginous choroiditis. Eye 2003. 17: 563–566
58. Kishore, K., Conway, M. D. and Peyman, G. A., Intravitreal clindamycin and dexamethasone for toxoplasmic retinochoroiditis. Ophthalmic Surg Lasers 2001. 32: 183–192
59. Park, S. S., Vallar, R. V., Hong, C. H., von Gunten, S., Ruoff, K. and D'Amico, D. J., Intravitreal dexamethasone effect on intravitreal vancomycin elimination in endophthalmitis. Arch Ophthalmol 1999. 117: 1058–1062

Chapter 2

Intraocular Corticosteroid Implants

David Callanan

Core Messages

- Sustained release of corticosteroids inside the eye has the inherent advantages of eliminating systemic side effects and providing long-term, continuous control of inflammation.
- The fluocinolone acetonide intravitreal implant developed by Bausch & Lomb is approved by the US Food and Drug Administration and currently available in the USA. It demonstrates that local delivery can be effective in constantly controlling inflammation, reducing flare-ups, and maintaining vision.
- Several other implantable devices are currently under study.
- The anticipated side effects of cataract and glaucoma are produced by corticosteroid implants and must be carefully monitored.
- The benefits of local control and no systemic side effects must be weighed against the associated local side effects in each patient.

Contents

2.1	Introduction	17
2.2	Background	17
2.3	Implantable Corticosteroid Devices	18
2.4	Fluocinolone Acetonide Intravitreal Implant	18
2.4.1	Characteristics	18
2.4.2	Efficacy	18
2.4.3	Safety	19
2.4.4	Surgical Complications	20
2.4.5	Surgical Procedure	20
2.4.6	Patient Selection	20
2.5	Biodegradable Dexamethasone Implant	21
2.6	Nonbiodegradable Triamcinolone Acetonide Implant (I-vation®)	21
2.7	Summary	21
References		21

This chapter contains the following video clips on DVD: Video 2 and 3 show Insertion of Retisert Implant (Surgeon: David Callanan).

2.1 Introduction

The delivery of corticosteroids directly to the eye over a sustained period has long been a goal of clinicians [5]. The hope of controlling local inflammation without systemic side effects has been every patient's dream, and devices that can accomplish this are now becoming available. We will focus on three of these devices, two that are implanted and one that is injected.

2.2 Background

Numerous drugs are used by uveitis specialists to control inflammation in the eye [1]. Each of these has its own limitations and potential complications. Periocular or intraocular injections are often effective but have a limited duration and must be repeated often [8, 18]. Repetitive intraocular injections increase the risk of endophthalmitis, and the steroids administered may actually increase this risk [2, 18]. The devices we will discuss have a longer duration and reduce the number of interventions. Systemic medications that alter the immune response help control flare-ups and provide long-term maintenance but are accompanied by serious systemic side effects that can be permanent and in some cases fatal [6, 9]. The ability to provide local control and eliminate any systemic toxicity is a primary goal of corticosteroid implants.

2.3 Implantable Corticosteroid Devices

A surgically implanted, sustained-release device containing fluocinolone acetonide is now available in the USA and should be available shortly in Europe. The fluocinolone acetonide intravitreal implant is manufactured and marketed by Bausch & Lomb under the brand name Retisert®. It was approved by the US Food and Drug Administration in July 2005. An injectable, biodegradable dexamethasone implant made by Allergan (brand name Posurdex®) has been evaluated in phase II trials for macular edema. Two large, randomized trials are under way evaluating its use in uveitis. A nonbiodegradable helical device coated with triamcinolone (I-vation®) is manufactured by SurModics. It is currently under study in the USA.

2.4 Fluocinolone Acetonide Intravitreal Implant

2.4.1 Characteristics

The fluocinolone acetonide intravitreal implant is the first, and at this time the only, intravitreal drug implant approved for the treatment of chronic uveitis by the FDA. It is a flat device measuring 2.5 mm wide and 1.5 mm thick and is nonbiodegradable (Fig. 2.1). It is

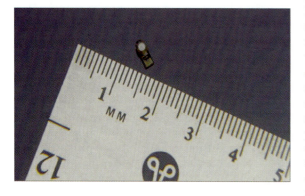

Fig. 2.1 Photo of a fluocinolone acetonide intravitreal implant next to ruler

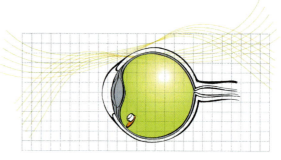

Fig. 2.2 Illustration of a fluocinolone acetonide intravitreal implant inside the eye, showing relative size and location

the only drug delivery device that has been studied in a completed, randomized, and multicenter trial specifically for uveitis. It is sewn into the posterior chamber and releases fluocinolone over a 30-month period (Fig. 2.2). The drug is slowly released through semipermeable membranes at a nominal initial rate of 0.6 µg/day, decreasing over the first month to a steady state of 0.3–0.4 µg/day. The implant contains a total of 0.59 mg fluocinolone acetonide; the implant itself remains intact when all of the drug has been released.

2.4.2 Efficacy

Jaffe et al. performed an initial safety study in rabbits, followed by a small trial in five patients using the fluocinolone acetonide implant [10, 11]. Their early report was quite promising and led to a larger trial. A three-year, multicenter, prospective, randomized, dose-masked clinical trial was performed in 278 patients with chronic and recurrent uveitis (Bausch & Lomb 415-001) [13]. Patients were randomized using a 2:3 ratio to receive the 0.59-mg or 2.1-mg fluocinolone acetonide intravitreal implant in one eye. Systemic medication for uveitis was tapered after implantation as per protocol. The primary clinical endpoints were uveitis recurrence rate, visual acuity, safety parameters, and adjunctive treatment. No significant differences were noted between the 0.59-mg and the 2.1-mg implants in terms of efficacy or complications. The 0.59-mg implant received FDA approval and is the only one marketed at present. Therefore, the following efficacy data refers only to those patients receiving the 0.59-mg dose. The rate of uveitis recurrence in implanted eyes was reduced from 54.6% preimplantation to 6.4% 34 weeks postimplantation ($p < 0.0001$); the recurrence rate in fellow nonimplanted eyes rose from

Table 2.1 Recurrence rate

	34 weeks prior	34 weeks post	2 years post
Implanted eye	54.6%	6.4% $p < 0.0001$	11.2%
Fellow eye	23.9%	41.3% $p < 0.0009$	50.0%

All data for 0.59-mg dose only. B&L 415-001

Table 2.2 Need for adjunctive treatment

		34 weeks prior	34 weeks post	2 years post
Periocular injections	Implanted eye	64.6%	2.7% $p < 0.0001$	9.7%
	Fellow eye	24.8%	32.1% $p < 0.1167$	45.3%
Systemic medications		47.2%	10.4% $p < 0.0001$	12.5%

All data for 0.59-mg dose only. B&L 415-001

Table 2.3 Cumulative ocular complications at 2 years

	% of implanted patients
Topical IOP medications	53.7
Filtering operations	30.6
Cataract[a]	89.4
Hypotony	6.1
Wound leak	3.2
Retinal detachment	2.9
Endophthalmitis	0.4
Explantation	3.6

[a] Includes only phakic patients at time of enrollment

23.9% preimplantation to 41.3% postimplantation ($p < 0.0009$) (Table 2.1). This effect was maintained at two years with a recurrence rate of 11.2% in implanted eyes and 50.0% in nonimplanted eyes (data in press). An improvement in visual acuity of three lines or more from baseline was observed at 34 weeks postimplantation in 21.0% of implanted eyes versus 6.0% of nonimplanted eyes ($p < 0.0001$, both doses). Mean acuity in implanted eyes increased from +0.54 logMAR (20/68) to +0.46 logMAR (20/55) at 34 weeks ($p < 0.001$). The percentage of patients using systemic corticosteroid and/or immunosuppressive therapy or periocular steroids was decreased from 47.2% and 64.6% respectively preimplantation to 10.4% and 2.7% 34 weeks postimplantation ($p < 0.0001$) (Table 2.2). In nonimplanted eyes, the rate of periocular injections increased from 24.8% to 45.3% at two years.

Long-term follow-up of the original patients implanted by Jaffe shows continued control of inflammation over an extended period of time [12]. A second multicenter, randomized trial in Europe has also been conducted and confirms the significant reduction in flare-ups and improved control of inflammation in implanted patients. The results of this trial will be published soon. The combined data from these trials shows that the fluocinolone acetonide intravitreal implant is effective in controlling inflammation in patients with uveitis and helps reduce or eliminate the need for systemic medication.

2.4.3 Safety

The most common adverse events associated with the fluocinolone acetonide intravitreal implant were elevated intraocular pressure (IOP) and cataract. Both of these complications are known to occur in uveitis patients [14–16]. The rates of cataract formation and IOP elevation were not different when comparing the 0.59-mg implant to the 2.1-mg implant. Pooling of the data with both implants showed a significant increase in the use of topical IOP lowering medication in implanted eyes from 14.0% at enrollment to 53.7% at 2 years postimplantation ($p < 0.0001$). Usage of topical IOP lowering medication in nonimplanted eyes also increased from 10.9% at enrollment to 20.2% at 2 years ($p = 0.002$). Glaucoma filtration surgery was required in 30.6% of patients with an implant. Cataract formation leading to removal developed in 89.4% of phakic eyes by two years after implantation, while only 13.3 % of fellow eyes required cataract extraction. Table 2.3 lists all significant complications. No detectable level of fluocinolone can be found in the serum of implanted patients. No systemic side effects are known to occur with its use.

2.4.4 Surgical Complications

Complications related to the surgical implantation include wound leakage (3.2%), ocular hypotony (6.1%), retinal detachment (2.9%), and endophthalmitis (0.4%). Hypotony and retinal detachment are known to occur in uveitis patients that have not had implantations, so the percentage attributable directly to the intravitreal implant may be smaller. Wound leaks accounted for half of the cases of hypotony. Wound leaks would also be expected to lead to a higher incidence of endophthalmitis. Early in the Bausch & Lomb 415-001 trial, investigators were allowed to sew the implant in place without placing a throw over the top of the strut. This leads to the strut being incarcerated in the wound and in some cases even exposed under the conjunctiva. By placing a throw of the anchoring suture over the top of the strut, the implant is anchored completely inside the eye. This keeps the strut out of the wound and allows the scleral wound to be fully closed. This should reduce the incidence of wound leaks, hypotony, and potentially endophthalmitis. A total of 3.6% of the patients had the implant removed because of adverse events. Other rare adverse events that resulted from the implant included choroidal detachment, temporary impairment in visual acuity, exacerbation of intraocular inflammation, and vitreous hemorrhage.

2.4.5 Surgical Procedure

The conjunctiva should be opened in the inferonasal or inferotemporal quadrant. This preserves the superior quadrants for possible glaucoma surgery. The fluocinolone acetonide intravitreal implant is preloaded with an 8-0 double-armed prolene suture through the hole in the strut. The sclera should be opened 3.5–4.0 mm posterior to the limbus in a circumferential fashion for a length of 3.5 mm. The implant is placed through the scleral opening, and a single throw knot is placed over the top of the strut. Each of the double-armed needles is passed in the appropriate direction through the full thickness of the sclera from the inside of the eye to the exterior. A triple throw knot is then tied to secure the implant (anchoring suture) and close the scleral opening. The ends of the 8-0 prolene knot are left long. Interrupted 9-0 prolene sutures are then placed on either side of the anchoring suture and used to simultaneously close the wound and capture the long ends of the anchoring suture under them. These 9-0 prolene sutures are then rotated so the knots are buried. The anchoring suture knot is the only knot on the surface. The conjunctiva is then pulled back over the area and closed with dissolvable gut sutures.

> **Take Home Pearls**
> - Make sure the inner edges of the scleral opening are incised full thickness to prevent the implant from catching any tissue.
> - After placing the implant through the sclera, gently depress the strut and wound and visualize the implant through the pupil to be sure that it is all the way into the posterior chamber.
> - Make sure that you place one throw over the top edge of the strut before you sew the implant in place. This assures that the strut is not in the wound and the sclera can be closed securely.
> - Leave the ends of the 8-0 prolene anchoring suture long so they can be tied down against the sclera.
> - Rotate the 9-0 prolene knots so they are buried.

2.4.6 Patient Selection

The decision of which uveitis patients should undergo implantation remains a strictly case-by-case judgment. It is, however, important to remember that uveitis is a potentially blinding condition. Even with our current immunosuppressant medications, patients can suffer visual loss [4, 16]. Some uveitis patients have a systemic condition such as Behçet's that requires systemic immunosuppression to control symptoms outside the eye. These patients can sometimes use lower systemic doses when the eyes are controlled locally. Patients that cannot be completely controlled with periocular or intraocular injections, oral corticosteroids, or systemic immunosuppressants should be considered candidates. Patients with significant systemic side effects from oral immunosuppressants should also be considered. The risks of cataract formation are higher in uveitic eyes in general, and the use of periocular or intraocular corticosteroids exacerbates this. Cataract formation following the use of a fluocinolone acetonide intravitreal implant is therefore easier to accept. Glaucoma, on the other hand, represents a serious morbidity and needs to be carefully explained to the patient. Glaucoma in patients with uveitis can be controlled using either topical medications or surgery [3, 7, 17]. Both the patient and physician, however, must be prepared to deal with this complication because of the frequent occurrence following implantation. The patient must be advised and educated in the decision to pursue this form of therapy.

Take Home Pearls

- All therapies in uveitis have complications.
- If a patient has already had glaucoma surgery, an implant is a good option.
- Patients with unilateral uveitis should be considered for a fluocinolone acetonide intravitreal implant.

2.5 Biodegradable Dexamethasone Implant

A biodegradable implant (Posurdex®) which delivers dexamethasone over an extended period of time inside the eye is being evaluated in both a 350-µg and 700-µg dose. The implant consists of a 400-µm cylinder made of polymers that incorporate the drug and release it for approximately 1 month, after which the polymers degrade, disappearing in 3–6 months. The biodegradable implant is injected into the posterior chamber of the eye through a 22-gauge needle at present, but a 25-gauge system is under development. Unlike the fluocinolone acetonide intravitreal implant, the biodegradable dexamethasone implant is not sutured into place, and no foreign body remains inside the eye when it finally degrades.

The safety and efficacy of the implant was tested in a controlled, prospective, randomized, multicenter, phase II clinical trial with 306 macular edema patients whose conditions were associated with diabetes, retinal vein occlusions, uveitis, or post-cataract surgery. Only 14 of the 306 patients had uveitic macular edema, so the number of uveitis cases studied with this device is currently small. The data has been submitted for publication. Large clinical trials evaluating the efficacy of the biodegradable implant in uveitis patients are currently under way.

2.6 Nonbiodegradable Triamcinolone Acetonide Implant (I-vation®)

Another sustained-release drug delivery implant is manufactured by SurModics. The implant is composed of a rigid, nonferrous metallic scaffold coated with a nonbiodegradable polymer and triamcinolone. It has a helical design to maximize the area available for drug delivery. The release of triamcinolone is controlled by the composition of the coating polymers. The implant's small diameter enables implantation through a pars plana needle stick less than 0.5 mm in diameter. This helical design feature also may ensure secure anchoring of the implant against the sclera and facilitate retrieval. However, the conjunctiva must be opened and then closed over the top of the implant, thus requiring a surgical procedure. Initial clinical trials are under way with the I-vation implant evaluating its use in diabetic macular edema, but its capabilities make it an interesting possibility for uveitis.

2.7 Summary

The advantage of these surgically implanted devices is sustained local control of inflammation. The fluocinolone acetonide intravitreal implant is the first approved device developed specifically for treating uveitis. These devices help eliminate systemic side effects that can have severe and lifelong implications for patients. As with all technology, further improvements will likely follow. All of these devices, however, contain corticosteroids. They are all likely to produce cataracts and glaucoma as unwanted side effects. In each case, these complications must be carefully weighed against the ability to control the ocular inflammation with other means such as systemic therapy or periocular injections. If other therapy can be developed to prevent cataracts or glaucoma caused by steroids, these implants will have even greater appeal.

Implants containing cyclosporine were evaluated, but they did not appear capable of adequately controlling inflammation. There are other medications that may be effective when delivered locally, but none have yet made it to the clinical trial stage. The fluocinolone acetonide intravitreal implant is now available and adds to the armamentarium that physicians treating uveitis can use. It has proven that local treatment can be successful in uveitis patients over an extended period of time, and it is likely that other delivery platforms and other medications will be developed for local inflammatory control.

References

1. Becker MD, Smith JR, Max R et al (2005) Management of sight-threatening uveitis: new therapeutic options. Drugs 65:497–519
2. Bucher RS, Hall E, Reed DM et al (2005) Effect of intravitreal triamcinolone acetonide on susceptibility to experimental bacterial endophthalmitis and subsequent response to treatment. Arch Ophthalmol 123:649–653

3. Ceballos EM, Beck AD, Lynn MJ (2002) Trabeculectomy with antiproliferative agents in uveitic glaucoma. J Glaucoma 11:189–196
4. Durrani OM, Tehrani NN, Marr JE et al (2004) Degree, duration, and causes of visual loss in uveitis. Br J Ophthalmol 88:1159–1162
5. Geroski DH, Edelhauser HF (2000) Drug delivery for posterior segment eye disease. Invest Ophthalmol Vis Sci 41:961–964
6. Hesselink DA, Baarsma GS, Kuijpers RW et al (2004) Experience with cyclosporine in endogenous uveitis posterior. Transplant Proc 36:372S–377S
7. Hill RA, Nguyen QH, Baerveldt G et al (1993) Trabeculectomy and Molteno implantation for glaucomas associated with uveitis. Ophthalmology 100:903–908
8. Jabs DA (2004) Treatment of ocular inflammation. Ocul Immunol Inflamm 12:163–168
9. Jabs DA, Rosenbaum JT, Foster CS et al (2000) Guidelines for the use of immunosuppressive drugs in patients with ocular inflammatory disorders: recommendations of an expert panel. Am J Ophthalmol 130:492–513
10. Jaffe GJ, Ben-Nun J, Guo H et al (2000) Fluocinolone acetonide sustained drug delivery device to treat severe uveitis. Ophthalmology 107:2024–2033
11. Jaffe GJ, Yang CH, Guo H et al (2000) Safety and pharmacokinetics of an intraocular fluocinolone acetonide sustained delivery device. Invest Ophthalmol Vis Sci 41:3569–3575
12. Jaffe GJ, McCallum RM, Branchaud B et al (2005) Long-term follow-up results of a pilot trial of a fluocinolone acetonide implant to treat posterior uveitis. Ophthalmology 112:1192–1198
13. Jaffe GJ, Martin D, Callanan D et al (2006) Fluocinolone acetonide implant (Retisert™) for noninfectious posterior uveitis: 34-week results of a multicenter randomized clinical study. Ophthalmology 113:1020–1027
14. Merayo-Lloves J, Power WJ, Rodriguez A et al (1999) Secondary glaucoma in patients with uveitis. Ophthalmologica 213:300–304
15. Panek WC, Holland GN, Lee DA et al (1990) Glaucoma in patients with uveitis. Br J Ophthalmol 74:223–227
16. Rothova A, Suttorp-van Schulten MS, Frits TW et al (1996) Causes and frequency of blindness in patients with intraocular inflammatory disease. Br J Ophthalmol 80:332–336
17. Towler HM, McCluskey P, Shaer B et al (2000) Long-term follow-up of trabeculectomy with intraoperative 5-fluorouracil for uveitis-related glaucoma. Ophthalmology 107:1822–1828
18. van Kooij B, Rothova A, de Vries P (2006) The pros and cons of intravitreal triamcinolone injections for uveitis and inflammatory cystoid macular edema. Ocul Immunol Inflamm 14:73–85

Chapter 3

Noncorticosteroid Intraocular Drug Therapy

Francine Behar-Cohen, Jean-Louis Bourges

Core Messages

- The use of noncorticosteroid anti-inflammatory agents opens a wide range of possibilities to regulating specific pathways involved in immune reactions, cytokine production or cell death.
- In order to achieve this specificity, drug delivery to the target tissue or cell is part of an efficient and safe ocular therapy. Particularly, for the treatment of recurrent intraocular inflammation, local and sustained delivery of the therapeutic agent is required to limit systemic side effects and reduce the need for repeated intraocular administration.
- Among the different strategies proposed, attention must be paid to minimize iatrogenic inflammation that might be caused by the material or the procedure used to deliver the therapeutic compounds.
- Most of the described technologies are still at the bench state, but they represent new and exciting potential for future clinical applications.

Contents

3.1	Introduction	24
3.2	Different Types of Drug Delivery Systems and Materials	24
3.2.1	Solid Drug Delivery Systems	24
3.2.1.1	Nonbiodegradable Solid Implants	24
3.2.1.2	Biodegradable Solid Implants	24
3.2.2	Semisolid and Viscous Polymers for Injectable DDS	25
3.2.2.1	Poly(ortho esters)	25
3.2.2.2	Other Injectable Materials	26
3.2.3	Particulate Drug Delivery Systems	26
3.2.4	Electrically Assisted Intraocular Drug Delivery	26
3.3	Applications of Intraocular Drug Delivery for Noncorticosteroid Treatments	27
3.3.1	Nonsteroidal Anti-Inflammatory Drugs	27
3.3.1.1	Indomethacin	27
3.3.1.2	COX-2 Inhibitors	27
3.3.2	Antiproliferative Drugs: 5-Fluorouracil, 5-Fluorouridine, Mitomycin, Taxol, Daunorubicin, EDTA and FGF-Saporin	27
3.3.2.1	An Adjunct to Filtering Surgery	27
3.3.2.2	Prevention of Posterior Capsule Opacification	27
3.3.2.3	Prevention of Proliferative Vitreoretinopathy	27
3.3.3	Immunosuppressive and Immunomodulatory Drugs: Cyclosporine A, Sirolimus, Tacrolimus and Tamoxifen	28
3.3.3.1	Treatment of Chronic Uveitis and Inflammatory Retinal Diseases	28
3.3.4	Antibiotics	28
3.3.4.1	Treatment of Endophthalmitis	28
3.3.4.2	Prevention of Proliferative Vitreoretinopathy	29
3.3.5	Ganciclovir in the Treatment of Cytomegalovirus Retinitis	29
3.3.6	Therapies Aimed at Regulating Expression of Specific Cytokines	30
3.3.6.1	Oligo(deoxy)nucleotides	30
3.3.6.2	Soluble Receptors for TNF-α	30
	References	30

3.1 Introduction

When inflammation is limited to the eye, local delivery of drugs is the option of choice. The eye is confined and isolated from the circulation by the inner and outer blood–retinal barriers, limiting the systemic diffusion of intraocular drugs. However, in the case of intraocular inflammation, ocular barriers are compromised at a very early stage of the ocular disease and for a prolonged period of time, most of the time after clinical resolution of the inflammation. This aspect should be taken into account as pharmacokinetic profiles are significantly influenced by ocular barrier rupture. At this stage of our strategic developments, it is apparent that no single drug delivery implant can fulfill all clinicians' expectations and needs. Thus, ocular implantable drug delivery systems need to be specifically designed and adapted to the targeted tissue or cell type, the physicochemical properties of the active compound to be used and the desired kinetic of intraocular release.

Nonbiodegradable implants offered in the early 1970s had the advantages of long-lasting release and reduced host response. Nowadays, new eroding polymers ensuring sustained release and limited induced inflammation have been designed. The erosion rate and spontaneous degradation of these polymers can be modulated to allow for the desired intraocular kinetics of drug release to take place. Biodegradable polymers can be used to form solid or injectable implants, or they can be used to encapsulate particular systems such as nano- and microparticles. Particulate systems can be injected through thin needles and have different behaviors and distribution in the ocular media associated with their size and composition. Other means to favor intraocular drug delivery use include physical methods such as electric current, ultrasounds, or lasers.

3.2 Different Types of Drug Delivery Systems and Materials

3.2.1 Solid Drug Delivery Systems

Solid drug delivery systems (DDS) can be divided into biodegradable and nonbiodegradable devices.

3.2.1.1 Nonbiodegradable Solid Implants

Polyvinyl alcohol (PVA) and ethylene vinyl acetate (EVA) combine to form nonbiodegradable solid implants that have been widely investigated for the long-sustained delivery of both steroidal and nonsteroidal anti-inflammatory drugs. PVA is a permeable polymer that acts as the framework of the implant and regulates the rate of release. EVA and silicon are permeable to certain lipophilic substances, but due to their hydrophobic character, they are relatively impermeable to hydrophilic drugs and can therefore limit the surface area for the release of this type of drug. EVA is mainly used as a membrane in reservoir systems. These polymers' mechanism of action is based on diffusion of a fluid (water) into the device, dissolving the drug pellet and creating a saturated solution released to the medium by diffusion out of the device. As long as the inside solution is saturated with the drug, the release rate is constant. The nonbiodegradable polymer devices do not produce an initial burst of the drug. Very long-lasting (more than a year) and controlled release has been achieved using this type of implant, with higher concentrations measured in the vitreous than in the aqueous humor and very low serum concentrations [1–3]. The major drawbacks for the use of this type of device are the need for surgical implantation and the possible need to remove it after it empties. Complications associated with the implantation of these devices have been observed and include vitreous hemorrhage, retinal detachment, endophthalmitis, cystoid macular edema and the formation of tenacious epiretinal membranes [2].

3.2.1.2 Biodegradable Solid Implants

Polymers and copolymers of polylactic acid (PLA) and poly(lactic-co-glycolic acid) (PLGA) are synthesized by condensation reaction at high temperature. Once implanted, bulk erosion occurs, causing a burst of encapsulated drug. This phenomenon takes place following the cleavage of the polymeric chains by enzymatic and nonenzymatic hydrolysis. The half-life of pure PLA is longer than that of the copolymers, while PLGA (50:50) has the shortest half-life in tissue. Drug release from these devices usually follows a triphasic pattern: initial drug burst, diffusive phase and a final drug burst. The last phase is generally uncontrollable, poorly predictable and, therefore, largely undesirable. The choice of polymers must thus be based on the drug characteristics and the foreseen duration of its release. Many attempts to improve the release pattern of these polymeric implants have been made. Minimizing the final burst, achieving a pseudo-zero-order kinetic of drug release and control of its speed was achieved by using two PLA polymers of different molecular weight at different ratios [4, 5]. These devices can be modulated into various shapes, including rods, plugs, pellets, discs and sheets. Accord-

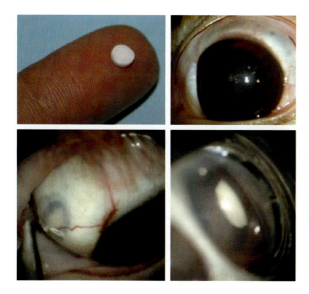

Fig. 3.1 PCL implant 18 months after intravitreous implantation

ingly, they can be implanted into the anterior chamber, the vitreous cavity through the pars plana or into the intrascleral space [4, 5].

Other polymers have been developed to improve the drug release profile and biocompatibility. Among those, polycaprolactone (PCL) is synthesized at high temperature by an open ring polymerization of the monomer ε-caprolactone. It is semicrystalline and hydrophobic compared to PLA. PCL degradation by cleavage of the ester bond produces small polymeric fragments, which diffuse from the matrix and undergo phagocytosis. Drug release with the PCL porous reservoir can be obtained for more than 250 days with a zero-kinetic order. PCL has an excellent tolerance and biocompatibility. Figure 3.1 shows a 0.4-mm-diameter PCL implant, still present in the vitreous cavity of rabbits 18 months after implantation.

Polyanhydrides can be synthesized by melt polycondensation, dehydrochlorination and dehydrative coupling. The most studied polyanhydride is 1,3-bis(carb oxyphenoxypropane) (PCPP) with sebatic acid (SA), a more hydrophilic polymer. Pure PCPP has an extremely long life (more than 3 years), whereas after copolymerization with 80% SA, it is reduced to a few days. The rate of hydrolysis can be controlled by modulating the ratio of the two polymers. These polymers are degraded by surface erosion and have very good biocompatibility.

3.2.2 Semisolid and Viscous Polymers for Injectable DDS

3.2.2.1 Poly(ortho esters)

Poly(ortho esters) (POE) are hydrophobic polymers degraded by surface erosion confined to the polymer–water interface that follow a zero-order kinetic when placed in a biological environment. Since the 1970s, four families of POE have been synthesized; POE III and IV have interesting characteristics valuable for ophthalmic therapeutic applications. They have a gel-like conformation, allowing for the incorporation of therapeutic agents by simple mixing without the need for solvents, and can be injected directly into the eye with an appropriate needle. The degradation rate of the polymer can be controlled by incorporating acidic substances into the polymer matrix to increase the erosion rate, or, conversely, basic ones to stabilize the polymer backbone. Biocompatibility of POE III and IV to ocular tissues has been extensively investigated. Advantages of POE IV include a relatively easy synthesis process, the possibility to produce large quantities and the ability to carry out irradiation sterilization [6]. Figure 3.2 shows POE IV forming a mobile bubble after an intravitreous injection of 100 μl of polymer.

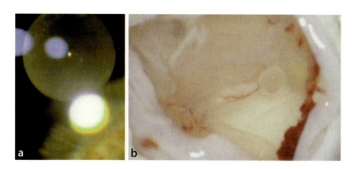

Fig. 3.2 **a** POE (100 μl) injected in the vitreous cavity. **b** Residual bubble of POE at 30 days after injection on macroscopic dissection of the posterior pole of the rabbit eye

3.2.2.2 Other Injectable Materials

Bioadhesive polymers are transparent and highly hydrophilic. Polyacrylic acid, chitosan or hyaluronic acid have been used for DDS. Hyaluronan is naturally present in the ocular tissues, especially in the vitreous. It is a glycosaminoglycan, which combines easily with hydrophilic drugs, modifying their properties of diffusion to the tissues.

3.2.3 Particulate Drug Delivery Systems

Particulate drug delivery systems (PDDS) include nano- and microparticles, nano- and microspheres, nano- and microcapsules, and liposomes. The biologically active agent can be combined or encapsulated in the material composing the particles. Nanoparticles can be obtained by (co)polymerization or by the formation of complexes by electrostatic forces using cationic peptides or by cationic polymers [7, 8]. Microparticles are spherical entities up to several hundred microns in diameter, whereas nanoparticles are smaller (< 1 μm). In micro- or nanospheres, the drug particles or droplets are entrapped in a polymeric membrane. Spheres are a polymer–drug combination where the drug is homogeneously dispersed in the polymeric matrix. In nanospheres, the drug is either incorporated within or attached to the surface. Capsules (micro or nano) have a central cavity surrounded by a polymeric membrane. To avoid opsonization and recognition by the host phagocytes, the surface of the particles can be modified by PEGylation.

PDDS have the advantage of intraocular delivery by injection. Their size and polymer composition influence markedly their biological behavior in vivo. Microparticles act as a reservoir after intravitreous injection and poorly diffuse in the vitreous gel [9]. PLA microspheres remain in the vitreous for 1.5 months in normal rabbit eyes and for 2 weeks in eyes after a vitrectomy. Nanoparticles, on the other hand, diffuse rapidly and are internalized in ocular tissues and cells of the anterior and posterior segment of the eye. They can be used as a reservoir of drugs within the retinal pigment epithelial cells [10, 11]. PLA or PLGA particles can induce some inflammatory reaction by the (co)polymers [11]. Functionally, however, the nanoparticles administered by intravitreous injections do not affect the electroretinogram. Figure 3.3 represents the fate of PDDS after injection in the vitreous cavity, depending on size (nano- or microparticulate).

Liposomes have a diameter ranging between 50 nm to a few micrometers. Liposomes are vesicular lipid biocompatible and biodegradable and are composed of lipids similar to those present in biological membranes. It is possible to produce them industrially. Using liposomes, hydrophilic, lipophilic or amphiphilic drugs can be encapsulated. They allow the encapsulation of a wide variety of drug molecules such as proteins, nucleotides, and even plasmids. Their membranes are stable and may undergo severe deformation without disruption. The vesicles can also be injected under a liquid dosage form, thus a 27- or 30-gauge needle may be used for injection, even though the liposomal diameter may be greater than the lumen of the needle. Finally, they can provide a convenient way of obtaining slow drug release from a relatively inert depot without changing the intrinsic characteristics of the encapsulated agents [12, 13].

3.2.4 Electrically Assisted Intraocular Drug Delivery

One proposed method of achieving sustained therapeutic protein delivery into the eye, such as antibodies or soluble receptor entrapping proinflammatory cytokines, is electrotransfer of the plasmid DNA encoding these proteins. Electrotransfer is a physical gene delivery method relying on the application of electric pulses to the targeted tissue, increasing gene transfection ability. Devices required for electrotransfer are a pulse generator and electrodes. Electrode geometry must be adapted to the geometry of the targeted tissue since it determines the orientation, shape and homogeneity of the electric field. For eye gene delivery, plate surface electrodes, contact-lens-type electrodes, needle electrodes

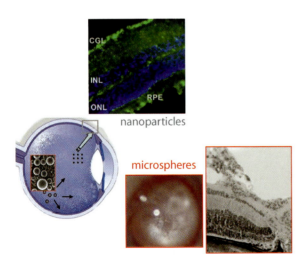

Fig. 3.3 Fate of intravitreous PDDS as a function of their size

for deeper tissues, tweezer-type electrodes and custom devised electrodes have been used successfully. Recently, electrotransfer of the ciliary muscle has been successful in producing efficient therapeutic levels of the soluble receptor for TNF-a in the ocular media, thus reducing experimental uveitis. Production of proteins after a single treatment is achieved for at least 6 months [14].

3.3 Applications of Intraocular Drug Delivery for Noncorticosteroid Treatments

3.3.1 Nonsteroidal Anti-Inflammatory Drugs

3.3.1.1 Indomethacin

PLGA disks implanted in the capsular bag and containing 7 mg of indomethacin allow drug release for 3 weeks with a significant reduction in inflammation observed postsurgery, but without any reduction in capsular opacification [15].

3.3.1.2 COX-2 Inhibitors

Biodegradable PLGA microparticles coupled with celecoxib, a selective cyclooxygenase-2 (COX-2) inhibitor, release the loaded nonsteroidal anti-inflammatory drug (NSAID) for 49 days. Subconjunctivally administered, they sustained retinal and other ocular tissue celecoxib levels during the 14-day study in rats and inhibited the diabetes-induced oxidative stress in the ocular tissues [16].

3.3.2 Antiproliferative Drugs: 5-Fluorouracil, 5-Fluorouridine, Mitomycin, Taxol, Daunorubicin, EDTA and FGF-Saporin

3.3.2.1 An Adjunct to Filtering Surgery

DDS-releasing antiproliferative agents have been widely investigated for the prevention of excessive wound healing after filtering surgery, which may be a concern in uveitis eyes. 5-fluorouracil (5-FU) was incorporated into nonbiodegradable PVA–EVA copolymer Elvax discs of 4 mm diameter containing 12 mg of 5-FU, which was released over 2 weeks. A subconjunctival implantation led to a constant 1 mg/day release of 5-FU for 10 days and reduced intraocular pressure for more than 3 months in monkeys [17]. These implants were also used subconjunctivally in four patients undergoing high-risk trabeculectomies with a mean follow-up of 2.5 years. In three of the four studied patients, intraocular pressure remained low with stabilization of the visual field and without any unwarranted events [18].

Using small PLGA cylinders, more constant release rates were achieved [19]. In the rabbit eye, a release rate of 1.2 µg/h for more than 18 days was recorded. Total degradation of the implant was achieved around 86 days after implantation. No infection or inflammatory reactions were detected during the study period.

Polyanhydridic polymers, because of their surface erosion and excellent biocompatibility, also have been evaluated for this indication. More hydrophobic drugs may be preferred as their release is less rapid. In vitro, release of taxol (50 µg) occurred at concentrations exceeding its LD50 for at least 100 days, and etoposide (1 mg) was released for 31 days. Following the subconjunctival implantation in the monkey of these two types of polymer discs, only the taxol discs allowed long-term reduced intraocular pressure with satisfactory appearance of the filtration bleb [20]. Daunorubicin release by a polyanhydride disc implanted subconjunctivally significantly reduced the bleb failure rate from 91% in control eyes to 22% in treated eyes.

POE, a viscous polymer loaded with 5-FU, led to decreased intraocular pressure and persistence of the filtering bleb in the rabbit eye with a reduced corneal toxicity compared to 5-FU tamponade [21] and is now under evaluation in high-risk filtering surgery in humans. The ocular tolerance of POE in the human eye is good without any inflammatory reaction.

3.3.2.2 Prevention of Posterior Capsule Opacification

An open-loop hydrogel ring releasing 5-FU (0.25 µg/h) was implanted in the capsular bag of the lens of rabbit eyes after lens phacoemulsification to prevent posterior capsule opacification (PCO). No beneficial effect on the formation of PCO associated with the release of 5-FU was observed in the treated eyes [22].

3.3.2.3 Prevention of Proliferative Vitreoretinopathy

Retinal detachment complicating uveitis may require additional pharmacologic intervention to reduce proliferative vitreoretinopathy (PVR) occurrence or recurrence. A cylindrical solid PLGA implant loaded with 1 mg of fluorouracil and placed in the vitreous cavity of rabbits allowed drug release for almost 3 weeks and reduced the incidence of tractional retinal detachment. No toxic or mechanical effects were observed. However, as the device is free in the vitreous cavity, it can cause trauma to the retina. Therefore, scleral plugs fixed at the pars plana were developed. When these plugs were loaded with 1% doxorubicin, drug release at therapeutic levels was observed in the vitreous of rabbit eyes during 1 month with reduction of the incidence of tractional retinal detachment. In 1998, Zhou et al. developed a multidrug PLGA implant made of three cylindrical segments, each containing one drug: 5-fluoroudine (5-Furd), triamcinolone and recombinant tissue plasminogen activator (rtPa). This device can easily be inserted through a syringe needle in the vitreous. In vitro kinetic studies showed release of 5-Furd and triamcinolone at 1 μg/day for more than 4 weeks and at 10–190 μg/day for 2 more weeks. An active rate of rtPa release was detected after a lag time of 2 days and during a shorter period of 2 weeks. However, this drug-releasing implant has not been, as yet, evaluated in vivo. Two types of PLGA scleral implants (PLGA 65/35 and PLGA 50/50) were combined for the release of cis-4-hydroxyproline (CHP), releasing the drug for 4 and 7 weeks respectively in a triphasic release profile. Delivery of both PLGA 65/35 and PLGA 50/50 implants led to synergistic therapeutic effects.

Polycaprolactone (PCL) has been also been used to deliver intravitreal 5-FU. This device allowed slow release of the drug and led to a 100% protection against tractional retinal detachment. Mild vitreous hemorrhage was observed in a few of the treated eyes, but no other significant complications were detected.

The kinetics of PDDS loaded with 5-fluorouracil were also tested in rabbit and monkey eyes. PLA or PLGA microspheres cleared after 48 days from the rabbit vitreous and were still detectable in the eye of monkeys 11 days after injection.

Although efficient in experimental PVR models, none of these systems have ever been evaluated in clinical practice [23, 24].

3.3.3 Immunosuppressive and Immunodulatory Drugs: Cyclosporine A, Sirolimus, Tacrolimus and Tamoxifen

3.3.3.1 Treatment of Chronic Uveitis and Inflammatory Retinal Diseases

A sustained and constant release of 500 ng/ml of cyclosporine A (CsA) was obtained for more than 6 months by intravitreal implantation of PVA–EVA nonbiodegradable implants in rabbit and monkey eyes. The very slow CsA release rate provided sustained intravitreal drug levels for up to 9 years. However, lens opacities were observed in the implanted rabbit eyes [25]. A PVA bioerodible implant designed as a matrix reservoir loaded with 10% CsA also reduced equine recurrent uveitis after implantation in the vitreous or in the sclera lamellae in horses.

A PVA–EVA device releasing both dexamethasone and CsA was also studied. Both drugs were released for 10 weeks at similar rates to devices containing a single drug without any evident clinical toxic effects. The potential therapeutic synergistic effect of this device remains to be assessed.

More recently, a glycolide-co-lactide-co-caprolactone copolymer (PGLC) implant loaded with 2 mg of CsA was evaluated. In rabbit eyes with experimental uveitis, therapeutic CsA levels were measured in the aqueous humor up to 14 weeks postimplantation, and efficient anti-inflammatory effects were observed in the CsA–PGCL-treated eyes. Reduced systemic toxicity was noted with the CsA–PGCL-treated rabbits compared to those receiving systemic CsA treatment. In rabbit eyes with uveitis, significant reduction of inflammation, a preserved architecture of the eye and no detectable CsA levels in the blood were recorded. Therapeutic levels of CsA within the vitreous were observed in the implanted eyes for at least 6 months.

Rod-shaped devices with a drug coating made of polybutylmethacrylate and polyethylene-co-vinyl acetate were developed and implanted in the subretinal space [26]. These implants were used to deliver sirolimus. During a follow-up period of 4 weeks, although good retinal tolerance was observed, cataract and corneal edema developed in some implanted eyes.

PLGA scleral plugs loaded with tacrolimus reduced significantly the incidence and extent of uveitis in rabbit eyes.

De Kozak et al. used polyethylene-glycol-coated cyanoacrylate nanoparticles loaded with tamoxifen for the inhibition of intraocular inflammation in a rat model of experimental autoimmune uveitis (EAU). After intravitreal injection, these nanoparticles induced a significant inhibition in the expression and extent of the uveitis in the treated eyes without any detectable ocular toxicity [27].

3.3.4 Antibiotics

3.3.4.1 Treatment of Endophthalmitis

PLA or PLGA intraocular implants loaded with ciprofloxacin were used for the treatment of experimental endophthalmitis in rabbit eyes. This antibiotic was released in the vitreous at therapeutic levels up to 4 weeks after implantation. Scleral implants loaded with fluconazole released the antifungal drug within three weeks. The implants were reabsorbed 4 months after implantation [12].

Liposomes have widely been studied for intravitreal delivery [12, 13]. Interestingly, after intravitreal injection, drugs encapsulated within liposomes (antibiotics, antiviral, antifungal, antimetabolic agents, etc.) are less toxic than the free forms. The decrease of toxicity can be explained by the limited amount of drug being in a free form, directly in close contact with the tissues. This beneficial effect results from the sustained release of the molecule from the liposomes. In addition, liposomes significantly increase drug half-life in the vitreous, showing their stability in this medium. However, the residence time of liposomes is shorter in infected eyes than in normal eyes. This might result from an increased rate of diffusion of liposomes through liquefied vitreous, enhanced uptake by macrophages recruited, and/or a breakdown of the blood–retinal barrier in infected eyes.

3.3.4.2 Prevention of Proliferative Vitreoretinopathy

Moritera et al. tested PLA microspheres containing 10 µg of Adriamycin and significantly reduced the rate of PVR formation.

3.3.5 Ganciclovir in the Treatment of Cytomegalovirus Retinitis

PVA–EVA polymer implants were developed in 1992 for the release of ganciclovir in cytomegalovirus retinitis and led to long-term (more than 80 days) drug delivery in the rabbit eye with no toxic effects [1]. Studies in experimental animals and in humans [28, 29] were conducted and led to the device's approval for clinical use by the Food and Drug Administration in 1996 (Vitrasert®).

Advantages of the Vitrasert® approach include convenience, reduced cost and lack of systemic toxicity. This strategy, however, also has potential disadvantages, including endophthalmitis and other surgical complications. It allows also for the development of nonocular cytomegalovirus disease and cytomegalovirus retinopathy in uninvolved fellow eyes. The Vitrasert® device showed a long median time of CMV retinitis control. However, postoperative complications occurred in 12% of the procedures and were associated with decreased visual acuity. Thus, recommendations of the International AIDS society for Vitrasert® use in combination with antiretroviral therapy were made [30].

Sustained release of ganciclovir was also obtained with 10%-loaded PLA/PLGA (75/25) scleral implants for more than 3 months in the retina and more than 5 months in the choroid of rabbit eyes. Long-term release for 12 weeks was also obtained with PLGA scleral plugs containing 25% ganciclovir with no significant toxicity. Scleral implants made of two different PLA sizes allowed for constant drug release of ganciclovir over the course of 6 months without a significant burst release in the late phase. One advantage of these biodegradable implants is the minimal sclerotomy required for implantation, which minimizes surgical complication risks [31].

PDDS loaded with ganciclovir have also been tested after intraocular injections in animal CMV retinitis models. In a CMV rabbit model, a single injection of PLGA microspheres loaded with 10 mg of ganciclovir was found as efficient as the direct injection of 130 µg of ganciclovir every 4 days. In these experiments, the microspheres were still detected within the eye 8 weeks after their injection. Localized foreign body reaction has been observed after injection of microspheres loaded with ganciclovir. Negatively charged albumin nanoparticles loaded with ganciclovir were injected in normal rat eyes. These particles showed a two-week-residence time within the vitreous but did not induce any noticeable inflammatory reaction in the retina tissue and did not influence the organization of the surrounding ocular tissues. Almost 40% of the loaded drug was released within 1 h with a slower release rate during the following 10 days [32].

Akula et al. evaluated the potential of liposomes to treat CMV retinitis in AIDS patients [12]. The patients received an intravitreal injection of liposome-encapsulated ganciclovir in the right eye. The left eye served as a control, receiving intravitreal free ganciclovir. The right eye showed no retinal hemorrhages or detachment; however, vision declined initially, stabilizing later. Indeed, the major clinical changes after intravitreal injection of liposomes consisted of vitreal bodies (i.e., small, white, sparkling opacities mainly located in the lower part of the eye), vitreal condensations and retinal abnormalities. The liposome formulations spread diffusely within the vitreous cavity and caused cloudiness, interfering with the patient's visual acuity and the ability of the ophthalmologist to examine the fundus until complete resorption of the formulation had occurred 14–21 days after administration. Despite this drawback, weekly examination showed neither progression of the CMV retinitis nor new lesions in the eye treated with liposomes, whereas eyes injected with the solution of ganciclovir showed reactivation of old CMV retinitis. Liposome-encapsulated ganciclovir also reduced the number of intravitreal injections.

3.3.6 Therapies Aimed at Regulating Expression of Specific Cytokines

3.3.6.1 Oligo(deoxy)nucleotides

An interesting study was conducted with an 8.4% phosphorothioate-oligodeoxynucleotide-loaded PLGA intravitreal implants, which led, in vitro, to an initial 20% release of the oligodeoxynucleotides (ODN) followed by a pseudo-zero-kinetic order of release for more than 20 days [13]. Liposomes also protect poorly stable drugs from degradation as shown with phosphodiester antisense oligonucleotides and peptides [33].

More recently, polyethylenimine–oligonucleotide complexes forming nanoparticles were injected in the rat vitreous to evaluate the possibility to inhibit TGFb2 expression. Interestingly, these complexes localized in retinal Müller glial cells [34].

3.3.6.2 Soluble Receptors for TNF-α

A novel electroporation technique for specific transfection of ocular ciliary muscle has recently been developed in our laboratory. This strategy aimed at using the ciliary muscle as a reservoir for high and long-standing intraocular expression and secretion of therapeutic proteins [14]. Due to their accessibility, size, shape and morphology, skeletal muscles are workable targets for electrotransfer strategy. In the eye, the ciliary muscle is a smooth muscle with some characteristics of skeletal muscle. Thus, theoretically, the ciliary muscle might be an ideal "reservoir" of plasmids encoding for therapeutic molecules for the treatment of both anterior and posterior segment diseases. To this purpose, electric pulses were delivered to the rat eye by a specifically designed needle cathode electrode inserted through a corneal tunnel, and a contact anode was positioned on the sclera overlying the ciliary body. This strategy led to effective expression localized to the ciliary muscle after electrotransfer of a GFP plasmid. We then used this technique to deliver various plasmids, including a TNF-α-soluble receptor. The therapeutic potential of this strategy was further evaluated in an endotoxin-induced uveitis (EIU) model in the rat eye by electrotransfer of a plasmid construct encoding a TNF-α-soluble receptor (TNFR-Is, P55). High levels of TNFR-Is were found in the ocular media and led to strong inhibition of both clinical and histological signs of the uveitis in the treated eyes. At 8 days after electrotransfer, $1,070 \pm 202$ pg/m of chimeric protein were detected in the aqueous humor, which resulted in a significant reduction of TNF-α in the aqueous humor. This neutralization was correlated with the clinical efficacy of the treatment. No TNFR-Is was detected in the blood circulation [14]. Thus, using this technique, a local therapeutic effect can be achieved within the eye, and secondary, unwarranted side effects of systemic administration of the drug can be avoided. Other types of receptors or antibodies can efficiently be produced directly into the eye for a period of at least 6 months. Moreover, when using specific plasmids, controlled and inducible production of the therapeutic proteins can be achieved.

References

1. Smith TJ, Pearson PA, Blandford DL, Brown JD, Goins KA, Hollins JL, Schmeisser ET, Glavinos P, Baldwin LB and Ashton P. Intravitreal sustained-release ganciclovir, Arch Ophthalmol 110 (1992), pp. 255–8
2. Lim JI, Wolitz RA, Dowling AH, Bloom HR, Irvine AR and Schwartz DM. Visual and anatomic outcomes associated with posterior segment complications after ganciclovir implant procedures in patients with AIDS and cytomegalovirus retinitis, Am J Ophthalmol 127 (1999), pp. 288–93
3. Driot JY, Novack GD, Rittenhouse KD, Milazzo C and Pearson PA. Ocular pharmacokinetics of fluocinolone acetonide after Retisert intravitreal implantation in rabbits over a 1-year period, J Ocul Pharmacol Ther 20 (2004), pp. 269–75
4. Yasukawa T, Ogura Y, Sakurai E, Tabata Y and Kimura H. Intraocular sustained drug delivery using implantable polymeric devices, Adv Drug Deliv Rev 57 (2005), pp. 2033–46
5. Merkli A, Tabatabay C, Gurny R and Heller J. Biodegradable polymers for the controlled release of ocular drugs, Prog Polym Sci 23 (1998), pp. 563–580
6. Einmahl S, Ponsart S, Bejjani RA, D'Hermies F, Savoldelli M, Heller J, Tabatabay C, Gurny R and Behar-Cohen F. Ocular biocompatibility of a poly(ortho ester) characterized by autocatalyzed degradation, J Biomed Mater Res A 67 (2003), pp. 44–53
7. Mainardes RM and Silva LP. Drug delivery systems: past, present, and future, Curr Drug Targets 5 (2004), pp. 449–55
8. Mainardes RM, Urban MC, Cinto PO, Khalil NM, Chaud MV, Evangelista RC and Gremiao MP. Colloidal carriers for ophthalmic drug delivery, Curr Drug Targets 6 (2005), pp. 363–71
9. Khoobehi B, Stradtmann MO, Peyman GA and Aly OM. Clearance of sodium fluorescein incorporated into microspheres from the vitreous after intravitreal injection, Ophthalmic Surg 22 (1991), pp. 175–80

10. Sakurai E, Ozeki H, Kunou N and Ogura Y. Effect of particle size of polymeric nanospheres on intravitreal kinetics, Ophthalmic Res 33 (2001), pp. 31–6
11. Bourges JL, Gautier SE, Delie F, Bejjani RA, Jeanny JC, Gurny R, BenEzra D and Behar-Cohen FF. Ocular drug delivery targeting the retina and retinal pigment epithelium using polylactide nanoparticles, Invest Ophthalmol Vis Sci 44 (2003), pp. 3562–9
12. Ebrahim S, Peyman GA and Lee PJ. Applications of liposomes in ophthalmology, Surv Ophthalmol 50 (2005), pp. 167–82
13. Bochot A, Fattal E, Boutet V, Deverre JR, Jeanny JC, Chacun H and Couvreur P. Intravitreal delivery of oligonucleotides by sterically stabilized liposomes, Invest Ophthalmol Vis Sci 43 (2002), pp. 253–9
14. Bloquel C, Bejjani R, Bigey P, Bedioui F, Doat M, BenEzra D, Scherman D and Behar-Cohen F. Plasmid electrotransfer of eye ciliary muscle: principles and therapeutic efficacy using hTNF-alpha soluble receptor in uveitis, FASEB J 20 (2006), pp. 389–91
15. Nishi O, Nishi K, Morita T, Tada Y, Shirasawa E and Sakanishi K. Effect of intraocular sustained release of indomethacin on postoperative inflammation and posterior capsule opacification, J Cataract Refract Surg 22 (1996), pp. 806–10
16. Ayalasomayajula SP and Kompella UB. Subconjunctivally administered celecoxib-PLGA microparticles sustain retinal drug levels and alleviate diabetes-induced oxidative stress in a rat model, Eur J Pharmacol 511 (2005), pp. 191–8
17. Blandford DL, Smith TJ, Brown JD, Pearson PA and Ashton P. Subconjunctival sustained release 5-fluorouracil, Invest Ophthalmol Vis Sci 33 (1992), pp. 3430–5
18. Smith TJ and Ashton P. Sustained-release subconjunctival 5-fluorouracil, Ophthalmic Surg Lasers 27 (1996), pp. 763–7
19. Wang G, Tucker IG, Roberts MS and Hirst LW. In vitro and in vivo evaluation in rabbits of a controlled release 5-fluorouracil subconjunctival implant based on poly(D,L-lactide-co-glycolide), Pharm Res 13 (1996), pp. 1059–64
20. Jampel HD, Thibault D, Leong KW, Uppal P and Quigley HA. Glaucoma filtration surgery in nonhuman primates using taxol and etoposide in polyanhydride carriers, Invest Ophthalmol Vis Sci 34 (1993), pp. 3076–83
21. Einmahl S, Behar-Cohen F, D'Hermies F, Rudaz S, Tabatabay C, Renard G, et al. A new poly(ortho ester)-based drug delivery system as an adjunct treatment in filtering surgery, Invest Ophthalmol Vis Sci 42 (2001), pp. 695–700
22. Pandey SK, Cochener B, Apple DJ, Colin J, Werner L, Bougaran R, et al. Intracapsular ring sustained 5-fluorouracil delivery system for the prevention of posterior capsule opacification in rabbits: a histological study, J Cataract Refract Surg 28 (2002), pp. 139–48
23. Yasukawa T, Ogura Y, Sakurai E, Tabata Y and Kimura H. Intraocular sustained drug delivery using implantable polymeric devices, Adv Drug Deliv Rev 57 (2005), pp. 2033–46
24. Sun JK and Arroyo JG. Adjunctive therapies for proliferative vitreoretinopathy, Int Ophthalmol Clin 44(3) (2004), pp. 1–10
25. Pearson PA, Jaffe GJ, Martin DF, Cordahi GJ, Grossniklaus H, Schmeisser ET, et al. Evaluation of a delivery system providing long-term release of cyclosporine, Arch Ophthalmol 114 (1996), pp. 311–7
26. Beeley NR, Stewart JM, Tano R, Lawin LR, Chappa RA, Qiu G, Anderson AB, de Juan E and Varner SE. Development, implantation, in vivo elution, and retrieval of a biocompatible, sustained release subretinal drug delivery system, J Biomed Mater Res A 76 (2006), pp. 690–8
27. de Kozak Y, Andrieux K, Villarroya H, Klein C, Thillaye-Goldenberg B, Naud MC, et al. Intraocular injection of tamoxifen-loaded nanoparticles: a new treatment of experimental autoimmune uveoretinitis, Eur J Immunol 34 (2004), pp. 3702–12
28. Anand R, Nightingale SD, Fish RH, Smith TJ and Ashton P. Control of cytomegalovirus retinitis using sustained release of intraocular ganciclovir, Arch Ophthalmol 111 (1993), pp. 223–7
29. Martin DF, Parks DJ, Mellow SD, Ferris FL, Walton RC, Remaley NA, et al. Treatment of cytomegalovirus retinitis with an intraocular sustained-release ganciclovir implant: a randomized controlled clinical trial, Arch Ophthalmol 112 (1994), pp. 1531–9
30. Martin DF, Dunn JP, Davis JL, Duker JS, Engstrom RE Jr, Friedberg DN, Jaffe GJ, Kuppermann BD, Polis MA, Whitley RJ, Wolitz RA and Benson CA. Use of the ganciclovir implant for the treatment of cytomegalovirus retinitis in the era of potent antiretroviral therapy: recommendations of the International AIDS Society-USA panel, Am J Ophthalmol 127 (1999), pp. 329–39
31. Yasukawa T, Kimura H, Kunou N, Miyamoto H, Honda Y, Ogura Y and Ikada Y. Biodegradable scleral implant for intravitreal controlled release of ganciclovir, Graefes Arch Clin Exp Ophthalmol 238 (2000), pp. 186–90
32. Veloso AA Jr, Zhu Q, Herrero-Vanrell R and Refojo MF. Ganciclovir-loaded polymer microspheres in rabbit eyes inoculated with human cytomegalovirus, Invest Ophthalmol Vis Sci 38 (1997), pp. 665–75
33. Yamakawa I, Ishida M, Kato T, Ando H and Asakawa N. Release behavior of poly(lactic acid-co-glycolic acid) implants containing phosphorothioate oligodeoxynucleotide, Biol Pharm Bull 20 (1997), pp. 455–9
34. Gomes dos Santos AL, Bochot A, Tsapis N, Artzner F, Bejjani RA, Thillaye-Goldenberg B and Behar-Cohen F. Oligonucleotide-polyethylenimine complexes targeting retinal cells: structural analysis and application to anti-TGFbeta-2 therapy, Pharm Res 23 (2006), pp. 770–81

II Surgery to Modify Uveitic Activity

Chapter 4

Therapeutic Vitrectomy for Noninfectious Uveitis

Kathrin Greiner, Andrew D. Dick

Core Messages

- Noninfectious uveitides are systemic (auto)immune disorders mediated by activation of antigen-specific T-lymphocytes and, in the main, tissue destruction orchestrated by nonspecific mononuclear cells. Disease remission is achieved by systemic immunosuppression, whilst control of chronic ocular inflammation can be achieved by a local or systemic suppression of the immune response.
- Given current evidence, the clinical efficacy of immunosuppressive and immunomodulatory drugs underlines their role as a first-line therapy for uveitis.
- Vitrectomy is indicated in patients with uveitis to manage complications and improve visual acuity. There is only scant evidence supporting a therapeutic effect of vitrectomy for noninfectious uveitis.
- Vitreous opacities in patients with Fuchs uveitis syndrome and intermediate uveitis refractory to medical treatment are indications for a therapeutic vitrectomy.

Contents

4.1	Introduction	35	4.4	Therapeutic Vitrectomy	41
4.1.1	Immunopathological Rationale		4.4.1	Perioperative Immunosuppression	41
	for Therapeutic Vitrectomy	36	4.4.2	Vitreoretinal Surgery	41
4.1.1.1	Ocular Immunology	36	4.4.3	Follow-up and Complications	41
4.1.1.2	Changes in Ocular Compartments		4.5	Specific Disease Entities	42
	During Uveitis	36	4.5.1	Intermediate Uveitis	42
4.1.2	Vitreous Body	38	4.5.2	Fuchs Uveitis Syndrome	42
4.2	Diagnostic Procedures	38	4.5.3	Behçet's Disease	43
4.3	Patient Selection	39	4.5.4	Eales Disease	43
4.3.1	Clinical Benefits and Risks	40	4.6	Conclusions	43
4.3.2	Indications for Therapeutic Vitrectomy	41	References		44

This chapter contains the following video clips on DVD: Video 4 shows Insertion of 23G trocar (Surgeon: Marc de Smet).

4.1 Introduction

The differentiation between infectious and noninfectious forms of intraocular inflammation is the first important decision in the management of uveitis. If an infectious agent, e.g., candida, is identified, the treatment is mostly determined by established standards, which may include vitrectomy. The term noninfectious uveitis is used when no overt infectious agent can be associated with the disease. These forms of uveitis are presumed immune-mediated or autoimmune. They occur in association with systemic diseases or are restricted to the eye or parts thereof (idiopathic uveitis) [12]. In approximately 50% of posterior uveitis, no nonocular site of inflammation can be detected [11].

Clinical studies are less clear, but experimental models suggest that noninfectious uveitis is generated by a breakdown of immunological tolerance to ocular antigens, thus inducing the activation and ocular infiltration of autoreactive T-lymphocytes and associated nonspecific mononuclear effector cells. In addition, a tightly controlled array of regulatory molecules, e.g., cytokines, modulates the immune response. Anatomical subtypes of uveitis can be distinguished by specific immunological mechanisms which influence the course of the disease as well as the response to treatment. Because of the large phenotypic array of uveitic conditions, the role of therapeutic vitrectomy has to be informed by immunological rationale and is thus likely to be confined to conditions largely involving the vitreous, e.g., intermediate uveitis.

4.1.1 Immunopathological Rationale for Therapeutic Vitrectomy

4.1.1.1 Ocular Immunology

The development of ocular inflammation is unquestionably multifactorial, involving genetic susceptibility, stimuli such as injury or concomitant ocular or systemic infection. Moreover, epidemiological studies have revealed distinct differences of patterns of uveitis between various geographic regions. All risk factors appear to contribute to a breakdown of immunological tolerance which normally prevents the maturation and activation of autoreactive lymphocytes. The specific regulatory network of the eye protects the ocular tissues against cell and cytokine-mediated immunoreactivity and preserves normal function of the eye. However, breakdown of regulatory mechanisms may lead to inflammation and subsequent destruction of ocular tissues. As a result, uveitis is a leading cause of blindness in industrialized countries [37].

A current paradigm is that central tolerance mechanisms, i.e., negative selection in the thymus to delete autoaggressive T-lymphocytes recognizing retinal antigens, are insufficient to maintain the ocular immune privilege [8]. Specialized anatomical structures in the eye suppress potentially destructive immune reactions by separating ocular antigens and immune cells and, thus, maintain peripheral tolerance. The blood–retinal barrier (BRB) is composed of the endothelium of retinal blood vessels and the retinal pigment epithelium (RPE) characterized by intercellular tight junctions. Consequently, breakdown of these barriers and exposure of previously sequestered retinal proteins to antigen-presenting cells (APC) after trauma or surgery can break T-lymphocyte ignorance and provoke an autoimmune response. The BRB, however, is not sufficient to prevent a systemic immune attack as demonstrated in patients with sympathetic ophthalmia. Here, intact eyes are damaged by the immune system after the previously sequestered antigens of the injured fellow eye were exposed to the immune system [7].

In the absence of overt inflammation, the evidence for immune privilege in man is:

- The intraocular presence of Fas ligand (CD95L) as an important mechanism for the deletion of T-lymphocytes entering the eye.
- Anterior chamber immunomodulatory cytokines and neuropeptides, including α-melanocyte-stimulating hormone (α-MSH) and transforming growth factor β (TGFβ), exert an immunoregulatory role.
- Resident tissues in the eye, notably the RPE, seem to exhibit a key role in controlling immunoreactivity. This function is orchestrated by interactions with the cellular and molecular components of the adaptive immune system.

Local mechanisms of immune privilege alone cannot provide sufficient protection against immunological challenges against ocular tissues. Thus, a state of systemic immune deviation must exist. Mechanisms for an active systemic tolerance induction for eye-derived antigens are illustrated by the anterior chamber-associated immune deviation (ACAID) model, although this has not been confirmed in man. ACAID is demonstrated experimentally by the inability of anterior chamber-antigen-inoculated mice to display antigen-specific, delayed-type hypersensitivity responses in the periphery on rechallenge with the same antigen [21]. After arrival of APC from the eye in the spleen, natural killer T-lymphocytes are stimulated to produce IL-10, which induces regulatory CD8+ T-lymphocytes suppressing delayed hypersensitivity [36]. The APC carrying the antigenic signal are primed in the ocular compartment with high levels of immunosuppressives like TGFβ and are induced to present HLA class I [10]. A mechanism similar to ACAID was also described for the vitreous body, presumably involving hyalocytes, which are the only cells so far detected in the normal vitreous [33].

4.1.1.2 Changes in Ocular Compartments During Uveitis

Features of T-lymphocytes and cytokine expression patterns were extensively studied in patients to elucidate the immunological mechanisms of human uveitis:

- Immunohistological studies of human ocular tissues, albeit few in number, have identified activated CD4+ T-lymphocytes expressing the IL-2 receptor as a major component of inflammatory foci in the retina in various forms of posterior, intermediate or panuveitis, such as sympathetic ophthalmia, Vogt-Koyanagi-Harada disease (VKH), sarcoidosis and the white dot syndromes [7].
- Large numbers of CD4+ T-lymphocytes were detected in the vitreous of patients with multifocal chorioretinitis [23]. Immunosuppressive therapies directed against T-lymphocytes led to a complete and persistent remission in a substantial number of patients with uveitis.
- Elevated levels of IL-1, IL-6, IL-8 and IL-12 in ocular fluids are part of the immunological response pattern in uveitis [10].
- Increased concentrations of the proinflammatory cytokine TNFα were found in the sera and aqueous humor of patients [30]. However, Perez et al. [27] could not detect TNFα and IL-2 in the vitreous of patients with active posterior uveitis.
- Cytokine expression in the aqueous humor of patients with clinically inactive uveitis was studied by RT-PCR [19]. A Th1-like cytokine profile was found in the majority of patients.

Uveitis is associated with an infiltration of ocular tissues and compartments by inflammatory cells. Infiltration of the vitreous body by these cells, mostly CD4+ T-lymphocytes and macrophages, and deposition of cellular debris at a variable degree are cardinal features of several forms of uveitis [12]. The immunological mechanisms regulating ocular inflammation appear to change during disease progression with cytokine-mediated tissue destruction dominating the chronic stages of uveitis (Fig. 4.1). Remission of uveitis appears to be induced by the intraocular conversion of Th1 cells into T regulatory cells [20].

Chronic inflammation can also induce proliferative vitreoretinopathy and retinal gliosis. The formation of epiretinal membranes (ERM) occurs at the vitreoretinal interface and is a frequent cause of declined visual acuity in uveitis patients [32]. The ERM is composed of various cell types, such as RPE cells, fibroblasts, endothelial cells and glial cells, originating from underlying tissue layers. These cells secrete proinflammatory cytokines, e.g., TNFα, and growth factors, which may stimulate the further development of ERMs in an autocrine or paracrine way [14]. On the other hand, the extracellular matrix of the ERM contains thrombospondin 1, which could be involved in the ocular immune privilege [15].

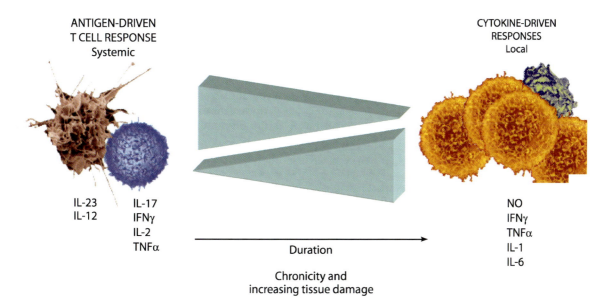

Fig. 4.1 Changes in immune response during progression of uveitis

4.1.2 Vitreous Body

Major anatomical features of the vitreous body are [4]:

- The human vitreous body occupies a volume of approximately 4.5 ml. Most parts of the vitreous are acellular.
- The vitreous can be divided into distinct anatomical regions: the central vitreous, the basal vitreous, the vitreous cortex, the vitreoretinal interface and the zonule. The basal vitreous is characterized by a strong adhesion to the retina and ciliary epithelium of the pars plana. In contrast, the posterior part of the vitreous is less firmly attached to the retina, so that a posterior vitreous detachment is observed in a substantial part of the population.
- The cortex of the vitreous body represents a thin layer which surrounds the central gel. It contains a small amount of cells (hyalocytes) whose major function seems to be the maintenance of vitreous transparency.
- The vitreous gel is a hydrated extracellular matrix with a water content of more than 98% which liquefies during ageing.
- The architecture of the vitreous body is maintained by a network of collagen fibrils of various subtypes, such as collagen types II, XI and IX. The glycosaminoglycan hyaluronan is a major component occupying the space between collagen fibrils. Various ocular disorders can induce perturbations of the macromolecular structure of the vitreous gel, thus causing alterations of the optical properties of the vitreous body as well as of the functional and anatomical characteristics of the neighboring tissues.
- Several extracellular matrix proteins are associated with the collagen fiber network. Opticin is a glycoprotein that can modulate cell proliferation, e.g., by the binding of retinal growth hormone [29].

Hyalocytes appear to contribute to vitreoretinal interface diseases such as epiretinal membrane formation and diabetic macular edema. They were shown to be derived from bone marrow cells with a fast turnover rate [28]. These phagocytic cells probably belong to the monocyte/macrophage lineage, although they differ from macrophages in other tissues [17]. They express leukocyte-associated antigens CD45, CD11a and S-100 and HLA class I and II, but do not express CD68, CD11b, CD14, glial fibrillary acidic protein (GFAP) or cytokeratin [17, 22]. Hyalocytes can be stimulated to proliferate and migrate by platelet-derived growth factor [22]. They are also thought to possess antigen-presenting capabilities [33] and, therefore, may contribute to the regulation of immunological processes in the eye with the natural state being immunosuppressive. The specific role of hyalocytes for uveitis still remains to be elucidated.

> Noninfectious uveitis is a systemic immune disorder mediated by autoreactive T-lymphocytes overriding the immunosuppressive mechanisms of the eye. The processes activated during this disease involve cellular and molecular components of the immune system and occur within ocular compartments and tissues. Therapeutic interventions are aimed at redressing immunological tolerance within the eye. Since the vitreous body has the potential to participate in proinflammatory as well as in anti-inflammatory processes, the consequences of its removal remain elusive from an immunological perspective.

4.2 Diagnostic Procedures

The general assessment of patients with uveitis includes a comprehensive history and ophthalmic and physical examination. Concomitant systemic diseases are identified by the medical history, clinical and radiological examination and laboratory tests. The exclusion of infectious conditions or masquerade syndromes, as well as the distinction between certain subtypes of uveitis, influence the selection of the treatment regimen and can be performed by diagnostic vitrectomy.

Major diagnostic parameters to assess in uveitis patients are:

- Visual acuity (VA) is the most reliable single parameter to monitor uveitic activity involving posterior segments of the eye. Thus, changes of best corrected VA indicate progression or remission of uveitis. A significant change can be assumed if the log minimum angle of resolution (logMAR) changes by at least 0.2. This threshold ensures reliability of changes and was set in accordance with epidemiological studies involving large populations.

- Specific signs of ocular tissue inflammation should be monitored with standardized methods. Anterior chamber cells and flare, the absence or presence of a hypopyon, are evaluated by slit lamp examination according to the Standardization of Uveitis Nomenclature (SUN) working group [16].
- Clinical activity of vitreal inflammation can be assessed by a binocular indirect ophthalmoscopy (BIO) score of vitreous haze (Table 4.1).
- Fundus evaluation of chorioretinal lesions, neovascularizations and retinal vessels for signs of vasculitis should be performed according to Forrester et al. [12].
- The presence of cystoid macular edema (CME) is determined by fundoscopy. The extent of macular edema can be evaluated by fluorescein angiography and optical coherence tomography (OCT). OCT also provides the opportunity to obtain information on the internal architecture of the macular edema.
- Other complications of uveitis can be assessed by standardized techniques. Cataract formation is monitored quantitatively with the Lens Opacity Classification System (LOCS). ERM formation is reported as present or absent. Neovascularizations at various sites should be confirmed by angiography [16].

The detection and identification of systemic inflammatory diseases associated with uveitis may determine the long-term management strategy of patients. If the clinical examination does not lead to an unequivocal diagnosis, additional examinations, including microbiological and serological tests, may become necessary. Notably, connective tissue diseases can be identified by characteristic patterns of autoreactive antibodies, e.g., ANA and ANCA. In addition to standard panels of laboratory screening tests for systemic immunoreactivity, specific surrogate markers for the pathophysiological processes involved in idiopathic uveitis have the potential to guide diagnostic as well as management decisions during treatment. However, several promising markers, such as IL-8, have been evaluated only in small trials. The predictive value with respect to diagnostic accuracy and disease activity, hence, remains to be confirmed by larger studies.

4.3 Patient Selection

Clinical studies indicate a role of pars plana vitrectomy (PPV) for the treatment of noninfectious uveitis with additional procedures performed in a substantial number of patients [2]. In these reports, the largest subgroup with a specific uveitic diagnosis consists of patients with Behçet's disease. Intermediate uveitis was the most frequently identified anatomical subtype followed by panuveitis and anterior uveitis. Whereas vitreoretinal surgery is indicated for the management of complications arising from intraocular inflammation, the evidence for vitrectomy as a means to control inflammatory activity is less strong. Several authors suggested the existence of a vitreous compartment where autoreactive lymphocytes are protected against pro-apoptotic stimuli. The presence of cellular debris and macromolecular complexes in the vitreous was hypothesized to (co-)stimulate inflammation [32]. Moreover, the vitreous body might contain a significant quantity of proinflammatory mediators, such as cytokines. Thus, the removal of the vitreous could possibly decrease inflammatory activity. Evidence from animal models and patients, however, suggests that immune-mediated uveitis is a systemic disease and regulated by the circulation of effector and regulatory cells as well as molecular mediators from and into the eye. Although PPV might alleviate acute symptoms of uveitis, the long-term course of this chronic disease appears to be determined by the immune system and not by surgery [6]. One might speculate that the replacement of the altered vitreous gel by newly produced ocular fluids after PPV may lead to the exposure of ocular tissues to the immunoregulatory factors of the aqueous humor. The immunosuppressive effects of these factors are illustrated by experiments showing that the aqueous humor inhibits proliferation and cytokine secretion of T-lymphocytes and IFNγ-dependent macrophage activation.

Table 4.1 Grading of vitreous haze through the binocular indirect ophthalmoscope [24]

Score	Description	Clinical findings
0	Nil	None
1	Minimal	Posterior pole clearly visible
2	Mild	Posterior pole details slightly hazy
3	Moderate	Posterior pole details very hazy
4	Marked	Posterior pole details barely visible
5	Severe	Fundal details not visible

4.3.1 Clinical Benefits and Risks

There is only scant clinical evidence that demonstrate a reduction in inflammation induced by PPV. This is mainly due to the following reasons:

- Most surgical interventions were combined with systemic and local administration of immunosuppressives modulating uveitic activity.
- PPV removes vitreous infiltrates which served as a surrogate marker for intraocular inflammation. Only a few papers included ancillary testing, such as fluorescein angiography [2]. The set of standardized quantitative parameters for grading specific signs of inflammation is still incomplete [16]. Documenting changes of immunosuppressive doses in patients after PPV suffers from observer bias.
- No controlled clinical trial on PPV aimed at assessing uveitic activity has been conducted yet. A recent randomized study was focused on CME [38].

PPV clearly induces clinical effects in uveitis patients. However, they often cannot be unequivocally assigned to the removal of the vitreous causing remission of inflammation. The immediate amelioration of visual acuity demonstrated in numerous studies [2] is mainly due to the clearance of this compartment from cellular infiltrates and debris, cataract surgery and reduction of CME [38]. ERM peeling has also shown beneficial effects on visual acuity [2]. How far such surgical interventions can influence proinflammatory signaling pathways involving specific cell groups is unclear. Concerning the photoreceptor function of the inflamed retina, Ahn et al. reported that ERG parameters did not change after PPV in patients with Behçet's disease [1].

The quantitative assessment of intraocular inflammation is a difficult task, since most parameters used in clinical practice are only surrogate markers. Tranos et al. [38] could not find significant differences in anterior chamber activity but documented a marked decline in vitreous activity 6 months after removal of the vitreous. The strongest evidence so far for a specific modulation of inflammatory activity by PPV comes from the comparison of relapse rates before and after surgery [39]. Scott et al. [32] investigated 38 patients with endogenous posterior uveitis and found an overall reduction of uveitic exacerbations during a 12-month period after surgery. Interestingly, the frequency of anterior chamber relapses increased, whereas acute exacerbations at the other anatomical locations were rare after PPV. These findings might be due to differences in the immunological mechanisms controlling tolerance and inflammation in different parts of the eye. It seems possible that PPV provided access for the aqueous humor to posterior ocular tissues, which are still receptive for its immunoregulatory factors. In contrast to these findings, Nolle and Eckhardt [23] could not find a long-term benefit of PPV for visual acuity or the relapse rate in a selected group of patients with multifocal chorioretinitis, indicating that these hypothetical mechanisms could be overridden by proinflammatory stimuli in certain subtypes of uveitis.

In addition to objective measures of intraocular inflammation, such as visual acuity and vitreous haze, a subjective self-assessment of the vision-related quality of life sums up the consequences of the disease on patients' physical, mental and social functioning. Furthermore, it provides the opportunity to monitor the response to treatment. The quality of life after PPV for uveitis was only evaluated in very few studies [3]. The majority of patients expressed satisfaction with the overall result. This was due to the improvement of visual acuity and visual field as well as a decreased rate of relapse.

Vitreoretinal surgery is characterized by a profile of complications and side effects which could be especially harmful in uveitis. The rates of complications after PPV for uveitis patients were estimated as 8% for cataract and between 2% and 5% for retinal detachment, secondary glaucoma, hypotony, ERM formation, and vitreous hemorrhage [3]. Tissue damage inflicted by surgical procedures could stimulate the immune systems, leading to an increased recruitment of leucocytes and elevated local concentrations of proinflammatory cytokines. These mechanisms may cause a bystander activation of autoreactive lymphocytes. The immunosuppression required to prevent these processes or reduce their activity might increase the risk for infections. Furthermore, surgery frequently has to be performed in the context of severely altered tissue structures. The impact of these conditions on the anatomical and functional outcomes of vitreoretinal surgery still has to be determined.

PPV for uveitis was introduced in a time period when the armamentarium of immunosuppressives consisted of corticosteroids. Research into the immunological mechanisms of uveitis revealed major cellular and molecular components orchestrating the systemic and ocular immune response. Consequently, new pharmacological strategies could be introduced to specifically target these components. This development led to a markedly improved control of uveitic activity in most patients. Clinical trials with well-selected groups of patients and controls as well as a standardized follow-up are necessary to determine the place for PPV and associated interventions, such as the administration of intraocular drugs, for the control of inflammatory activity in uveitis. An algorithmic approach of pharmacological treatment regimes appears to be reasonable [2]. Furthermore, some forms of uveitis, e.g., Fuchs uveitis syndrome, might be more responsive to surgical interventions than others.

4.3.2 Indications for Therapeutic Vitrectomy

The decision to perform PPV solely for reducing uveitic activity in the absence of anatomical complications to treat or indications to obtain diagnostic samples is difficult due to the lack of evidence-based guidelines [3]. When choosing between surgery and/or a possible escalation or modification of immunosuppressive drug therapy, we must consider the needs of the individual patient. Current data support the surgical removal of the vitreous in such patients where vitreous opacities compromise visual function, especially in intermediate uveitis [35] or Fuchs uveitis syndrome [40]. Thus, the major indication for PPV is a decline of visual acuity. Apart from Fuchs uveitis syndrome, current evidence supports that PPV should only be performed after optimal medical treatment failed to sufficiently restore visual acuity due to the persistence of vitreous opacities. There is no evidence supporting the use of PPV for modifying inflammatory activity. Active inflammation compromising the transparency of anterior segment structures or access to the vitreous, e.g., in pars planitis, is a relative contraindication for PPV. When urgent vitreoretinal surgery is required in patients with active uveitis, it should be accompanied by an intensive systemic and local immunosuppression regimen, i.e., by intravitreal administration of triamcinolone acetonide [13].

4.4 Therapeutic Vitrectomy

Since the indications for PPV to modify inflammatory activity do not constitute an emergency, there is time for a careful preparation of patients.

4.4.1 Perioperative Immunosuppression

Surgical interventions in patients with uveitis can exacerbate ocular inflammation. Thus, adequate immunosuppression is an important factor for the outcome of surgery in these patients, e.g., by preventing the onset or progression of postsurgical macular edema. Data on the benefit of steroids for cataract surgery in uveitis patients support the administration of immunosuppressives for vitreoretinal surgery, too. However, the adequacy of immunosuppression has to be assessed individually. Whereas data exist for the usefulness of steroids and steroid-sparing agents, e.g., cyclosporine A (CsA) or mycophenolate mofetil (MMF), there is a lack of experience for new immunomodulatory drugs in this setting. Thus, immunosuppression should not be changed when PPV is planned and the inflammatory activity is controlled.

Uveitis should have been quiescent for several weeks before surgery. There is no standardized approach to preoperative immunosuppression. For patients not previously given steroids, oral prednisolone at a daily dose of 40 mg should be commenced 2 weeks before surgery. If the history of individual patients includes frequent and intensive relapses of uveitis, 100 mg of intravenous methylprednisolone can be administered perioperatively to prevent flare-ups. Steroids should be continued after surgery according to clinical symptoms and tapered over 3–5 weeks to adjust to preoperatively given doses. Postoperative immunosuppression also includes topical steroids administered between 6 times daily and hourly for up to 1 week.

4.4.2 Vitreoretinal Surgery

In a major part of the patient population with uveitis, vitreoretinal surgery is performed to manage structural complications of ocular inflammation or to obtain diagnostic samples. Even in the absence of ocular comorbidities, PPV undertaken to clear the vitreous and to modulate uveitic activity requires care to avoid surgical complications which might further enhance immunological reactivity. Standard equipment for PPV and surgical procedure, ensuring posterior hyaloid separation (posterior vitreous detachment) whenever possible, can be used in this setting.

4.4.3 Follow-up and Complications

The follow-up after PPV must include:

- Best corrected visual acuity
- Intraocular pressure measurement
- Biomicroscopy of the anterior segment and the fundus

The assessment of inflammatory activity should be based on standardized grading schemes. Due to the removal of the vitreous, an important surrogate marker of ocular inflammation is absent. Thus, special attention has to be paid to other signs of uveitis, notably vasculitis, macular edema and tissue infiltrates. Ancillary testing, such as angiography or OCT, should be performed to evaluate uveitic activity in a quantitative way. The overall function of the retina can be assessed by electroretinography.

Complications of PPV include:

- Cataract formation
- Macular edema
- Retinal detachment
- Vitreal hemorrhage
- Hypotony
- Hypertension
- ERM formation
- Infections

The risk of inflammatory exacerbation with the induction or progression of macular edema is especially high for uveitis patients. Cataract and CME are frequent causes for the long-term decline of visual acuity after PPV. Some of these complications give rise to other ocular pathologies. Retinal detachment can induce PVR and ERM. CME can lead to macular holes. Phthisis occurs in extreme cases of uncontrolled complications. The incidence of these complications can only be estimated from a small number of retrospective studies, with the median number of patients with complications after PPV being 23% [3].

The risk of complications is correlated with the immunological and anatomical situation before surgery. Thus, adequate immunosuppression and a thorough preoperative examination of the posterior segments contribute to the outcome of vitreoretinal surgery. After PPV, patients should be carefully monitored to adjust immunosuppression and correct complications as early as possible. Wound leakage or retinal detachment must be ruled out in postsurgical hypotony. Since this condition could be caused by an inflammation-induced decline of aqueous humor production, oral steroids are useful. Topical therapy is often sufficient to manage transient hypertension. Vitreal hemorrhages can be monitored for a certain period of time, since the blood is often cleared from the vitreous without further intervention. Retinal tears or newly formed vessels have to be excluded as sources of the hemorrhage.

4.5 Specific Disease Entities

The group of noninfectious uveitis comprises several entities which share common pathophysiological features but also differ with respect to certain immunological mechanisms. Most significantly, anterior and posterior forms of uveitis appear to be based on different pathways of immunological reactivity. Patients with intermediate uveitis were found to have a larger fraction of CD4+ lymphocytes in the vitreous than patients with Fuchs uveitis syndrome [18]. These differences between uveitis entities could cause variation of the response to specific medical as well as surgical treatments. The first studies on PPV in uveitis involved mixed patient populations; more recent studies, however, focused on patients with specific disorders, e.g., Behçet's disease. In fact, these investigations revealed varying success rates for different disease entities [3].

4.5.1 Intermediate Uveitis

Intermediate uveitis is an intraocular inflammation involving the anterior vitreous, peripheral retina and pars plana. This chronic relapsing disease is bilateral in 80% of the patients [5]. It is frequently associated with systemic diseases, such as multiple sclerosis or sarcoidosis. Intravitreal "snowballs" and retinal "snowbanking" are the hallmarks of pars planitis. Macular edema and retinal vasculitis are other manifestations of intermediate uveitis. Cataract and glaucoma are frequent complications. Treatment of intermediate uveitis is primarily based on steroids and other immunosuppressives with CsA being a first-line steroid-sparing agent.

PPV is indicated in patients with vitreous opacities compromising visual acuity and being refractory to medical treatment. Complications of intermediate uveitis, such as CME, tractional retinal detachment or vitreous hemorrhage, are other indications for vitreoretinal surgery. Patients with intermediate uveitis constitute the largest subgroup reported in the literature [2]. Stavrou et al. [35] investigated 32 patients. The clinical course improved in 44% after PPV. Immunosuppressive therapy could be discontinued in seven patients. PPV combined with cataract surgery led to an increased or stable visual acuity in almost all patients. In another study, PPV induced regression of CME refractory to medical therapy [41].

4.5.2 Fuchs Uveitis Syndrome

Fuchs uveitis syndrome is characterized by iridocyclitis, iris atrophy, keratic precipitates and heterochromia. Vitritis is a common finding which causes floaters. CME is absent despite chronic inflammation. Cataract is the most common complication. No immunosuppressive treatment, including steroids, is known to influence the course of the disease. Thus, PPV is indicated to remove vitreous opacities which can be increased after posterior vitreous detachment or by cataract surgery. Two studies investigating the outcome after PPV described an improvement of visual acuity in all 25 patients [31, 40]. Moreover, PPV is a safe procedure and did not appear to induce exacerbation of this disease. Thus, PPV is recommended early in the course of Fuchs uveitic syndrome when visual perception is restricted by vitreous infiltrates [3].

4.5.3 Behçet's Disease

Behçet's disease represents a multisystem disorder with recurrent panuveitis. Features of ocular inflammation are occlusive retinal vasculitis and vitritis. Complications include CME, ERM, and tractional retinal detachment. Conventional immunosuppression is frequently insufficient to control ocular inflammation. In the literature on PPV in uveitis, patients with Behçet's disease have been the largest subgroup with a specific disease entity described so far [2]. A report on seven patients with vitreous hemorrhage and infiltrates first suggested that PPV might induce severe complications in eyes affected by Behçet's disease [25]. Other studies, however, showed that the relapse rate is reduced after PPV [26, 34]. Ahn et al. [1] investigated the outcome of PPV in patients with Behçet's disease and persistent panuveitis. These authors also demonstrated a decrease in the relapse rate. However, the majority of surgical interventions were assisted by intravitreal administration of triamcinolone. A subgroup of patients exhibiting optic disc neovascularization were identified whose inflammatory activity was not improved by PPV. Summarizing these findings, there is suggestive evidence that PPV should be contemplated for uveitis in Behçet's disease when currently available medical treatment fails. PPV should be accompanied by intravitreal triamcinolone injection.

4.5.4 Eales Disease

Eales disease presents as a retinal vasculitis with a still unknown etiology. Dehghan et al. [9] reported a benefit of PPV to induce regression of retinal neovascularization that is refractory to laser photocoagulation.

4.6 Conclusions

> Noninfectious uveitis is associated with an activation of the adaptive immune system. Thus, the prospects of a single local treatment to modulate disease activity are limited. Currently, there is no evidence that the pattern of regulatory molecules expressed in ocular tissues is changed by vitrectomy in a way that induces immunosuppression. Moreover, experiments in animals indicate that the regulatory immune system in the eye responsible for maintaining tolerance can be overridden by external stimuli.

The advent of new and more effective medical treatment options which also have fewer side effects than conventional immunosuppressives restricts the indications of PPV to control uveitic activity. Medical treatment constitutes the first-line therapy for uveitis and has to be continued even after PPV. Vitreoretinal surgery is clearly indicated to manage complications of uveitis. A collateral impact on inflammatory activity cannot be ruled out, especially in patients with macular edema. There is only scant evidence in the literature that indicates a beneficial effect of the removal of the vitreous for immune reactivity. Several studies describe positive outcomes of PPV in patients with distinct disease entities. The removal of vitreous opacities clearly improves visual function in patients with intermediate uveitis and Fuchs uveitis syndrome. PPV also demonstrated an effect on the relapse rate in some patients with Behçet's disease. In the latter case, however, prognostic factors have to be defined for patient selection. To collect further evidence for the role of PPV in uveitis, controlled trials have to be performed which involve patient populations being homogeneous with respect to the disease entity and concomitant immunosuppression as well as standardized procedures to assess uveitic activity.

Take Home Pearls

- The treatment of immune-mediated uveitis requires an ongoing control of immunological reactivity.
- Vitrectomy is not an established method to control intraocular inflammation.
- Vitrectomy may alter the course and prognosis of patients with Fuchs or Eales disease.

> ■ Correcting structural complications of ocular inflammation, including vitreous opacities, is the major indication for therapeutic vitrectomy in patients with uveitis.

References

1. Ahn JK, Chung H, Yu HG. Vitrectomy for persistent panuveitis in Behçet disease. Ocul Immunol Inflamm. 2005;13:447–53
2. Becker M, Davis J. Vitrectomy in the treatment of uveitis. Am J Ophthalmol. 2005;140:1096–105
3. Becker MD, Harsch N, Zierhut M, Davis JL, Holz FG. Therapeutic vitrectomy in uveitis: current status and recommendations. Ophthalmologe. 2003;100:787–95
4. Bishop PN. Structural macromolecules and supramolecular organisation of the vitreous gel. Prog Retin Eye Res. 2000;19:323–44
5. Bonfioli AA, Damico FM, Curi AL, Orefice F. Intermediate uveitis. Semin Ophthalmol. 2005;20:147–54
6. Bovey EH, Herbort CP. Vitrectomy in the management of uveitis. Ocul Immunol Inflamm. 2000;8:285–91
7. Boyd SR, Young S, Lightman S. Immunopathology of the noninfectious posterior and intermediate uveitides. Surv Ophthalmol. 2001;46:209–33
8. Caspi RR. Regulation, counter-regulation, and immunotherapy of autoimmune responses to immunologically privileged retinal antigens. Immunol Res. 2003;27:149–60
9. Dehghan MH, Ahmadieh H, Soheilian M, Azarmina M, Mashayekhi A, Naghibozakerin J. Therapeutic effects of laser photocoagulation and/or vitrectomy in Eales' disease. Eur J Ophthalmol. 2005;15:379–83
10. de Smet MD, Chan CC. Regulation of ocular inflammation – what experimental and human studies have taught us. Prog Retin Eye Res. 2001;20:761–97
11. Dick AD, Isaacs JD. Immunomodulation of autoimmune responses with monoclonal antibodies and immunoadhesins: treatment of ocular inflammatory disease in the next millennium. Br J Ophthalmol. 1999;83:1230–4
12. Forrester JV, Okada AA, BenEzra D, Ohno S. Posterior segment intraocular inflammation. The Hague: Kugler; 1998
13. Gutfleisch M, Spital G, Mingels A, Pauleikhoff D, Lommatzsch A, Heiligenhaus A. Pars-plana vitrectomy with intravitreal triamcinolone: effect on uveitic cystoid macular edema and treatment limitations. Br J Ophthalmol. 2007;91:345–8
14. Harada C, Mitamura Y, Harada T. The role of cytokines and trophic factors in epiretinal membranes: involvement of signal transduction in glial cells. Prog Retin Eye Res. 2006;25:149–64
15. Hiscott P, Paraoan L, Choudhary A, Ordonez JL, Al-Khaier A, Armstrong DJ. Thrombospondin 1, thrombospondin 2 and the eye. Prog Retin Eye Res. 2006;25:1–18
16. Jabs DA, Nussenblatt RB, Rosenbaum JT, Standardization of Uveitis Nomenclature (SUN) Working Group. Standardization of uveitis nomenclature for reporting clinical data. Results of the First International Workshop. Am J Ophthalmol. 2005;140:509–16
17. Lazarus HS, Hageman GS. In situ characterization of the human hyalocyte. Arch Ophthalmol. 1994;112:1356–62
18. Muhaya M, Calder VL, Towler HM, Jolly G, McLauchlan M, Lightman S. Characterization of phenotype and cytokine profiles of T-lymphocyte lines derived from vitreous humor in ocular inflammation in man. Clin Exp Immunol. 1999;116:410–4
19. Murray PI, Clay CD, Mappin C, Salmon M. Molecular analysis of resolving immune responses in uveitis. Clin Exp Immunol. 1999;117:455–61
20. Namba K, Kitaichi N, Nishida T, Taylor AW. Induction of regulatory T-lymphocytes by the immunomodulating cytokines alpha-melanocyte-stimulating hormone and transforming growth factor-beta2. J Leukoc Biol. 2002;72:946–52
21. Niederkorn JY. See no evil, hear no evil, do no evil: the lessons of immune privilege. Nat Immunol. 2006;7:354–9
22. Noda Y, Hata Y, Hisatomi T, Nakamura Y, Hirayama K, Miura M, Nakao S, Fujisawa K, Sakamoto T, Ishibashi T. Functional properties of hyalocytes under PDGF-rich conditions. Invest Ophthalmol Vis Sci. 2004;45:2107–14
23. Nolle B, Eckardt C. Vitrectomy in multifocal chorioretinitis. Ger J Ophthalmol. 1993;2:14–9
24. Nussenblatt RB, Palestine AG, Chan CC, Roberge F. Standardization of vitreal inflammatory activity in intermediate and posterior uveitis. Ophthalmology. 1985;92:467–71
25. Ozdemir O, Erkam N, Bakkaloglu A. Results of pars plana vitrectomy in Behçet disease. Ann Ophthalmol. 1988;20:35–8
26. Ozerturk Y, Bardak Y, Durmus M. Vitreoretinal surgery in Behçet disease with severe ocular complications. Acta Ophthalmol Scand. 2001;79:192–6
27. Perez VL, Papaliodis GN, Chu D, Anzaar F, Christen W, Foster CS. Elevated levels of interleukin 6 in the vitreous fluid of patients with pars planitis and posterior uveitis: the Massachusetts eye & ear experience and review of previous studies. Ocul Immunol Inflamm. 2004;12:193–201
28. Qiao H, Hisatomi T, Sonoda KH, Kura S, Sassa Y, Kinoshita S, Nakamura T, Sakamoto T, Ishibashi T. The characterisation of hyalocytes: the origin, phenotype, and turnover. Br J Ophthalmol. 2005;89:513–7

29. Sanders EJ, Walter MA, Parker E, Aramburo C, Harvey S. Opticin binds retinal growth hormone in the embryonic vitreous. Invest Ophthalmol Vis Sci. 2003;44:5404–9
30. Santos Lacomba M, Marcos Martin C, Gallardo Galera JM, Gomez Vidal MA, Collantes Estevez E, Ramirez Chamond R, Omar M. Aqueous humor and serum tumor necrosis factor-alpha in clinical uveitis. Ophthalmic Res. 2001;33:251–5
31. Scott RA, Sullivan PM, Aylward GW, Pavesio CE, Charteris DG. The effect of pars plana vitrectomy in the management of Fuchs heterochromic cyclitis. Retina. 2001;21:312–6
32. Scott RA, Haynes RJ, Orr GM, Cooling RJ, Pavesio CE, Charteris DG. Vitreous surgery in the management of chronic endogenous posterior uveitis. Eye. 2003;17:221–7
33. Sonoda KH, Sakamoto T, Qiao H, Hisatomi T, Oshima T, Tsutsumi-Miyahara C, Exley M, Balk SP, Taniguchi M, Ishibashi T. The analysis of systemic tolerance elicited by antigen inoculation into the vitreous cavity: vitreous cavity-associated immune deviation. Immunology. 2005;116:390–9
34. Soylu M, Demircan N, Pelit A. Pars plana vitrectomy in ocular Behçet disease. Int Ophthalmol. 2001;24:219–23
35. Stavrou P, Baltatzis S, Letko E, Samson CM, Christen W, Foster CS. Pars plana vitrectomy in patients with intermediate uveitis. Ocul Immunol Inflamm. 2001;9:141–51
36. Streilein JW. Immunoregulatory mechanisms of the eye. Prog Retin Eye Res. 1999;18:357–70
37. Suttorp-Schulten MS, Rothova A. The possible impact of uveitis in blindness: a literature survey. Br J Ophthalmol. 1996;80:844–8
38. Tranos P, Scott R, Zambarajki H, Ayliffe W, Pavesio C, Charteris DG. The effect of pars plana vitrectomy on cystoid macular edema associated with chronic uveitis: a randomised, controlled pilot study. Br J Ophthalmol. 2006;90:1107–10
39. Trittibach P, Koerner F, Sarra GM, Garweg JG. Vitrectomy for juvenile uveitis: prognostic factors for the long-term functional outcome. Eye. 2006;20:184–90
40. Waters FM, Goodall K, Jones NP, McLeod D. Vitrectomy for vitreous opacification in Fuchs heterochromic uveitis. Eye. 2000;14:216–8
41. Wiechens B, Nolle B, Reichelt JA. Pars-plana vitrectomy in cystoid macular edema associated with intermediate uveitis. Graefes Arch Clin Exp Ophthalmol. 2001;239:474–81

Chapter 5

Cryotherapy and Laser for Intermediate Uveitis

Javier A. Montero, Jose M. Ruiz-Moreno

Core Messages

- Pars plana exudates in intermediate uveitis (IU) are associated with more severe vitreous disease and increased incidence of cystoid macular edema (CME).
- Cryotherapy and laser photocoagulation are used in the treatment of the pars planitis variant of corticosteroid resistant IU.
- Cryotherapy should be avoided in retinal detachment or marked peripheral vitreoretinal adhesions. A B-scan ultrasound may be needed.
- Technique for cryotherapy:
  - Peribulbar or sub-Tenon anesthesia.
  - "Freeze-thaw-freeze" or "double row single freeze" of inferior snowbank.
  - Treat contiguous, uninvolved retina (one third width of snowbank) and area with dense exudates.
  - Average of 20 freezes per eye.
  - Postoperative posterior sub-Tenon injection of long-acting corticosteroids and topical steroids.
- Technique for laser photocoagulation:
  - Topical anesthesia is preferred for office treatment.
  - Endophotocoagulation may be performed during pars plana posterior vitrectomy, under peribulbar, retrobulbar or general anesthesia.
  - Nonconfluent, grayish laser marks, 300–500-μm wide, 0.2 s duration.

Contents

5.1	Introduction	47
5.2	Definition of Intermediate Uveitis	48
5.3	Epidemiology	48
5.4	Signs and Symptoms	48
5.5	Clinical Course	49
5.6	Diagnostic	50
5.6.1	Laboratory Tests	50
5.6.2	Imaging Studies	50
5.6.2.1	Fluorescein Angiography	50
5.6.2.2	Optical Coherence Tomography	50
5.6.2.3	B-Scan Ultrasonography	50
5.6.2.4	Magnetic Resonance Imaging	50
5.7	Complications	50
5.8	Treatment	50
5.8.1	Medical Therapy	51
5.8.2	Surgical Therapy	51
5.8.2.1	Cyclocryotherapy	52
5.8.2.2	Retinal Cryotherapy	52
5.8.2.3	Retinal Laser Photocoagulation	54
5.8.2.4	Vitrectomy	56
References		56

5.1 Introduction

The management of intermediate uveitis often involves not only medical treatment with corticosteroids and immunosuppression, but also a surgical approach including vitrectomy, laser and cryotherapy. Laser photocoagulation and cryotherapy applied to the peripheral retina and the ciliary body are useful tools to reduce intraocular inflammation in patients who have not responded fully to medical therapy or wish to avoid it. In addition to reduction of intraocular inflammation, regression of peripheral and optic disk neovascularization may also be achieved.

5.2 Definition of Intermediate Uveitis

Intermediate uveitis (IU) is an intraocular inflammatory syndrome involving primarily the anterior vitreous, peripheral retina and pars plana. The term IU was introduced by the International Uveitis Study Group in 1987 [6] and revised by the Standardization of Uveitis Nomenclature (SUN) Working Group in 2005. IU was retained as the preferred term for uveitis in which the vitreous is the major anatomic site of inflammation. Pars planitis was reserved for *idiopathic* IU in which there is snowball or snowbank formation. Cases secondary to systemic disease with snowbanks should be classified as IU [18].

Despite attempts to standardize nomenclature, confusion between IU and pars planitis (PP) occurs in the medical literature. Some authors use PP when there are pars plana exudates and collagen bands (snowbanks) over the pars plana. Other authors consider PP to be an idiopathic form of IU not associated with systemic diseases, with cells in the anterior vitreous and exudates over the pars plana or peripheral retina that may be associated with neovascularization in the vitreous base. Snowbanking is not required for the diagnosis of IU, but it is associated with worse vitreous inflammation and macular edema [17].

5.3 Epidemiology

PP is the most common variant of IU. It represents approximately 4–16% of all uveitis cases seen in *referral practices* and 16–33% of all uveitis cases in children. Approximately two thirds of IU patients will have PP [17, 35].

PP usually affects children and young adults and is relatively rare in the elderly and aged population. Cryotherapy and laser will therefore occasionally need to be performed under general anesthesia. Early onset is not common and is seen in about 10% of affected patients [1]. The mean age of onset occurs in the third decade of life with 80% of cases presenting bilaterally, quite frequently in an asymmetrical manner.

The age of onset correlates inversely with the severity of expression: in cases symptomatic within the first decade of life, the severity of inflammation, the resulting vitreous opacification and the resistance to therapy are significantly greater than when the onset occurs in the second to fourth decades.

5.4 Signs and Symptoms

The initial symptoms of IU are usually blurred vision and floaters with only a mild decrease of visual acuity (VA). More severe visual loss may appear at later stages, secondary to chronic CME, uveitic glaucoma, retinal detachment, or epiretinal membrane.

The anterior segment usually shows mild inflammation. Synechiae are infrequent, and the pupil usually dilates well. Cataracts and glaucoma are less common than in anterior uveitis. Cyclitic membranes may form in severe disease, eventually causing traction on the ciliary body leading to hypotony and phthisis bulbi. Retinal and pars plana exudates can form membranes that contract and cause peripheral tractional detachment. Peripheral serous detachments are quite common in active inflammation.

Posterior vitreous detachment (PVD) is common in young patients with IU and may be the presenting symptom. Vitritis is the most consistent sign of IU and is troublesome for patients even in whom it is of little clinical consequence. However, it may become dense and obscure the retina entirely. Clusters of lymphocytes and macrophages may coalesce to form intravitreal snowball opacities or debris. These are best seen with the Goldmann three-mirror lens or with a +20 D lens and scleral indentation. These "snowballs," also described as "ants' eggs," can be seen in the inferior peripheral vitreous, close to the retina. Snowballs are not specific for PP and may occur with any kind of inflammation of the peripheral fundus or with an extensive and diffuse uveitis. The vitreous may show degenerative changes with cylindrical condensations of coarse vitreous strands at later stages.

Snowbanks are preretinal, peripheral and typically inferior but may also be superior or divided into multiple foci or extend 360° over the entire pars plana (Fig. 5.1). Snowbanking is not always present. Its presence is indicative of the likelihood of a more severe and chronic course with a higher incidence of CME and consequently a poorer prognosis.

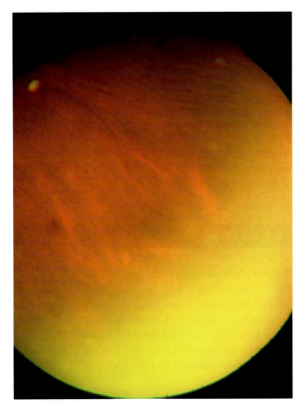

Fig. 5.1 Inferior pars plana collagen band in a patient with pars planitis

Inflammation may be associated with patchy peripheral retinal vasculitis, which is best appreciated by fluorescein angiography. Neovascularization of the peripheral retina is infrequent and may cause vitreous hemorrhage.

CME may appear in 28–50% of cases. Angiographic or Optical Coherent Tomography (OCT) studies are often necessary for a diagnosis, especially if the edema is subtle or if the media are hazy.

> Retinal detachment is rarely seen. However, the association of vitreous hemorrhage and vitreous fibrosis may cause a tractional retinal detachment, which may become complete, leading to phthisis bulbi.

The optic nerve is usually normal but can be slightly hyperemic and swollen, especially in late stages. Severe optic disc swelling is unusual. Neovascularization of the disc may appear in cases of severe inflammation or ischemia.

5.5 Clinical Course

The clinical course of IU is usually self-limited or chronic with one or more episodes of exacerbation and can be bilateral in 80% of cases. The disease usually lasts for about 5–10 years. However, durations of active disease up to 15–20 years are not uncommon. Eighty percent of patients are expected to retain a VA of 20/40 or better in at least one eye, but IU may also result in visual disability. Courses type 2 and 3 may be treated by laser and cryotherapy if not responsive to steroidal therapy.

> Patterns of disease of pars planitis [38]:
> - Self-limiting course, characterized by gradual improvement without exacerbation and low-grade activity (10%).
> - Prolonged course without noticeable exacerbations (59%).
> - Chronic course with one or more episodes of exacerbation (31%).

The prognosis for vision is related to the severity of the inflammation rather than to the duration. CME and postinflammatory macular degeneration are the most important causes for visual loss. Pars plana exudates indicate a higher risk of more severe vitreous disease and an increased incidence of CME [17]. Permanent spontaneous resolution of IU is uncommon, and vision loss can occur before the disease "burns out."

> IU classification [2]:
> - Type 1: Inflammatory membranes covering the inferior pars plana and peripheral retina over approximately 90°, with exudative foci on the peripheral retina and pars plana.
> - Type 2: Similar findings as type 1. The inflammatory membrane covers 180° or more.
> - Type 3: Similar to type 2 with neovascularization of the pars plana extending from the anterior portion of the pars plana and from the peripheral retina.

Type 3 of IU, which is associated with neovascularization of the pars plana, is more amenable to treatment by cryotherapy and laser photocoagulation.

5.6 Diagnostic

Since IU has been described in association with several systemic disorders, the initial diagnostic evaluation should serve to exclude masquerade syndromes and infectious diseases in which immunosuppression may be ineffective or contraindicated. The diagnostic approach to IU should center on the history and clinical examination.

5.6.1 Laboratory Tests

A minimum workup for IU should include a serum ACE, chest X-ray, syphilis test (FTA-ABS and VDRL), and CBC. The laboratory workup can be expanded, depending upon the clinical history and physical findings.

5.6.2 Imaging Studies

5.6.2.1 Fluorescein Angiography

The most important investigation for the presence of CME in patients with IU is fluorescein angiography. Most early reports have noted this complication in 28–50% of cases. Staining of the vessel walls and/or leakage indicates perivasculitis. Peripheral areas of ischemia and neovascularization are potential indications for laser therapy.

> The angiogram provides information about the integrity of the retinal vasculature, areas of ischemia and neovascularization.

5.6.2.2 Optical Coherence Tomography

Optical coherence tomography (OCT) is a useful, noninvasive tool to monitor the presence of CME, even in the presence of moderately dense vitreous opacities.

5.6.2.3 B-Scan Ultrasonography

In cloudy media, B-scan ultrasonography can be useful to document vitreous debris, retinal detachment, and cyclitic membranes. Ultrasound biomicroscopy may also show features that are not clinically obvious, such as uveal thickening, the nature of inflammatory condensations in the vitreous and vitreoretinal adhesions with traction.

> Peripheral retinal cryotherapy should be avoided in patients with traction retinal detachment or areas of strong vitreoretinal adhesion.

5.6.2.4 Magnetic Resonance Imaging

Neurological symptoms or a history of optic neuritis justify performing magnetic resonance imaging (MRI) of the brain to rule out multiple sclerosis.

5.7 Complications

The most common complications are cataract formation (42%), CME (28%), and, in order of decreasing incidence, band keratopathy, glaucoma, retinal detachment, retinoschisis, vitreous hemorrhage, retinitis-pigmentosa-like changes, and dragged disc vessels [38]. Retinal and optic disk neovascularization are less common and usually appear associated to ischemia [13].

> Neovascularization without apparent retinal ischemia may be due to angiogenic factors released by the retina in chronic intraocular inflammation [13, 24, 37]. Neovascularization seems to be associated with exacerbations of inflammation; therefore, therapy should be oriented toward controlling the inflammation.

Vitreous hemorrhages have been found in two thirds of the cases with optic disk neovascularization [22]. Most of these hemorrhages are relatively mild and clear quickly, allowing photocoagulation and cryotherapy. Vitreous hemorrhages and vitreous fibrosis can cause traction on the peripheral retina and lead to retinal detachment. The frequency of this complication ranges from 3 to 22%. Retinal detachment and cyclitic membranes may lead to phthisis bulbi.

5.8 Treatment

Indications for treatment of IU are:

- CME
- VA below 20/40

- Severe floaters in patients with a VA of 20/40 or better
- Underlying systemic disease requiring treatment

5.8.1 Medical Therapy

Corticosteroids administered topically, periocularly by injection or orally, are the mainstay of therapy. The treatment protocol most commonly accepted is based on the four-step algorithm proposed by Kaplan [23] and modified by Bonfioli et al. [7] (Fig. 5.2). Unilateral forms may be treated first by an injection of sub-Tenon corticosteroids such as methylprednisolone acetate or triamcinolone acetonide (TA). Retrobulbar (not sub-Tenon) injections may have a high risk of complications and poorer intraocular penetration of the drug. Since a single injection is often highly effective in controlling inflammation for 6–8 months, repeating injections in a short interval of time is controversial. Lack of effect of the initial injection may indicate the need to consider other therapy such as systemic corticosteroids or local therapy with laser or cryotherapy.

> VA less than 20/40 associated with snowbanks and/or lack of response to periocular injections may be treated by laser or cryotherapy.

Bilateral cases may be treated initially by systemic corticosteroid therapy to avoid bilateral injections. Unilateral and bilateral recurrences should be treated as if they were new unilateral or bilateral episodes.

Immunosuppression is most commonly used when no response is achieved after systemic or periocular steroid therapy, or when steroids cause severe side effects. Azathioprine, cyclosporine, and methotrexate are frequently used agents [29].

Corticosteroids given as high-dose intravenous pulses daily for 3 days are a useful alternative when systemic immunosuppressants are contraindicated and in one-eyed patients in whom local injections and surgeries may be less desirable.

Intraocular corticosteroids have been used as an effective short-term treatment for resistant CME in uveitis, in association with cataract surgery in uveitic children and to reduce the dosage of oral corticosteroids [4, 25, 41].

Fluocinolone acetonide intravitreal implants have effectively controlled intraocular inflammation, reducing the need for systemic, topical and periocular anti-inflammatory medications [19]. Intraocular steroids and implants are described in another chapter.

Low-dose acetazolamide can be a useful therapeutic option for chronic CME in uveitis, though recurrences are frequent after discontinuation of the drug [36].

5.8.2 Surgical Therapy

Indications for surgical therapy are:

- VA under 20/40
- Eyes with snowbanking or extensive vasculitis or neovascularization
- Complaint of severe floaters [7]

> Peripheral retinal neovascularization or ischemia are absolute indications of laser and/or cryotherapy. Persistent inflammation would be an additional, relative indication of laser/cryotherapy.

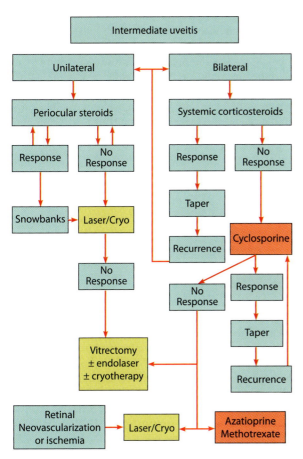

Fig. 5.2 Treating algorithm for intermediate uveitis. (Modified from [7])

5.8.2.1 Cyclocryotherapy

Gills described the use of cyclodiathermy to treat peripheral inflammation and exudation [15]. Kwrawicz reported cryocoagulation of the peripheral retina and ciliary body to treat uveitis in 1967 [26]. Inflammation subsided in 75% of 200 cases by the 10th day after the treatment and persisted after the 15th day only in 5 cases of 200. The type of uveitis was not specified. His results were later confirmed by other authors [2, 10, 20].

In this obsolete treatment for uveitis, freezing induces destruction of the ciliary processes, followed by atrophia and replacement by fibroplastic tissue [34]. Changes occur in the aqueous fluid, mainly in the concentrations of immunoglobulins [26].

Technique

> Cyclocryotherapy is performed transconjunctivally under sub-Tenon or peribulbar injection of lidocaine. However, general anesthesia may be performed in children, and topical anesthesia with cocaine drops may also be used in cooperative patients.

Cyclocryotherapy was generally administered through the conjunctiva at −70°C, allowing the probe to freeze for 10–14 s. Approximately 10 applications were performed. Quigley [34] studied the histological and physiological effects of cyclocryotherapy. He demonstrated in vivo that, regardless of the duration of the freezing, the lowest temperature reached in the pars plicata is −10°C when the probe reached −70°C, and the internal temperature remained below 0°C for 10–20 s after the end of the application.

Complications

Among the possible complications of cyclocryotherapy were persistently decreased IOP, transitory worsening of inflammation, sustained rupture of the blood–aqueous barrier with flare, hyphema, vitreous hemorrhage, cataract progression, damage to the trabecular meshwork, iris retraction and atrophia [34].

5.8.2.2 Retinal Cryotherapy

Retinal cryotherapy was also developed in the 1960s and rapidly supplanted cyclocryotherapy as a surgical treatment for uveitis [26]. Initially it was used to treat toxoplasmosis in an attempt to clear inflammation and reduce recurrences by destroying the parasites but was found to be ineffective in this regard [12]. In the following decades, the principal use for retinal cryotherapy in the treatment of uveitis was pars planitis that had failed to respond to corticosteroid therapy. The first reports of the use of cryotherapy to treat peripheral exudation and neovascularization in pars planitis began to appear in 1973 [1, 3, 9].

The mechanism of cryotherapy is not known, although it is unlikely that it treats the actual cause of peripheral uveitis. By analogy to the histological studies of cyclocryotherapy [34], ablation of the peripheral retina destroys compromised vasculature and ischemic tissue, eliminating both the source for inflammatory mediators and the stimulus for neovascularization. This may lead to a decrease of the inflammatory process, accumulation of exudates and organization of the vitreous base, reducing the risk of traction or rhegmatogenous retinal detachment [30].

Cryotherapy is also indicated in patients with snowbanking who have not responded to steroid therapy for 6 months. It is also a useful alternative to immunosuppressants in patients who show intolerance to steroid therapy. Patients with retinal neovascularization may benefit from cryotherapy applied directly to areas of neovascularization. Some authors advocate the use of cryotherapy only for patients with peripheral retinal neovascularization and a history of vitreous hemorrhage. Others consider it to be a useful procedure early in the course of disease before resorting to systemic corticosteroids.

Technique

> Transconjunctival cryotherapy is performed under topical anesthesia with cocaine drops; subconjunctival is performed under sub-Tenon or peribulbar anesthesia. General anesthesia may be necessary in children.

Cryotherapy is generally administered directly over areas of neovascularization utilizing a freeze, thaw and refreeze technique (after a brief period of thawing, it is refrozen to the same intensity) [2], or by applying two rows of single freeze. Under direct visualization, generally using a +20 D lens and an indirect ophthalmoscope (Fig. 5.3), the area covered with the new vessels and the gelatinous exudates is frozen for 10–15 s, or until ice formation is evident for 1–2 s [5]. On average, 10–20 freezes are performed per eye (8–12 cryotherapy spots in each quadrant), just posterior to the ora serrata. The

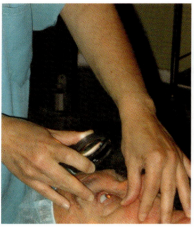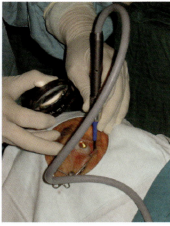

Fig. 5.3 Cryotherapy procedure. Identification of the pars plana exudates and cryoapplications under indirect ophthalmoscopy control

margins of the freeze are extended one or two freezes (one clock hour) width beyond visible neovascularization. The areas of dense exudates are also included in the treated zone. Because of the known complications of cyclocryotherapy, treatment is rarely extended anterior to the ora serrata.

The precipitation of inflammatory material to the lower half of the eye has engendered the idea that the inflammation is centered in the inferior periphery. However, inflammation may involve the entire periphery, leading some authors to recommend cryotherapy superiorly as well [5].

> Cryotherapy applications are usually followed by a sub-Tenon corticosteroid injection and topical corticosteroids. Cryotherapy usually reduces the need for systemic corticosteroid treatment for a prolonged period.

The effect of cryotherapy may take several weeks to develop and usually lasts 3–6 months. Though it may need to be repeated, it should not be done before 3 months after the last application. When no response is observed, 2–3 months are allowed before subsequent treatments, which can be performed in the same area or in the areas of new snowbank formation. More than two sessions are rarely applied.

Results

> Prognosis after cryotherapy may be better if less than 60° of the periphery is affected [7].

In 1973, Aaberg et al. [2] reported cryotherapy in the treatment of vitreous base exudation and neovascularization. In their experience, 35% of treated eyes showed a complete quiescence of inflammation while an additional 57% showed a marked reduction in inflammatory activity. Only 61% of these eyes had definite pars plana neovascularization. A follow-up study by Devenyi et al. [9] reported on the use of cryotherapy in eyes with pars plana neovascularization unresponsive to corticosteroid therapy. In this study, neovascularization regressed in all 27 treated eyes, the inflammation remained quiescent in 78% of the eyes and VA improved an average of three Snellen lines.

Mieler et al. [30] described their results after performing cryotherapy of the vitreous base on 30 eyes from 21 patients with peripheral uveitis. All patients had previously undergone topical, periocular and systemic corticosteroid therapy with persistence of the inflammation and active neovascularization of the vitreous base. Of the eyes, 87% required only one session of cryotherapy, 10% of eyes required two sessions and 3% required three sessions. Regression of neovascularization was achieved in all cases. At the final follow-up visit, 80% of eyes showed no active inflammation in the anterior chamber or vitreous cavity and 67% of the total had improved VA an average of three Snellen lines. However, one eye progressed into atrophia bulbi 9 years after the initial therapy. Two further eyes lost VA caused by preretinal membrane formation and cataracts progression. Six eyes required vitreous surgery for retinal detachment, vitreous hemorrhage, preretinal membrane and vitreous opacification.

Berg et al. described in 1990 their results after treating 185 uveitic eyes by cryoapplications [5]. Of the eyes, 174 were treated once, 10 eyes were treated twice and one eye was treated three times. Sixteen eyes underwent an additional vitrectomy due to lack of sufficient effect of the cryotherapy, and 33 eyes had been previously vitrectomized. Of the eyes, 38% were treated for IU. Cryo-applications achieved improvement in VA in 45.8% of the eyes, and vision was unchanged in 31.3% of the eyes. Anterior chamber inflammation decreased from 31.9% of the eyes before cryotherapy to 7% after the treatment (78% success). Recurrences appeared in 51 of 151 eyes (37.5%) after an average 1.3 years, in nine cases bilaterally. The course of these recurrences seemed to be milder than the previous inflammations. The need for systemic corticosteroid therapy decreased from 56.8% before surgery to 24.1% after surgery. Additionally, the presence of CME decreased from 31.5% to 20.7% of the eyes.

Prieto et al. [33] described a retrospective series of 44 patients with PP, seven of them undergoing cryotherapy associated to periocular corticosteroids. In six of them the pharmacological treatment was decreased and was followed by a subsequent average time of inactivity of 11.5 months (SD 8.9).

In another study of mixed uveitis in a pediatric population, cryotherapy was the most frequent surgical approach. It was performed in 22.5% of the children with PP, compared to cataract extraction (14.3%), and lensectomy and anterior vitrectomy (2%) [21].

Complications

Possible complications of cryotherapy are transitory worsening of inflammation (17%), hyphema, persistent CME (37%), preretinal membrane formation (20%), retinoschisis and development or acceleration of a traction retinal detachment (3%) [30]. Cataract progression has been described in 17% of the eyes as the only complication of cryotherapy [5]. Exudative retinal detachment was described to appear after cryotherapy [11].

5.8.2.3 Retinal Laser Photocoagulation

Indications

Laser photocoagulation was initially reserved for patients with recurrent vitreous hemorrhages and significant capillary closure. The procedure was performed when the eye was quiet [16]. However, the role of laser photocoagulation for preretinal and optic disc neovascularization in chronic uveitis and IU has become clearer in the past 20 years.

> Medical treatment is initiated first to control inflammation. Laser photocoagulation is justified if the neovascularization persists or medical therapy is insufficient [14].

As described for cryotherapy, ischemic and inflammatory mechanisms have been postulated for the production of the retinal, iris and optic disc neovascularization. Destruction of ischemic tissue reduces the release of angiogenic factors, inducing regression of new vessels. Medical therapy in cases of chronic inflammation without ischemia has resulted in the regression of the retinal and disc neovascularization [13].

Laser photocoagulation of the peripheral retina is useful mainly in patients who develop neovascularization of the vitreous base associated with ischemia. It is also used in cases with nonischemic neovascularization not responsive to periocular injections and in patients developing severe side effects from corticosteroids [27]. In these cases, regression of neovascularization and remission of intraocular inflammation has been achieved [14].

> Peripheral photocoagulation is considered at least as useful as peripheral cryotherapy to treat neovascularization of the vitreous base associated with pars planitis [31]. Laser photocoagulation is thought to cause less disruption of the blood–ocular barrier and induce less vitreous gel contraction than cryotherapy, reducing the risk of retinal detachment.

Technique

Argon, diode and doubled-Nd:YAG lasers can be used to perform panretinal photocoagulation (Fig. 5.4). The lenses more commonly used include the wide field and the conventional Goldmann three-mirror lenses. We prefer the frequency doubled-Nd:YAG laser emitting 532-nm-wavelength visible light for office-based photocoagulation under topical anesthesia, using a Super Quad 160 lens. We usually set the laser spot at 250–300 µm with 0.2 s exposure and energy sufficient to cause a grayish burn. Photocoagulation can also be performed using a binocular indirect laser delivery system.

Endolaser photocoagulation for vitreous base neovascularization may be performed during pars plana vitrectomy, especially in cases with nonresolving vitreous hemorrhage, or with extensive vitreous opacities. In this situation, we prefer to use a curved diode laser probe with coaxial illumination. Coaxial illumination of the probe avoids the need to use two instruments very close to the lens, reducing the risk of iatrogenic cataracts.

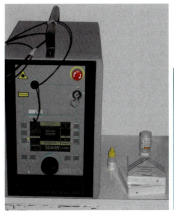
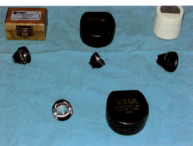

Fig. 5.4 Frequency doubled-Nd:YAG laser device and lenses used for retinal photocoagulation in office

> Two techniques have been used for laser therapy:
> - Local, confluent photocoagulation over the areas of nonelevated retinal neovascularization is the classical approach, usually achieving regression of the areas of neovascularization.
> - If additional areas of neovascularization appear, confluent, panretinal, full-scatter photocoagulation may be performed.

Results

> Laser photocoagulation seems to be as effective as cryotherapy with less risk of inflammation and retinal detachment.

Park and colleagues evaluated the use of peripheral-scatter photocoagulation in 10 eyes with steroid-resistant PP. Photocoagulation appeared to be as effective as cryotherapy in controlling intraocular inflammation and neovascularization of the vitreous base. Laser therapy induced a regression of neovascularization and a complete resolution of the clinical signs of ocular inflammation [31]. Regression of the neovascularization after photocoagulation alone has been reported in eyes with PP [13]. Kalina et al. [22] reported the use of argon laser photocoagulation, in two cases to treat neovascularization of the disc in PP. Panretinal photocoagulation was performed in one case, and the second patient, who also presented iris neovascularization, received focal peripapillary photocoagulation associated with peripheral cryotherapy. VA in the first eye remained stable at 20/20 and decreased in the second eye from 20/50 to no light perception due to chronic smoldering inflammation resulting in phthisis bulbi.

Other situations not related to neovascularization in which laser photocoagulation has been attempted are the treatment of CME and retinoschisis associated with IU.

CME is the first cause of VA loss in patients with IU. Different therapeutic approaches have been proposed for CME and diffuse macular edema, such as systemic, periocular and intraocular steroids, acetazolamide, vitrectomy and photocoagulation.

> CME has been described to disappear after grid-pattern photocoagulation. However, visual acuity recovery is usually very limited [40].

In 1981, Brockhurst described the association of pars planitis and retinoschisis [8] (Fig. 5.5), which was later reported by other groups in the form of a Coats-like ex-

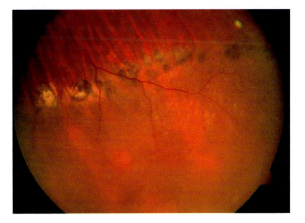

Fig. 5.5 Inferior retinoschisis in a case of pars planitis delimited by argon laser photocoagulation

udative detachment [39]. Peripheral photocoagulation has been occasionally performed in an attempt to limit or at least to evaluate its progression [28].

> Due to the probable exudative origin and the lack of progression, most retinoschisis associated with IU are managed by observation or by treatment of the leaking vessels [32].

Complications

Complications of photocoagulation include immediate vitreous hemorrhage, peripheral field loss, choroidal neovascularization, preretinal hemorrhage, vitreoretinal traction and retinal detachment.

> The appearance of epiretinal membranes secondary to both laser therapy and chronic inflammation is not uncommon and may cause a late reduction of VA.

5.8.2.4 Vitrectomy

> Lack of response to laser or cryotherapy may be treated by vitrectomy with endolaser and/or cryotherapy.

Pars plana vitrectomy (PPV) is being used more and more commonly as a diagnostic and therapeutic modality in IU. Its use is described in another chapter.

Take Home Pearls

Management of IU is based on a step-by-step approach. Corticosteroids are the usual first stage of therapy. Other therapeutic approaches such as cryotherapy and laser photocoagulation may reduce inflammation, the need for corticosteroids and complications.

Modalities and indications of cryotherapy:
- Cryotherapy to the ciliary body may be used in cases of intense ocular inflammation. However, it is associated with more complications than other procedures.
- Cryotherapy to the snowbank is indicated in cases with reduced visual acuity (below 20/40), nonresponsiveness to steroidal therapy, retinal ischemia and neovascularization. Cryotherapy usually decreases the inflammatory reaction and neovascularization. Reduction of CME may improve VA.

Modalities and indications of laser therapy:
- Local photocoagulation of new vessels in cases of neovascularization limited to 1–2 clock hours, with flat retina.
- Panretinal photocoagulation for retinal ischemia, neovascularization and inflammation. Retinal photocoagulation may be performed as an office procedure or during vitrectomy.
- Photocoagulation to the borders of retinoschisis to limit and verify progression of retinoschisis.

Common complications of the procedures:
- Complications of cryotherapy to the ciliary body: decrease in intraocular pressure, phthisis bulbi, retinal detachment, hyphema, vitreous hemorrhages and macular pucker
- Complications of cryotherapy to the snowbank: phthisis bulbi, macular pucker, retinal detachment and vitreous hemorrhages
- Complications of local photocoagulation: vitreoretinal hemorrhages, retinal detachment, recurrences of neovascularization and epiretinal membranes
- Complications of panretinal photocoagulation: visual field defects, epiretinal membranes, vitreoretinal hemorrhages and retinal detachment
- Complications of photocoagulation to the borders of retinoschisis: progression of retinoschisis, retinal holes and epiretinal membranes.

References

1. Aaberg TM (1987) The enigma of pars planitis. Am J Ophthalmol 103:828–830
2. Aaberg TM, Cesarz TJ, Flickinger RR (1973) Treatment of peripheral uveoretinitis by cryotherapy. Am J Ophthalmol 75:685–688
3. Aaberg TM, Cesarz TJ, Flickinger RR Jr (1977) Treatment of pars planitis I. Cryotherapy. Surv Ophthalmol 22:120–125

4. Androudi S, Letko E, Meniconi M et al (2005) Safety and efficacy of intravitreal triamcinolone acetonide for uveitic macular edema. Ocul Immunol Inflamm 13:205–212
5. Berg P, Kroll P, Busse H (1990) Operative Therapie bei Uveitis. Klin Monatsbl Augenheilkd 197:373–377
6. Bloch-Michel E, Nussenblatt RB (1987) International Uveitis Study Group recommendations for the evaluation of intraocular inflammatory disease. Am J Ophthalmol 103:234–235
7. Bonfioli AA, Damico FM, Curi AL et al (2005) Intermediate uveitis. Semin Ophthalmol 20:147–154
8. Brockhurst RJ (1981) Retinoschisis. Complications of peripheral uveitis. Arch Ophthalmol 99:1988–1989
9. Devenyi RG, Mieler WF, Lambrou FH et al (1988) Cryopexy of the vitreous base in the management of peripheral uveitis. Am J Ophthalmol 106:135–138
10. Dijkman JHP, Notting G, Deutman AF (1976) Possibilities of treatment of peripheral uveitis (pars planitis). Ophthalmologica 173:401
11. Dinning WJ (1984) Therapy-selected topics. In: Kraus-Mackiw E, O'Connor GR (eds) Uveitis. Thieme, Stuttgart
12. Dobbie JG (1968) Cryotherapy in the management of toxoplasma retinochoroiditis. Trans Am Acad Ophthalmol Otolaryngol 72:364–373
13. Felder KS, Brockhurst RJ (1982) Neovascular fundus abnormalities in peripheral uveitis. Arch Ophthalmol 100:750–754
14. Franklin RM (1992) Laser photocoagulation of retinal neovascularization in intermediate uveitis. Dev Ophthalmol 23:251–260
15. Gills JPJ (1968) Combined medical and surgical therapy for complicated cases of peripheral uveitis. Arch Ophthalmol 80:747–753
16. Graham EM, Stanford MR, Shilling JS et al (1987) Neovascularisation associated with posterior uveitis. Br J Ophthalmol 71:826–833
17. Henderly DE, Haymond RS, Rao NA et al (1987) The significance of the pars plana exudate in pars planitis. Am J Ophthalmol 103:669–671
18. Jabs DA, Nussenblatt RB, Rosenbaum JT (2005) Standardization of Uveitis Nomenclature (SUN) Working Group. Standardization of uveitis nomenclature for reporting clinical data. Results of the first international workshop. Am J Ophthalmol 140:509–16
19. Jaffe GJ, Ben-Nun J, Guo H et al (2000) Fluocinolone acetonide sustained drug delivery device to treat severe uveitis. Ophthalmology 107:2024–2033
20. Jünemann G, Küchle HJ (1981) Zur Kryotherapie bei peripherer Uveitis. Ber Dtsch Ophthalmol Ges 78:273
21. Kadayifcilar S, Eldem B, Tumer B (2003) Uveitis in childhood. J Pediatr Ophthalmol Strabismus 40:335–340
22. Kalina PH, Pach JM, Buettner H et al (1990) Neovascularization of the disc in pars planitis. Retina 10:269–273
23. Kaplan HJ (1984) Intermediate uveitis (pars planitis, chronic cyclitis): a four step approach to treatment. In: Saari KM (ed) Uveitis update. Medica, Amsterdam
24. Kelly PJ, Weiter JJ (1980) Resolution of optic disk neovascularization associated with optic disk neovascularization. Am J Ophthalmol 90:545–548
25. Kok H, Lau C, Maycock N et al (2005) Outcome of intravitreal triamcinolone in uveitis. Ophthalmology 112:1916
26. Krwawicz T (1977) Erfahrung mit der Kryotherapie der Iridozyklitis. Klin Monatsbl Augenheilkd 170:852–854
27. Lai WW, Pulido JS (2002) Intermediate uveitis. Ophthalmol Clin North Am 15:309–317
28. Lesnoni G, Rossi T, Nistri A et al (1999) Nanophthalmic uveal effusion syndrome after prophylactic laser treatment. Eur J Ophthalmol 9:315–318
29. Malik AR, Pavesio C (2005) The use of low dose methotrexate in children with chronic anterior and intermediate uveitis. Br J Ophthalmol 89:806–808
30. Mieler WF, Aaberg TM (1992) Further observations on cryotherapy of the vitreous base in the management of peripheral uveitis. Dev Ophthalmol 23:190–195
31. Park SE, Mieler WF, Pulido JS (1995) Peripheral scatter photocoagulation for neovascularization associated with pars planitis. Arch Ophthalmol 113:1277–1280
32. Pollack AL, McDonald HR, Johnson RN et al (2002) Peripheral retinoschisis and exudative retinal detachment in pars planitis. Retina 22:719–724
33. Prieto JF, Dios E, Gutierrez JM et al (2001) Pars planitis: epidemiology, treatment, and association with multiple sclerosis. Ocul Immunol Inflamm 9:93–102
34. Quigley HA (1976) Histological and physiological studies of cyclocryotherapy in primate and human eyes. Am J Ophthalmol 82:722–732
35. Rodriguez A, Calonge M, Pedroza-Seres M et al (1996) Referral patterns of uveitis in a tertiary eye care center. Arch Ophthalmol 114:593–599
36. Schilling H, Heiligenhaus A, Laube T et al (2005) Long-term effect of acetazolamide treatment of patients with uveitic chronic cystoid macular edema is limited by persisting inflammation. Retina 25:182–188
37. Shorb SR, Irvine AR, Kimura SJ (1976) Optic disk neovascularization associated with chronic uveitis. Am J Ophthalmol 82:175–178
38. Smith RE, Godfrey WA, Kimura SJ (1976) Complications of chronic cyclitis. Am J Ophthalmol 82:277
39. Suh DW, Pulido JS, Jampol LM et al (1999) Coats-like response in pars planitis. Retina 19:79–80
40. Tranos PG, Wickremasinghe SS, Stangos NT et al (2004) Macular edema. Surv Ophthalmol 49:470–490
41. Young S, Larkin G, Branley M et al (2001) Safety and efficacy of intravitreal triamcinolone for cystoid macular oedema in uveitis. Clin Experiment Ophthalmol 29:2–6

Part B
Surgical Treatment of Uveitic Complications

I Anterior Segment

Cornea / Chapter 6

Surgery for Band Keratopathy

Ruth Lapid-Gortzak, Jan Willem van der Linden,
Ivanka J. E. van der Meulen, Carla P. Nieuwendaal

Core Messages

- Most band keratopathies (BK) are calcific.
- Band keratopathy can cause decreased visual acuity, pain, and photophobia and can be cosmetically unfavorable.
- BK can be treated by chelation, superficial keratectomy, or phototherapeutic keratectomy (PTK).
- Healing of the ocular surface is compromised in these eyes and must be carefully monitored.

Contents

6.1	Introduction	63
6.2	Treatment Options	64
6.2.1	Chelation with EDTA	64
6.2.2	Phototherapeutic Keratectomy	64
6.3	Indications for Surgery	64
6.3.1	EDTA Chelation of Calcific Band Keratopathy—Surgical Procedure	64
6.3.2	Phototherapeutic Keratectomy for Band Keratopathy	65
6.4	Postoperative Care	65
References		65

6.1 Introduction

Band keratopathy is a degenerative condition of the cornea. It was first described in 1848 by Dixon [1]. There are two types of band keratopathies. The calcific type is associated with hypercalcemia or chronic ocular inflammation. The noncalcific type is associated with gout, in which crystals of urate form a pigmented band on the cornea [2]. The most common type is the calcific type, and when referring to a band keratopathy, the calcific type is usually meant. It is characterized by deposition of a grayish plaque in the superficial layers of the cornea. The deposited material presents as granules, which are in fact intracellular deposits of calcium. The deposition is interspersed with clear areas that are thought to be the places where the corneal nerves penetrate the Bowman layer [3]. In hypercalcemia or in renal failure, the calcium is deposited extracellularly as calcium-phosphate salts [3].

The pathophysiology of calcific band keratopathy has not yet been elucidated, and several mechanisms, including localized hypercalcemia, increased tissue pH, decreased tear breakup time, and increased tear evaporation have been implicated in the formation of band keratopathy. Dry eye conditions have been known to accelerate band keratopathy formation [3, 4].

Most of the band keratopathies are most dense in the interpalpebral zone of the cornea. They start at the 9 and 3 o'clock positions and spread centrally to cover the visual axis [5]. Clinically, band keratopathy may cause decreased visual acuity by obscuration of the visual axis. Pain and photophobia are related to recurrent epithelial defects. The ocular surface is compromised, and these patients are at risk for epithelial healing problems and are more prone to corneal infections. Calcific bands may also rarely become visible on keratoprostheses [6]. Band keratopathy with bulky calcific plaques may induce giant papillary conjunctivitis [7]. Some medication may induce band keratopathy; mostly these are medications containing phosphates [8].

Ocular and systemic diseases associated with band keratopathy are: congenital hereditary endothelial dystrophy (CHED), chronic uveitis, discoid lupus, dry eye syndromes, hyperparathyroid states, increased or decreased serum phosphate states, ichthyosis, interstitial keratitis, intraocular silicone oil, lithium therapy, mercury poisoning, metastatic carcinoma to the bone, milk-alkali syndrome, multiple myeloma, nephropathic cystinosis, Norrie disease, Paget disease, phthisis, prolonged corneal edema, prolonged glaucoma, sarcoidosis, spheroid degeneration of the cornea, Still disease, thiazides, trachoma, tuberous sclerosis, tumoral calcinosis, uremia, phosphate-containing viscoelastics, and vitamin D toxicity.

If the patient's history does not clarify the etiology of the band keratopathy, a limited workup, including serum calcium, phosphate, urea, and renal functions, may be performed. If the index of suspicion is high enough, parathyroid functions and serum ACE (angiotensin-converting enzyme) can also be checked.

6.2 Treatment Options

The treatment options described in the literature are: EDTA (Ethylene diamine tetraacetic acid) chelation of the calcific plaque, lamellar or superficial keratectomy, or phototherapeutic keratectomy (PTK) with an excimer laser [5, 9, 10]. Alternatives described in the literature but not often used are Nd:YAG-laser-assisted keratectomy [11], amniotic membrane transplantation after primary surgical management [12], and the use of a diamond burr [13].

6.2.1 Chelation with EDTA

EDTA $[(HO_2CCH_2)_2NCH_2CH_2N(CH_2CO_2H)_2]$ is an amino ester widely used to sequester di- and trivalent metal ions. Most EDTA is used in industrial cleaning (paper, agrochemical, and textile industries) for the complexation of Ca^{2+} and Mg^{2+} ions and the binding of heavy metals. It is approved by the FDA as a food preservative.

Medically, it is mainly used in acute hypercalcemia, lead and mercury poisonings, in the measurement of glomerular filtration rates, and as an anticoagulant in blood samples. In ophthalmology, it is used as a preservative in eyedrops in addition to its obvious use as a chelating agent in calcific band keratopathy.

Chelation is done with a 0.05 mol/l solution of EDTA [5]. Ninety-eight percent of patients in the study of Najjar et al. reported symptomatic relief after EDTA chelation of their band keratopathy. Vision improved in 35.2%. Recurrence was seen in 17.8% with a mean time of 17.7 years till the recurrence [5]. Calcific plaques respond to EDTA, while the noncalcific and mixed plaques do not respond to chelation [5].

6.2.2 Phototherapeutic Keratectomy

PTK is done with an excimer laser. Excimer lasers have been available for corneal surface ablations since the mid-1980s. The 193 nm laser ablates the tissue without thermal effect on the surrounding tissues, allowing for a controlled removal of the superficial tissue layers [10].

PTK can remove the superficial diseased layer and at the same time create a more smooth surface of the cornea, enhancing comfort and visual function [10]. The central part of the cornea is minimally ablated, just as deep as the band keratopathy is. In case of large, bulky calcific plaques, it is advisable to debulk the band keratopathy mechanically before ablating the corneal surface with an excimer laser. O'Brart et al. reported visual acuity improvement in 88% of patients treated with PTK for BK. Glare was reduced in 88%, and 95% had an improvement in ocular comfort. Hyperopic shift with a mean of +1.4D was observed. This is related to the depth and centrality of the laser ablation. Recurrence was seen in 8% with a mean recurrence time of 12 months [10].

6.3 Indications for Surgery

Indications for surgery include:

- Decreased visual acuity
- Central opacification of the cornea
- Tearing, photophobia, and pain
- Cosmesis

6.3.1 EDTA Chelation of Calcific Band Keratopathy—Surgical Procedure

1. After topical anesthesia, disinfection, and surgical draping, an eyelid speculum is inserted, and the ocular surface is then rinsed with 10 cc of balanced salt solution (BSS).
2. With a LASEK alcohol cup, 20% alcohol is applied to the cornea epithelium for 30 s and rinsed with BSS (optional to facilitate epithelial removal).
3. The epithelium is then removed from the ocular surface. If possible, it is retained in a sheet with a superior corneal hinge.
4. A cellulose sponge soaked in an EDTA 0.05 mol/l solution is applied to the involved subepithelial layer.
5. Between 15 and 30 minutes of intermittent EDTA application is performed.
6. With forceps, large plaques of the keratopathy can be removed. This will also enhance the contact of the EDTA with the remaining plaque to be chelated.

7. After the central cornea is deemed clear enough, the EDTA is rinsed with BSS.
8. A cycloplegic drop (cyclopentolate 1%) is applied.
9. The eye can be patched either with an antibiotic ointment, or a bandage contact lens (CL) can be applied.

6.3.2 Phototherapeutic Keratectomy for Band Keratopathy

1. The ablation depth and zone are set on the computer before the patient comes into the operating room. For example: depth of 10 μm or up to 70 μm. Remember that the deeper ablations have more effect on the spherical equivalent refraction postoperatively.
2. After disinfection and surgical draping, an eyelid speculum is inserted, and the ocular surface is then rinsed with 10 cc of BSS.
3. With a LASEK alcohol cup, 20% alcohol is applied to the cornea epithelium for 30 s. Alternatively, the epithelium can be removed with the excimer laser ablation itself.
4. The epithelium is then removed from the ocular surface. If possible, it is retained in a sheet form with a superior corneal hinge.
5. The band keratopathy is ablated; treatment zones and depth are to the discretion of the surgeon and depend on the type of laser used.
6. The ablated cornea is rinsed with cold BSS.
7. A drop of nonpreserved prednisolone 0.5% is applied.
8. A cycloplegic drop (cyclopentolate 1%) is applied.
9. The eye can be patched either with an antibiotic ointment, or a bandage contact lens can be applied with prophylactic topical antibiotic treatment.

6.4 Postoperative Care

Cycloplegic drops and preservative-free antibiotic drops are applied immediately postoperatively. After surgery, preservative-free antibiotic eyedrops are administered four times daily with a bandage contact lens or ointment without a CL. We most commonly use a combination of oral paracetamol, 500–1,000 mg, four times daily and 400 mg of diclofenac three times daily for analgesia.

Day 1: Check position of CL, check for corneal infiltrates, check for corneal healing, and monitor patient's analgesic needs.

Days 3–4: If the epithelial defect has healed, the contact lens is removed, and antibiotic ointment is prescribed for four more days four times daily.

In cases of prolonged or difficult healing, the bandage lens can remain in situ, with prophylactic, preservative-free antibiotic drops like tobramycin, under frequent supervision. Drops that can cause the formation of corneal deposits, like ciprofloxacin, should be avoided. After healing has occurred, follow-ups are adjusted to the underlying ocular condition.

Take Home Pearls

- Ensure a limited search for the etiology of the band keratopathy.
- Preoperatively, the procedure and expected results should be discussed thoroughly with the patient. Avoid treating the patient with unrealistic expectations.
- Excimer laser procedures are expensive. If there are no facilities for PTK, a chelation with EDTA is a good alternative.
- Do not perform a PTK for a band keratopathy that is not causing complaints of pain in an eye with severe loss of visual acuity due to reasons other than the corneal opacity.

References

1. Dixon J (1848) Diseases of the eye. Churchill, London, p 114
2. Ferry AP, Safir A, Melikian HE (1985) Ocular abnormalities in patients with gout. Ann Ophthalmol 17:632–635
3. Cursino JW, Fine BS (1976) A histologic study of calcific and noncalcific band keratopathies. Am J Ophthalmol 82:395–404
4. Lemp MA, Ralph RA (1977) Rapid development of band keratopathy in dry eyes. Am J Ophthalmol 83:657–659
5. Najjar DM, Cohen EJ, Rapuano CJ, Laibson PR (2004) EDTA chelation for calcific band keratopathy: results and long-term follow-up. Am J Ophthalmol 137:1056–1064
6. Wapner FJ, Srinivasan BD (1993) Calcific band keratopathy on a keratoprosthesis. Cornea 12:72–73

7. Heidemann DG, Dunn SP, Siegal MJ (1993) Unusual causes of giant papillary conjunctivitis. Cornea 12:78–80
8. Taravella MJ, Stulting RD, Mader TH, Weisenthal RW, Forstot SL, Underwood LD (1994) Calcific band keratopathy associated with the use of topical steroid-phosphate preparations. Arch Ophthalmol 112:608–613
9. Najjar DM (2004) Combined treatment for band keratopathy. J Korean Med Sci 19:915; author reply 915–916
10. O'Brart DP, Gartry DS, Lohmann CP, Patmore AL, Kerr Muir MG, Marshall J (1993) Treatment of band keratopathy by excimer laser phototherapeutic keratectomy: surgical techniques and long term follow up. Br J Ophthalmol 77:702–708
11. Baltatzis S, Papaefthimiou J (1992) Treatment of calcific band keratopathy by Nd:YAG laser. Eur J Ophthalmol 2:27–29
12. Anderson DF, Prabhasawat P, Alfonso E, Tseng SC (2001) Amniotic membrane transplantation after the primary surgical management of band keratopathy. Cornea 20:354–361
13. Bokosky JE, Meyer RF, Sugar A (1985) Surgical treatment of calcific band keratopathy. Ophthalmic Surg 16:645–647

Cornea / Chapter 7

Surgical Management of Diffuse Corneal Opacities

Thomas John

Core Messages

- Surgical management of corneal opacities secondary to inflammatory diseases usually help restore vision and improve the cosmetic appearance of the eye, especially when the opacities are large and diffuse. In the acute stage, such intervention helps preserve the globe, as in cases of corneal perforation, and at a later stage, visual restoration can be attempted using the appropriate technique described in this chapter.
- The corneal surgeon should be experienced in doing lamellar corneal surgery to successfully perform procedures such as total anterior lamellar keratoplasty and descemetorhexis with endokeratoplasty.
- The surgeon has many options, and the patient can benefit greatly from the advanced and improved surgical techniques that are currently available.

Contents

7.1	Introduction	67
7.2	Corneal Involvement in Inflammatory Diseases	67
7.3	Types of Surgery	73
7.3.1	Surgical Management in the Acute Stage	76
7.3.2	Surgical Management in the Chronic Stage	77
References		83

7.1 Introduction

Corneal inflammatory diseases can result in corneal opacities, necessitating corneal replacement surgery or corneal transplantation. Selective tissue corneal transplantation (STCT) [1–3] describes a new concept of the selective removal of the diseased portion of the cornea and its replacement with anatomically similar healthy donor corneal tissue [2]. In cases where the corneal opacities are confined to the corneal stroma, with healthy endothelium, only the portion of the cornea with the opacity is removed. This lamellar corneal surgery preserves the corneal endothelium and eliminates the possibility of endothelial graft rejection. If there is corneal edema from inflammatory damage to the endothelium without associated corneal opacity or with only mild corneal opacity that does not involve the visual axis, then posterior lamellar keratoplasty may be the preferred surgery, by maintaining corneal integrity without full-thickness corneal wounds or corneal sutures. Full-thickness corneal scarring with endothelial decompensation requires standard penetrating keratoplasty (PKP) for visual rehabilitation.

This chapter addresses surgical techniques to manage corneal opacities secondary to inflammatory diseases.

7.2 Corneal Involvement in Inflammatory Diseases

Inflammatory diseases can involve the cornea during either the acute phase or the chronic phase.

- Acute stage (Fig. 7.1)
  - Corneal melt, descemetocele formation, with or without perforation
- Chronic stage (Figs. 7.2–7.5)
  - Corneal opacities
- Superficial
- Deep

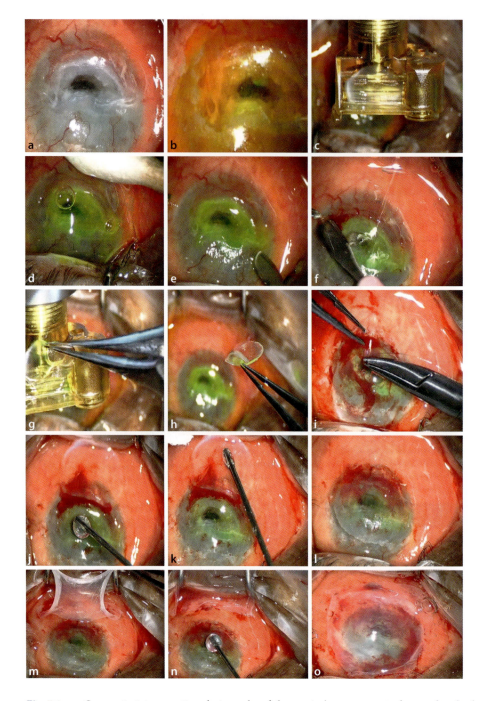

Fig. 7.1a–o Composite intraoperative photographs of the surgical management of corneal melt, descemetocele, with corneal perforation. Procedure: ALK, AMT, and use of tissue adhesive. **a** Sterile corneal melt, large descemetocele, with corneal perforation. **b** Fluorescein stain shows positive Seidel test. **c** Disposable Moria CB microkeratome with lamellar donor corneal disc. **d** Topical anesthesia, using Xylocaine 2% jelly on the ocular surface with MAC. **e,f** Removal of surrounding corneal epithelium using a straight crescent blade. **g,h** Removal of donor lamellar corneal disc. **i** Anchoring 10-0 nylon suture at 6 o'clock position. **j** Tissue adhesive component 1 applied to host cornea. **k** Tissue adhesive component 2 applied to donor corneal disc. **l** Donor lamellar disc attached to host cornea with tissue adhesive. **m** Surface of donor corneal disc and amniotic membrane are seen. **n** Tissue adhesive component 1, being applied to donor corneal surface. **o** Amniotic membrane attached to donor corneal and ocular surface after applying tissue adhesive, component 2 to the stromal surface of the amniotic membrane

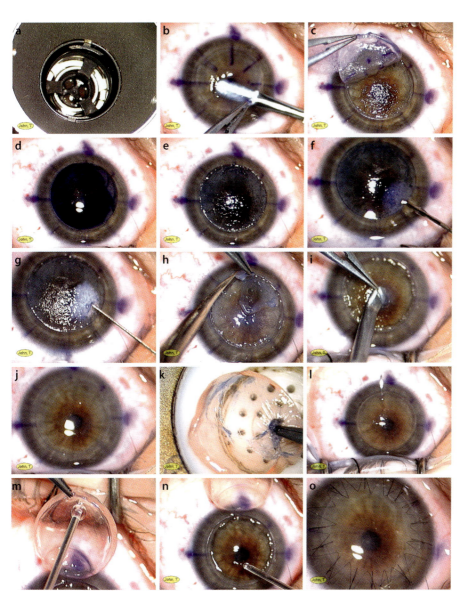

Fig. 7.2a–o Composite intraoperative photographs of TALK/John-Malbran classification of lamellar keratoplasty [4]. **a** Trephination of host cornea using the Hanna trephine with a preset dept. **b** First layer of host lamellar dissection. **c** Reflection of the lamellar layer exposes the host stroma. **d** Exposed stromal bed is bathed with VisionBlue. **e** Excess VisonBlue is removed using a Merocel sponge, showing the blue coloration of the exposed host corneal stroma without any staining of the surrounding uncut host cornea with intact epithelium. **f** Forced hydrodissection (John technique) separates the host stromal layer, which is clearly visible due to the blue–white coloration. **g** Second layer of lamellar, forced hydrodissection in a combination of onion-peel, and divide-and-conquer techniques. **h** Segmental removal of lamellar layers using sharp dissection of the separated stromal layers—notice the adjacent island of stroma yet to be excised. **i** Pre–descemet dissection of separated stromal layers at the visual axis. **j** Fully exposed DM. **k** Donor endothelial layer removal after staining the endothelium with VisionBlue for enhanced visualization of the endothelial layer. **l** Anchoring 10-0 nylon suture at 6 o'clock position, attaching the full-thickness donor cornea devoid of endothelium to the peripheral recipient cornea. **m** Component 1 of the Tisseel tissue adhesive (fibrin sealant) being applied uniformly to the stromal surface of the donor corneal button. **n** Component 2 of the tissue adhesive Tisseel tissue adhesive being applied uniformly to the recipient corneal bed. **o** Completed view of TALK, with clear donor corneal button lined on the inside by patient's DM and endothelial layer. Also seen are the running and interrupted 10-0 nylon sutures, with all knots buried within the recipient cornea

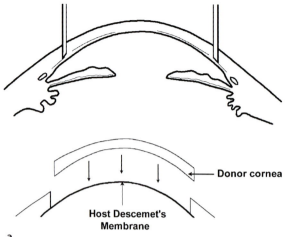

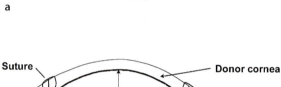

Fig. 7.3a,b Schematic representation of TALK procedure. Top schematic cross-sectional view of deep, nonperforating, recipient corneal trephination. **a** Donor corneal button is devoid of endothelium, to be attached to the patient's Descemet's membrane (DM). **b** Recipient DM uniformly attached to the donor corneal stroma, devoid of the endothelium and DM. (Reproduced with permission from Jaypee Brothers Medical Publishers, Ltd., New Delhi, India)

Surgical Management of Diffuse Corneal Opacities — Chapter 7

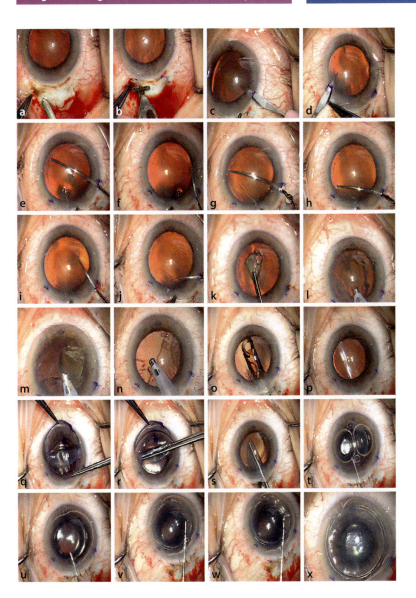

Fig. 7.4a–x Intraoperative comprehensive, composite photographs of Descemetorhexis (DX) with endokeratoplasty (DXEK), temporal approach, surgeon's view. **a** Hemostasis, using cautery. **b** Fixed-depth (350 μm) diamond blade is being used to create a scleral, perilimbal wound of fixed depth of 350 μm and chord length of 5.0 mm. **c** Anterior chamber (AC) entry using a superblade at the 2 o'clock position, right of the temporal groove. **d** Anterior chamber (AC) entry at 5 o'clock position, left of scleral groove, using the same blade. **e–j** Use of John DX-EKDSAEK Dexatome Spatula (patent pending) to complete the DX 360° and complete detachment of the DM, without exiting the AC. **k** John DXEK/DSAEK insertion forceps with the DM that was removed as a single disc. **l** Phacoemulsification of the cataractous nucleus in a triple procedure using the Infinity phacoemulsifier unit (Alcon). **m** Phacoemulsification being continued in the AC, without any concern as to the patient's endothelium, since the host corneal endothelium will be replaced. **n** Lens cortical remnants being removed using the I/A unit (Alcon). **o** Foldable, acrylic posterior chamber intraocular (IOL) being introduced into the intact, lens capsular bag. **p** Posterior chamber (PC) PC IOL almost completely unfolded. **q** Donor corneal cap is held with a 0.12 forceps, while the donor corneal disc is being folded into a 60/40 taco fold, using the John DXEK insertion forceps. **r,s** Donor taco lifted from the donor corneal cap and introduced into the recipient anterior chamber. **t,u** Unfolding of the donor taco using filtered air. **v,w** Moving the donor disc into a central position, using a reverse Sinskey hook over the convex surface of the air bubble filling the AC. **x** Well-centered donor corneal disc, with a uniform interface, without any macrofolds of the donor corneal disc, indicating a good end point for DXEK. (Reproduced with permission from Jaypee Brothers Medical Publishers, Ltd., New Delhi, India)

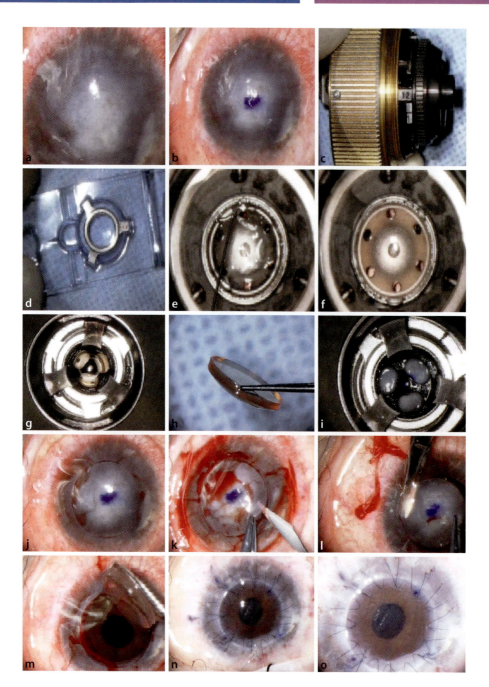

Fig. 7.5a–o Composite intraoperative photographs showing PKP procedure in a diffusely scarred cornea. **a** Intraoperative view of the diffusely scarred cornea. **b** Central cornea is marked with a marking pen after measuring with surgical calipers and using a sterile needle to focally disrupt the superficial stroma. **c** Hanna vacuum trephine without the outer encasing, exposing the central cylinder for mounting the trephine blade and the depth setting. **d** Hanna trephine blade within the sterile package. **e** Application of viscoelastic material to the artificial chamber. **f** Optisol GS solution fills the concavity of the central encasing ready to accept the donor cornea, with the endothelium facing down. **g** Trephination of the donor cornea from the epithelial surface using the Hanna trephine. **h** Evenly cut donor corneal disc. **i** Recipient corneal trephination using preset depth with a Hanna trephine. **j** Cut surface of the recipient cornea. **k** AC entry with a superblade at the 10 o'clock position. **l** Surgical excision of the recipient corneal disc. **m** Donor corneal disc placement. **n** Running 10-0 nylon suture almost completed. **o** Completed view of the PKP procedure, with all suture knots buried within the host corneal rim

7.3 Types of Surgery

The type of surgery is based on the location of the corneal opacity and the health of the corneal endothelium (Table 7.1). Anterior lamellar keratoplasty (LKP) is based on the John-Malbran classification (see below). Posterior lamellar keratoplasty (PLK) includes a number of procedures that vary in complexity in the procedures with different names and abbreviations such as descemetorhexis or descemet-stripping endokeratoplasty or endothelial keratoplasty, and automated endothelial keratoplasty (DLEK, DSEK, DXEK, DSAEK)]. Simpler, and currently preferred, techniques involve only removal of Descemet's membrane with the attached endothelium (DSEK, DXEK, DSAEK) rather than a lamellar button of posterior corneal stroma (DLEK). Table 7.2 shows the various abbreviations used for the surgical management of corneal opacities. Table 7.3 displays the normal thickness of the corneal layers in microns, which is important to consider in all types of lamellar corneal surgeries.

John-Malbran Classification of Optical Lamellar Keratoplasty (LKP) [4]

1. Anterior lamellar keratoplasty (ALK)
   a. Superficial (<160 μm) ALK (SALK)
   b. Mid (160–400 μm) ALK (MALK)
   c. Deep (400–490 μm) ALK (DALK)
   d. Total (>490 μm, and total stromal removal [almost 100% stroma], with retention of Descemet's membrane and endothelium) ALK (TALK)
2. Posterior lamellar keratoplasty (PLK)
   a. DLEK
      i. Without flap: DLEK, no corneal surface wound or corneal sutures
      ii. Flap-associated DLEK (FDLEK) with flap, corneal surface wound and corneal sutures are present
   b. DSEK, DSAEK, or DXEK
      i. Manual (DSEK or DXEK-M)
      ii. Automated: with microkeratome (DSAEK or DXEK-A)
      iii. Femtosecond laser-assisted PLK (DXEK-L)
   c. Descemet's membrane endothelial cell transplantation (DMEK or DECT)
   d. Endothelial cell transplantation (ECT). Not performed successfully in humans (ECT) at the time of writing.
   e. Endothelial cell activation (ECA). Not performed successfully in humans at the time of writing.

Table 7.1 Surgical management of corneal opacity

Location of corneal opacity	Endothelial status	Type of surgery (John-Malbran classification of optical lamellar keratoplasty)
Superficial	Healthy	Superficial anterior lamellar keratoplasty (SALK) (<160 μm)
Mid-stroma	Healthy	Mid-anterior lamellar keratoplasty (MALK) (160–400 μm)
Deep	Healthy	Deep anterior lamellar keratoplasty (DALK) (400–490 μm)
Very deep	Healthy	Total anterior lamellar keratoplasty (TALK) (>490 μm, total stromal removal [almost 100%] with retention of Descemet's membrane and endothelium)
None, or very mild opacity not involving the visual axis	Unhealthy	Descemetorhexis with endokeratoplasty (DXEK DSEK)
Full thickness	Unhealthy	Penetrating keratoplasty (PKP)

Table 7.2 Abbreviations used for surgical management of corneal opacities

Major surgical subdivision	Type of surgery (John-Malbran classification of optical lamellar keratoplasty)
ALK	• SALK • MALK • DALK • TALK

PLK	• DLEK
	  – No flap = DLEK
	  – FDLEK
	• DXEK
	  – DXEK-M, DSEK
	  – DXEK-A, DSAEK
	  – DXEK-L
	• DECT, DMECT, DMEK
	• ECT[a]
	• ECA[a]

ALK anterior lamellar keratoplasty, *PLK* posterior lamellar keratoplasty, *SALK* superficial ALK, *MALK* mid ALK, *DALK* deep ALK, *TALK* total ALK, *DLEK* deep lamellar endothelial keratoplasty, *FDLEK* flap-associated DLEK, *DXEK* descemetorhexis with endokeratoplasty, *DXEK-M* DXEK manual, *DSEK* descemet-stripping endothelial keratoplasty, *DXEK-A* DXEK automated, *DSAEK* descemet stripping with automated endothelial keratoplasty, *DXEK-L* DXEK laser (femtosecond laser), *DECT or DMECT* Descemet's membrane endothelial cell transplantation, *DMEK* Descemet's membrane endothelial keratoplasty, *ECT* endothelial cell transplantation, *ECA* endothelial cell activation

[a]Not performed successfully in humans at the time of writing

Table 7.3 Normal corneal thickness by layers of the cornea

Cornea	Central thickness (µm)	Paracentral thickness (µm)	Peripheral thickness (µm)
Normal	520	Av = 545 I = 520 S = 570	Av = 650 I = 630 S = 670
Epithelium	50		
DM[a]	Av = 11 A = 10–12 B = 3		
Endothelium	Av = 5 Range = 4–6		
Stroma	455		

I inferior, *S* superior, *DM* Descemet's membrane, *A* adults, *B* at birth
[a]Thickness increases as endothelium lays down a posterior, amorphous non-banded zone

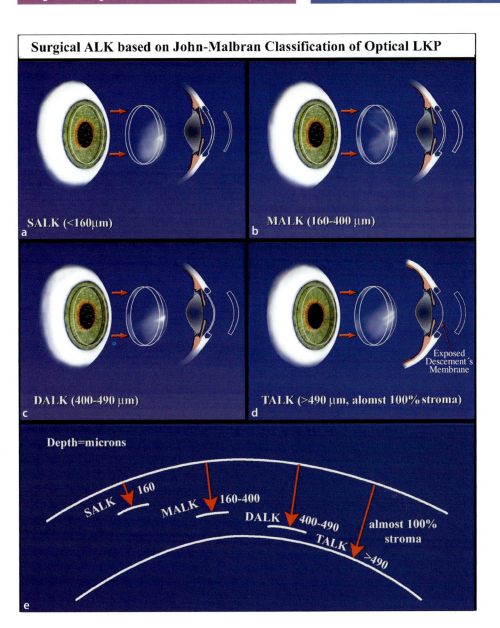

Fig. 7.6 Composite schematic representation of ALK based on John-Malbran classification of optical LKP. **a** SALK, **b** MALK, **c** DALK, **d** TALK, **e** schematic cross-sectional view of the cornea with varying corneal depths of lamellar keratoplasties. (Reproduced with permission from Jaypee Brothers Medical Publishers, Ltd., New Delhi, India)

7.3.1 Surgical Management in the Acute Stage

Surgical management may be necessary in corneal melt, or descemetocele, with or without perforation.

Surgery for Corneal Melt, with Descemetocele, with or without Perforation

Anesthesia used is (1) topical or peribulbar with monitored anesthesia care, or (2) general anesthesia.

There are two types of surgery recommended here, (1) anterior lamellar keratoplasty (ALK), with or without amniotic membrane transplantation (AMT), with or without use of Tisseel tissue adhesive (fibrin sealant, Baxter, Inc., Deerfield, IL.), and (2) multilayered AMT (perforation size <2.0 mm).

1. ALK, AMT, with tissue adhesive (Fig. 7.1)
   a. Donor corneal preparation
      The donor corneal button is obtained from the local eye bank. It is essential to request that the donor corneal rim has a uniform scleral width of 4.0 mm (>3.6 mm) in order to prevent potential donor button slippage within the artificial anterior chamber (AAC) [5]. Obtain a backup donor cornea, if the eye bank will provide it, which can be returned to the eye bank if not used. The donor corneal button may be prepared manually or by microkeratome-assisted automated preparation. For the automated dissection of the donor corneal disc, a Moria anterior lamellar therapeutic keratoplasty (ALTK) unit (Moria, Inc., Doylestown, PA), and a disposable 130-μm Carriazzo-Barraquer (CB) head (Moria) are required. The microkeratome pass is performed very slowly, resulting in a donor disc of about 160- to 170-μm thickness.
   b. Host corneal surgery
      During the intraoperative preparation and draping for the ocular surgery, it is important to avoid any undue pressure on the globe, especially in cases of extensive descemetocele formation with corneal perforation. Fluorescein staining will usually demonstrate a positive Seidel test (Fig. 7.1). Topical anesthesia with monitored anesthesia care (MAC) is preferred in cooperative patients; however, general anesthesia can be used if preferred. Xylocaine 2% jelly (lidocaine HCL, AstraZeneca, Wilmington, DE) is applied to the ocular surface with a sterile Q-tip (Fig. 7.1). It is important to remove the host corneal epithelium surrounding the ulceration to facilitate donor corneal disc adherence. A straight crescent blade (Alcon Surgical, Fort Worth, TX) is used (Fig. 7.1). The donor lamellar corneal disc of about 160- to 170-μm thickness is removed from the Moria disposable, 130-μm CB microkeratome head and attached to the host globe at the 6 o'clock position, using a single, 10-0 nylon suture (Fig. 7.1). The donor lamellar disc is then partially flipped to expose the stromal side of the disc (Fig. 7.1). Tissue adhesive component 1 is applied to the host corneal surface, and component 2 is applied to the stromal surface of the donor lamellar disc (Fig. 7.1). The lamellar donor corneal disc is then attached to the host cornea by flipping the disc back in place to cover the host corneal ulceration/perforation site and the area of descemetocele, using the anchoring suture to facilitate this motion of donor cap attachment (Fig. 7.1). Gentle, even pressure is then applied to the donor corneal surface to enhance approximation and donor–host corneal adhesion as the two components, fibrin and thrombin, interact.

Amniotic membrane use is by surgeon preference. The lamellar corneal disc will usually sufficiently correct the host cornea, and no additional surgery will be required. Amniotic membrane, as a single layer on the ocular surface, is used primarily to decrease ocular inflammation and help facilitate the healing process. The amniotic membrane is tacked at three points, as shown in Fig. 7.1, using interrupted 10-0 vicryl sutures. The amniotic membrane is then flipped on itself to expose the stromal connective tissue surface of the amniotic membrane (Fig. 7.1). Tissue adhesive component 1 is applied to the cornea and the surrounding conjunctiva, and component 2 is applied to the exposed stromal surface of the amniotic membrane (Fig. 7.1). The amniotic membrane is then flipped back to attach the amniotic membrane to the ocular surface as shown in Fig. 7.1. Excess amniotic membrane is trimmed using a Vannas or Westcott scissors (Fig. 7.1). Antibiotic–steroid combination ophthalmic ointment is applied to the ocular surface and the eye is patched, and a Fox eye shield is taped in place.

Postoperatively, topical corticosteroid and fluoroquine ophthalmic drop, Iquix (levofloxacin 1.5%, Vistakon Pharmaceuticals, Jacksonville, FL) are applied four times daily. For globe protection, the patient is asked to wear glasses or eye shield during the day and shield at night over the operative eye. Usual postoperative activity limitations in the immediate postoperative period are no bending over, no straining, and no lifting objects over 5 kg.

When the eye has fully healed and is no longer

inflamed, additional surgery may be planned for visual restoration if needed.

c. Multilayered AMT: principles of anatomic application of human amniotic membrane
   i. Cornea
   1. Important considerations
      AMT is useful in treating sterile corneal ulcers with or without corneal perforation. The shape of the corneal defect is important in choosing cases for AMT. AMT can be effectively used in sterile corneal ulcer with a crater or funnel-shaped configuration with a perforation size of 2 mm or smaller at the deepest part of the ulcer crater. If the edges are vertical, such as in a trephination wound, then AMT will not effectively seal the perforation, and other alternative surgical modalities should be considered.
   2. Surgical techniques
      Nonabsorbable sutures (NAS), namely 10-0 nylon, black monofilament sutures (Moria, or no. 8065-192101, Alcon), are preferred to attach human amniotic membrane (HAM) on to the cornea. NAS provide controlled removal of sutures, and the surgeon can decide the timing of sutures removal. This approach keeps the HAM on the corneal surface for the required period and avoids premature disruption of the membrane. A multilayered AMT can be performed to treat small corneal perforations and descemetoceles, as an alternative procedure to ALK. In this technique [8, 9], the HAM is used to fill or "plug" a corneal defect or perforation.

      A cellulose sponge is used to remove all cellular debris and exudates from the base and the walls of the ulcer. Loose epithelium surrounding the ulcer edge is removed mechanically using a fine forceps and a straight crescent blade (Alcon). The HAM may be used as a fluffed-up sheet of membrane or as a multilayer sheet. In the latter, the membrane is folded on itself twice, which makes it four layered, or more if needed, much like folding a blanket ("blanket fold"), and then it is anchored to the cornea, using 10-0 nylon sutures. In either case, namely fluffed-up or blanket-fold, a second single sheet of HAM is placed over the entire cornea, and it is anchored to the peripheral cornea close to the limbus with a running or interrupted 10-0 nylon sutures or with a 10-0 vicryl sutures to the conjunctiva and limbus. A bandage soft contact lens is placed on the cornea to enhance patient comfort postoperatively.
   3. Conjunctiva
      Absorbable sutures (AS) are preferred to anchor HAM on to the conjunctiva [9]. 10-0 Vicryl, violet, monofilament sutures (polyglactin 910, no. V-450, Ethicon, Somerville, NJ) on an Ultima spatula needle (CS-160-8) may be used for this purpose.

7.3.2 Surgical Management in the Chronic Stage

Surgical management involves correction of superficial opacities, and deep opacities (via ALK, PLK, and PKP).

1. Total anterior lamellar keratoplasty (TALK) (John technique) (Figs. 7.2, and 7.3)
   At the time of writing this chapter, TALK is only performed by a manual technique. Various anterior lamellar techniques are currently available, namely, use of air, fluid, viscoelastic materials, and a combination of these techniques [6, 7]. The surgeon may use the technique of his choice. However, TALK requires the surgeon to be an experienced lamellar corneal surgeon to avoid or minimize potential complications associated with this surgical technique [6, 7]. This chapter will describe TALK using VisionBlue (trypan blue ophthalmic solution, Dutch Ophthalmic USA, Kingston, NH) and forced hydrodissection (John technique).
   a. Host corneal surgery with trypan blue and forced-hydrodissection (John technique)
      The central cornea is marked after measuring with Castroviejo calipers. A Hanna vacuum trephine (Moria) is centered over the corneal mark, using the built-in crosswires for proper centration. Suction is applied to the trephine, and partial-thickness trephination is carried out at a depth of about 400 μm, depending on the preoperative corneal thickness (Figs. 7.2, 7.3). The corneal markings help in proper suture placement (Fig. 7.2). The plane of stromal dissection is initiated using a crescent knife (Beaver™, Becton Dickinson, Franklin Lakes, NJ), angled 55°, bevel up, matte finish, and then switched to a Morlet lamellar knife/dissector (no. 6-607, Duckworth and Kent USA, St. Louis, MO) (Fig. 7.2). The lamellar corneal dissector (long arm of the dissector) is used to dissect the host corneal cap, which is about 70% corneal thickness from the anterior corneal surface. This exposes the remaining host corneal stromal bed (about 30% corneal thickness) (Fig. 7.2). A 15° superblade (Alcon ophthalmic knife) or the angled crescent knife then is used to make a partial cut into the remaining corneal stroma, taking care not

to perforate the recipient Descemet' membrane (DM). This stromal opening is used to place a smooth 30-G AC cannula (Alcon), with the opening of the cannula facing down, and balanced salt solution (BSS) is injected under pressure, using a 5-ml disposable syringe. This forced hydrodissection (John technique) further splits the remaining corneal stromal layers, and the superficial layer of the corneal stroma turns white in the immediate segmental area (Fig. 7.2). VisionBlue is used to fill the well (Fig. 7.2) created in the host cornea, with the trephination and dissecting off of the corneal cap. The excess VisionBlue is removed immediately using sterile Merocel eye spears (Medtronic Solan, Jacksonville, FL). The exposed host corneal stroma is blue, which facilitates further layer-by-layer stromal dissection, and the segmental area of hydrodissection turns whitish blue. The short arm of the Morlet lamellar knife/dissector, i.e., the Paufique knife, then is introduced gently into this focal pocket, and intrastromal lamellar dissection is carried out (Fig. 7.2) by a to-and-fro, 180° arc rotation on the vertical axis of the handle of the Morlet lamellar knife/dissector held perpendicular to the stromal bed. After segmental lamellar dissection of the corneal stroma, a Vannas scissor blade is introduced gently into the dissected pocket and cut vertically, while the anterior stromal layer is simultaneously lifted away from the remaining stromal bed (Fig. 7.2). This segmentally separated blue stromal layer exposes in sharp contrast the relatively transparent, unstained deeper stromal layers (Fig. 7.2). The separated, blue stained, segmental stromal layer is then excised with the Vannas scissors. This creates a transparent area in the region of the excised stromal layer, surrounded by blue stroma. This segmental hydrodissection and layered excision of the corneal stromal bed is repeated (Fig. 7.2) until all blue stroma is excised, and the entire circular area is transparent. The well is filled with VisionBlue (Fig. 7.2), and the excess VisionBlue is removed using Merocel eye spears (Fig. 7.2). VisionBlue stains the corneal stroma instantaneously. A vertical cut is again made, using a 15° superblade or the angled crescent knife on the remaining thin corneal stroma, and hydrodissection and layer-by-layer segmental excision of the remaining corneal stroma is performed (Fig. 7.2) until once again the circular bed is fully transparent. After this, a final layer of stroma is removed similarly (Fig. 7.2), exposing the smooth DM with no corneal stroma in the entire circular area (Fig. 7.2). There is a clearly demarcated light reflex on the smooth DM (Fig. 7.2). The presence of a clear, sharp light reflex on Descemet' membrane confirms visually that the bare DM has been reached with no stromal fibers. If there is residual stroma after the third layer is removed, then this dissection process can be repeated until bare DM is exposed without corneal stroma.

b. Donor corneal surgery with VisionBlue staining of endothelium
The donor corneal button is placed on a Teflon block with the endothelial side up, and the concavity in the corneal button is filled with VisionBlue, which stains the donor corneal endothelium and facilitates easy visualization of the endothelium during DM–endothelial complex removal (Fig. 7.2). Excess VisionBlue is removed with Merocel eye spears. Vacuum is applied to the epithelial side of the donor cornea, and trephination is carried out using the same diameter Hanna trephine blade that was used on the host cornea (Moria). The scleral rim with the attached peripheral donor cornea is removed. Vacuum is applied again to the epithelial side of the donor disc, and the donor DM with the blue-stained endothelium (Fig. 7.2) is peeled from the donor corneal stroma, which exposes the donor corneal stroma without any VisionBlue.

c. Donor disk transplantation
The interface is rinsed thoroughly with sterile BSS, i.e., the stromal side of the donor disc and the host DM. Tisseel tissue adhesive (Baxter) is applied to the interface, namely, component 1 on the stromal side of the donor corneal disc, and component 2 on the DM of the host corneal bed. The donor corneal disc is then placed over the smooth host DM and sutured in place with 10-0 nylon interrupted and a running 360° suture (Figs. 7.2, 7.3). The tissue adhesive evenly attaches the host DM to the donor corneal disc, without any wrinkles. Suture knots are buried within the host stroma. Astigmatism is controlled by intraoperative suture adjustments as needed. A collagen corneal shield (Proshield™ RD, Alcon) soaked in tobramycin–dexamethasone ophthalmic solution is placed over the cornea.

d. Postoperative findings and management
Biomicroscopic examination using the slit lamp on day 1 after surgery reveals no VisionBlue within the cornea and hence, there is no bluish coloration of the cornea. Additionally, the donor cornea is well approximated to the host DM without any DM folds, air pockets, or debris in the interface between the donor corneal stroma and the host DM. It is essential to take all precautions to prevent the surgical introduction of any debris within the corneal interface. The corneal interface between the donor corneal stroma and the host DM is smooth, well approximated, without any haze or opacity even on the day after surgery. This clarity is possi-

ble only because the DM is fully exposed surgically without any stromal remnants. Both topical corticosteroid ophthalmic suspension (e.g., prednisolone acetate 1% [Pred Forte 1%, Allergan, Inc., Irvine, Calif.]) and a broad-spectrum fluoroquinolone ophthalmic solution (e.g., Iquix (Visakon Pharmaceuticals) are used initially four times a day and subsequently discontinued. Ocular lubrication is used as needed to sustain an optimal corneal surface.

In this surgical technique of VisionBlue-stained forced hydrodissection of the host cornea (John technique), 100% of the host corneal stroma is removed, up to the smooth DM in the area of trephination, and there is retention of the recipient endothelium that prevents any subsequent corneal endothelial graft rejection (Figs. 7.2, 7.3). An alternative technique is the big-bubble technique using air to expose the DM.

2. Descemetorhexis with endokeratoplasty (DXEK) (Fig. 7.4)
DXEK, synonymous with Descemet stripping with endothelial keratoplasty (DSEK), Descemet stripping automated endothelial keratoplasty (DSAEK), is a new, evolving, and increasingly popular surgical technique that has largely replaced DLEK [2, 10–21], and it may replace PKP as the gold standard of corneal transplantation [2].
  a. Anesthesia
  The author's preferred anesthesia is topical with MAC on all cases, except those requesting general anesthesia (GA), or if there is an indication for the use of GA. The author uses topical Xylocaine 2% jelly (lidocaine HCL, AstraZeneca Inc., Wilmington, Del.) with MAC. Other choices include peribulbar and retrobulbar anesthesia.
  b. DXEK may be viewed as a three-step procedure:
    i. The first and most important step in DXEK is the proper selection of the corneal trephine diameter. The donor disc diameter will usually be within the range of 7.5–9.0 mm, commonly, 8.0 mm. Sometimes the trephine diameter may be outside these ranges. It is equally important to have proper surgical instruments to perform DXEK in a reproducible, effective, and timely manner, without any significant damage to the host corneal stroma, thus maintaining a superior donor–host corneal interface and contributing to a better quality of vision following surgery. Several instruments (Table 7.4) are surgeon friendly for this procedure.
    ii. Donor disc
      1. AAC
      An AAC and a microkeratome with a 300-μm CB head is used (Moria). A sterile syringe filled with the Optisol GS solution from the eye bank vial containing the donor corneal button is attached to a short single-use, sterile tubing with a stop valve, and the other end of the tubing is attached to the ALTK system.
      2. Cap cutting and staining with VisionBlue
      Gently inject the Optisol from the syringe such that the solution fills the central post. Place the donor corneal button with a large scleral rim (>3.6 mm) [5], with the endothelial side down on the central post, with the Optisol wetting the donor corneal endothelium. Place the cylindrical fixation ring and lock the ring in place. The plunger in the syringe is pushed in to get a tactile pressure on the cornea within the AAC greater than 65 mm, and the valve is closed. Remove the corneal epithelium with dry Weckcel sponges, which adds an additional 50-μm depth for the corneal cut. Place a central dot on the dome of the cornea with a marking pen and a linear mark on the periphery of the cornea. Moisten the microkeratome head with sterile BSS, slide the head onto the post, and manually cut the corneal cap with the CB microkeratome head in a curvilinear fashion. A free cap is then obtained on the microkeratome head, and the donor corneal stroma is exposed in a circular manner in the central opening of the ALTK system. Apply VisionBlue onto the exposed corneal stroma. Dry the excess VisionBlue with Merocel sponges.
      3. Cap replacement
      Remove the free cap from the microkeratome head and replace it onto the exposed donor corneal stroma, such that the marks are aligned. Remove the corneal button with the outer corneal cap in place and place it on a Hanna corneal punch with the epithelial side down.
      4. Punching donor disc ("double unit")
      Since there is a free cap that is replaced, this becomes a double-unit donor cornea. The outer corneal cap will protect the interface stroma from any unwanted debris. Center the double-unit donor cornea on to the Hanna corneal punch. The circular blade should land within the area of the blue coloration to obtain a properly cut, well-centered donor disc.
    iii. Host cornea
      1. Trephine marking of host corneal epithelium
      After trephination of the donor cornea from the endothelial side, ink mark the trephine blade edge, and mark the recipient corneal surface on the epithelium using the same diameter trephine as used on the donor cornea. The subsequent descemetorhexis DX is performed 0.5 mm within this circular mark.

2. Wound construction
   Conjunctiva and Tenon's capsule are cut in the temporal region to expose the bare sclera. It is essential to obtain complete hemostasis (Fig. 7.4). In the perilimbal sclera, two marks, 5.0 mm apart are made. Next, a curvilinear incision is made at the limbus, using a diamond blade with a fixed depth of 350 μm (Fig. 7.4). The AC is not entered at this time.
3. Healon in AC
   In a step to simplify DXEK procedure, viscoelastic, namely, Healon is used in the AC during DX (M. Terry's recommendation, personal communication, 2006). The author uses Healon for DX in all cases without any complications that are attributable to Healon use. Two stab incisions are made at the limbus, one to the right (about 2 o'clock position), and a second stab incision is made on the left side of the temporal incision (about 5 o'clock position,) using a 15° superblade (Fig. 7.4). These are the first two incisions to enter the anterior chamber (AC). The 2 o'clock incision is used to inject the Healon, and the 5 o'clock incision is used to inject air to unfold the taco-folded donor disc. These incisions can also be used to introduce other instruments such as a John Dexatome spatula (patent pending) (ASICO, Inc., Westmont, IL), reverse Sinskey hook, John super microscissors, John super microforceps, etc. The Healon canula is introduced through the 2 o'clock incision, and the AC is filled with Healon.
4. DX
   A John Dexatome spatula (ASICO) is then introduced through the 2 o'clock incision, and a complete 360° Descemet's scoring is followed by a 360° DX (Fig. 7.4). The design of the John Dexatome spatula permits a 360° DX, without exiting the AC, and without using a second instrument such as a descemet stripper. A John Dexatome spatula allows DM to be removed as a single, complete disc, almost all the time. During DX, it is essential to stay in the proper plane 360°, meaning, at the DM–stromal interface. If the Dexatome spatula tip is at this interface, then the surgeon can perform rapid scoring without any stromal damage (Fig. 7.4). While performing DX, if the surgeon encounters any resistance then the tip of the Dexatome spatula is too deep, namely, inside the stroma, and the surgeon should stop and reenter the DM–stromal interface to complete the DX.
5. Removal of DM
   The surgeon should make every effort to remove the DM as a single disc (Fig. 7.4), since this will eliminate the need to reenter the AC with other instruments to excise DM tags. Next, the AC is entered through the temporal premade groove, using a 3.2-mm keratome blade (Alcon). The detached DM disc is then removed from the AC using a John insertion forceps (ASICO) and quickly examined under the microscope to confirm the removal of the DM as a single disc (Fig. 7.4).
6. Stromal scrubbing
   Peripheral stromal scrubbing is performed within the epithelial circular mark to increase adhesion of the donor corneal disc to the exposed host corneal stroma (M. Terry, personal communication 2006). The author performs peripheral scrubbing of the host corneal stroma routinely, using a John scrubber (ASICO). During the scrubbing of the peripheral stroma, Healon remains in the AC to prevent AC collapse.
7. Healon removal and wound enlargement to 5.0 mm
   Healon is removed from the anterior chamber using an irrigation/aspiration (I/A) unit attached to the Alcon Infiniti (Alcon). It is important to remove completely all Healon from the anterior chamber. Make sure that the Healon is also removed from the inner corneal surface. Any Healon left behind in this region of the host cornea can cause nonattachment of the corneal disc and contribute to postoperative disc detachment. The temporal perilimbal wound is then enlarged to its full length of 5.0 mm, using the angled crescent blade, bevel up.
8. Taco insertion into AC
   There are two techniques for the introduction of the donor corneal disc into the AC
a. Push technique
i. Taco-fold insertion
   The donor corneal disc is brought to the surgical field and placed on the host cornea, such that the epithelial surface of the donor corneal disc is in contact with the host corneal epithelium. This position provides a magnified view for the surgeon looking through the operating microscope. A small amount of Healon is placed on the endothelial surface in the center of the donor disc. One edge of the donor corneal disc is held with the John insertion forceps, and the donor disc is folded on itself in the shape of a taco. The donor disc is folded into a 60/40 fold such that the VisonBlue–stained stromal surface is facing up. Once a 60/40 taco fold is completed, John insertion forceps is used to gently

pick up the folded donor disc along its vertical fold. To prevent endothelial damage, avoid any undue pressure on the folded taco. The folded taco is then picked up, while the outer donor cap is discarded. The 60/40 folded donor taco corneal disc is then introduced into the recipient AC in one continuous, smooth motion, and it is deposited on the iris surface, past the pupillary margins and the John insertion forceps is withdrawn from the AC.

b. Pull technique

In this technique, the donor corneal disc is not folded as a taco for AC insertion.

i. Suture pulling of donor disc

In this technique, a suture is attached to the margin of the donor corneal disc. The donor corneal disc is brought to the perilimbal wound, and the donor corneal disc is introduced into the AC by pulling the suture from the opposite site. The suture is removed, leaving the donor corneal disc in the anterior chamber with the endothelial side down.

ii. Instrumental introduction

In this technique, the donor corneal disc is introduced between the lips of the limbal wound with an instrument that keeps the donor corneal disc with the endothelium facing down. The disc is then pulled into the AC with a forceps, introduced from the opposite side. The disc lays on the iris surface with the endothelium facing down. Currently, research work is underway in trying to develop a cartridge delivery system to introduce the donor corneal disc into the recipient AC.

– Wound closure

The perilimbal wound is closed with three interrupted, 10-0 nylon sutures, and the surgical knots are buried.

– "Fork-lift" of the folded taco donor corneal disc

A 27-G sterile cannula attached to a 5-ml sterile syringe containing sterile BSS is introduced into the AC from the 2 o'clock stab incision, and the tip of the cannula is placed between the donor taco-folded disc and the iris surface, and BSS is gently injected, which results in raising the taco upward toward the inner stromal surface of the recipient cornea and partially attaching the taco to the recipient cornea. The upper fold of the taco is attached to the recipient cornea, while the posterior leaflet is partially open towards the iris surface.

– Air-bubble unfolding and attaching donor disc to host cornea

Air-bubble unfolding is used in the taco-folded insertion technique of the donor corneal disc. A 30-G sterile cannula is introduced from the previously placed stab incision at the 5 o'clock position, and the tip of the cannula is placed between the leaflets of the folded taco. Filtered air is gently injected in a gentle, steady stream, thus unfolding the taco completely, and attaching the stromal side of the donor disc to the stromal side of the recipient cornea. Additional air is injected to fill the AC. Avoid injecting excess air, since it will pass via the pupil into the posterior chamber and push the iris forward. If the donor corneal disc is decentered, then the centration of the donor disc is achieved using a reverse Sinskey hook.

– Waiting 8 to 10 min

Following good centration of the donor disc and filling the AC with filtered air, wait about 8 to 10 min. If there are any macrofolds in the donor disc, then they are removed or diminished by using the John glider (ASICO) and gently massaging the dome of the recipient cornea.

– Decreasing air-bubble size (bubble diameter > disc diameter)

After about 8 to 10 min, the air-bubble size is decreased by injecting a small quantity of sterile BSS into the AC, while simultaneously releasing some of the AC air by gently depressing the lip of the surgical wound. At the conclusion, the diameter of the air-bubble must be larger than the diameter of the attached donor corneal disc.

– Dilating pupil

It is essential to dilate the pupil with homatropine 5% eye drops to prevent postoperative pupillary block glaucoma attack.

▪ Antibiotics, patch and shield

– Apply steroid–antibiotic combination ophthalmic ointment after placing a few drops of fluoroquinolone ophthalmic solution and patch the eye. An eye shield is applied for protection.

3 PKP (Fig. 7.5)

Peribulbar/retrobulbar anesthesia with MAC or GA is used for the procedure. The central cornea is marked with a sterile needle and highlighted with a surgical marking pen (Fig. 7.5), which permits proper centration of the trephine. The author uses the Hanna suction trephine, which allows for depth setting (Fig. 7.5) in microns. This trephine can be used for partial thickness trephination as for ALK or for full-thickness PKP. Figure 7.5 shows the trephine disposable blade, the AAC, and the donor corneal trephination from the epithelial surface, namely

Table 7.4 Surgical instruments for DXEK surgery

Name	Manufacturer	Comments
John Dexatome DXEK/DSAEK spatula (AE-2872)	ASICO	To score and detach DM as a single disc without exiting the anterior chamber, usually no need for DM stripper
John DXEK/DSAEK Descemet's stripper (AE-2874)	ASICO	Used for stripping DM
John DXEK/DSAEK inserting forceps (AE-4227)	ASICO	For insertion of the folded donor disc into the recipient anterior chamber
John retrocorneal super microforceps (AE-4962)	ASICO	For holding tissues on the inner surface of the recipient cornea
John Super-Micro-Scissors (AE-5762)	ASICO	For cutting tissues on the inner surface of the recipient cornea
John DXEK/DSAEK fixation hook (AE-2182)	ASICO	To stabilize the donor corneal disc
John DXEK/DSAEK stromal scrubber (AE-2878)	ASICO	Used to roughen the host inner corneal stroma
John DXEK/DSAEK corneal glider (AE-2879)	ASICO	Used to smooth the macro-folds in the donor disc
John DXEK/DSAEK double ended marker 8–9 mm (AE-2712)	ASICO	Used to make corneal epithelial marks to facilitate DXEK surgery
ALTK AAC and CB Microkeratome	Moria	Donor disc preparation
Stripper, 45° and 90°	Moria	Stripping DM
Goosey forceps	Moria	Handling tissues
Price hook	Moria	To score DM
DSAEK marker	Moria	To mark host cornea
Terry scraper	Baush & Lomb[a]	Scraping peripheral stroma after Descemetorhexis
Melles PLK scraper, 45° and 90°	D.O.R.C.[b]	Stripping DM

[a]Baush & Lomb, Rochester, N.Y.
[b]D.O.R.C., Zuidland, The Netherlands

"front cutting," donor trephination. Viscoelastic material is layered on the central well and filled with Optisol GS to protect the donor endothelium during donor corneal trephination. The use of the Hanna trephine system results in a uniform cut edge of the donor corneal button (Fig. 7.5). The same Hanna trephine is used to trephine the host cornea. Since both the donor and host trephination are carried out in the same fashion from the epithelial side, there is usually a good match for seating the donor corneal button into the central corneal opening in the recipient cornea (Fig. 7.5). The suction holds the trephine in place and permits uniform cutting of the recipient cornea (Fig. 7.5).

The AC is entered at the 10 o'clock position, using a superblade (Fig. 7.5). Cohesive viscoelastic material is injected into the AC prior to excising the recipient cornea (Fig. 7.5). Acetylcholine chloride 1:100 is injected into the AC to constrict the pupil. Corneal microscissors and 0.12 forceps are used to excise the host cornea. Additional Viscoat is injected into the AC, and the donor corneal button is placed in position and sutured with eight interrupted and one continuous 10-0 nylon suture. All suture knots are buried within the host cornea (Fig. 7.5). Suture adjustments are made to control or diminish the amount of postoperative corneal astigmatism. Subconjunctival antibiotics and corticosteroid are injected, and an antibiotic–steroid combination ophthalmic ointment is applied to the eye. The eye is patched and a shield is applied for ocular protection. Postoperatively, topical antibiotic and corticosteroid eye drops are used four times a day.

Take Home Pearls

- Inflammatory corneal involvement with significant tissue loss is an ocular emergency that requires close medical and/or surgical management.
- Selective tissue corneal transplantation may provide great, long-term benefit to the patient.
- John-Malbran classification of optical LPK provides a overview of the types of surgery.
- Health of the corneal endothelium and the location of the corneal opacity determines the type of surgery to be performed.
- Supplementary procedures such as a bandage soft contact lens, punctual occlusion, amniotic membrane transplantation, or conjunctival flap may be required in some cases.

References

1. John, T., Descemetorhexis with endokeratoplasty. In: John, T. (ed), Surgical Techniques in Anterior and Posterior Lamellar Corneal Surgery. Jaypee Brothers Medical, New Delhi, India: 2006, pp 411–420
2. John, T. (editorial), Selective tissue corneal transplantation: a great step forward in global visual restoration. Expert Rev Ophthalmol 2006. 1: 5–7
3. John, T., Descemetorhexis with endokeratoplasty (DXEK). In: John, T. (ed), Step-by-step anterior and posterior lamellar keratoplasty. Jaypee Brothers Medical, New Delhi, India: 2006, pp 177–196
4. John, T., Malbran, E. S., Classification of lamellar corneal surgery. In: John, T. (ed), Surgical techniques in anterior and posterior lamellar corneal surgery. Jaypee Brothers Medical, New Delhi, India: 2006, pp 36–43
5. Selvadurai, D., John, T., Ruszkowski, E., Pivoney, C. J., McCoy, K., The ideal size of human donor corneoscleral explants from eye banks used in artificial anterior chambers. Presented at the Annual Meeting of ARVO, Ft. Lauderdale, Fla., 2005
6. John, T. (ed), Surgical techniques in anterior and posterior lamellar keratoplasty. Jaypee Brothers Medical, New Delhi, India: 2006
7. John, T. (ed), Step-by-step anterior and posterior lamellar keratoplasty. Jaypee Brothers Medical, New Delhi, India: 2006
8. John, T., Human amniotic membrane transplantation: past, present, and future. Ophthalmol Clin N Am 2003. 16: 43–65
9. John, T., Foulks, G. N., John, M. E., Cheng, K., Hu, D., Amniotic membrane in the surgical management of acute toxic epidermal necrolysis. Ophthalmology 2002. 109: 351–360
10. Melles, G. R. J., Wijdh, R. H. J., Nieuwendaal, C. P., A technique to excise the Descemet membrane from a recipient cornea (descemetorhexis). Cornea 2004. 23: 286–288
11. Price, Jr., F. W., Price, M. O., Descemet's stripping with endothelial keratoplasty in 50 eyes; a refractive neutral cornea transplant. J Refract Surg 2005. 21: 339–345
12. Price, Jr., F. W., Price, M. O., Descemet's stripping with endothelial keratoplasty in 200 eyes: Early challenges and techniques to enhance donor adherence. J Refract Surg 2006. 32: 411–418
13. Melles, G. R., Posterior lamellar keratoplasty: DLEK to DSEK to DMEK. Cornea 2006. 25: 879–881
14. Price, Jr., F. W., Price, M. O., Descemet's stripping with endothelial keratoplasty: comparative outcomes with microkeratome-dissected and manually dissected donor tissue. Ophthalmology 2006. 113: 1936–1942
15. Gorovoy, M. S., Descemet-stripping automated endothelial keratoplasty. Cornea 2006. 25: 886–889
16. Terry, M. A., Ousley, P. J., Deep lamellar endothelial keratoplasty in the first United States patients: early clinical results. Cornea 2001. 20:239–243
17. Terry, M. A., Endothelial keratoplasty: History, current state, and future directions. Cornea 2006. 25: 873–878
18. John, T., Use of indocyanine green in deep lamellar endothelial keratoplasty. J Cataract Refract Surg 2003. 29: 437–443
19. Koenig, S. B., Dupps, Jr., W. J., Covert, D. J., Meisler, D. M., Simple technique to unfold the donor corneal lenticule during Descemet's stripping and automated endothelial keratoplasty. J Cataract Refract Surg 2007. 33: 189–190
20. Cheng, Y. Y., Pels, E., Nuijts, R. M., Femtosecond-laser-assisted Descemet's stripping endothelial keratoplasty. J Cataract Refract Surg 2007. 33: 152–155
21. Culbertson, W. W., Descemet stripping endothelial keratoplasty. Int Ophthalmol Clin 2006. 46: 155–68

Lens / Chapter 8

Selection of Surgical Technique for Complicated Cataract in Uveitis

Mauricio Miranda, Jorge L. Alió

Core Messages

- Control intraocular inflammation before, during and after elective surgery.
- Perform surgery when inflammation is as controlled as possible.
- Ideal control of inflammation is no cells in the anterior chamber, no active retinal inflammation and no cystoid macular edema.
- Use topical or periocular steroids to reduce intraocular inflammation for several weeks before surgery.
- Use nonsteroidal anti-inflammatory drugs to reduce the risk of postoperative cystoid macular edema.
- Control intraocular pressure prior to surgery, avoiding cholinergic drugs.
- Prostaglandins analogs may be associated with a higher risk of cystoid macular edema.

Contents

8.1	Introduction	85	8.3.1.1	Algorithm Approach for Decision Making for Cataract in Uveitis (IOIS) 91
8.2	Preoperative Condition of the Patient Related to the Surgical Approach	87	8.3.2	Surgical Procedure 91
8.2.1	Inflammation	87	8.3.3	Viscoelastics 93
8.2.2	Slit Lamp Evaluation	87	8.3.4	Capsulorhexis 93
8.2.3	Management of Associated Glaucoma	88	8.3.5	Microincisional Cataract Surgery 94
8.2.4	Considerations Related to Type of Uveitis	89	8.3.6	Intraoperative Treatment 94
8.2.5	Preoperative Planning	90	8.3.7	Choice of Intraocular Lens 94
8.2.6	Visual Prognosis	90	8.4	Complications 95
8.3	Surgical Planning	91	8.5	Postoperative Follow-up 96
8.3.1	Patient Preparation	91	References	96

8.1 Introduction

Cataract is a common complication of chronic uveitis. In juvenile idiopathic arthritis associated iridocyclitis, cataracts occur in up to 83% of patients during long-term follow-up [31]. The incidence of cataract in pars planitis and Fuchs heterochromic iridocyclitis is approximately 50% [9]. Often, cataract is only one of a number of uveitic complications, each of which may influence the surgical approach. Results of cataract surgery can be difficult to assess in eyes with disparate presurgical morbidities that may lead to different responses to the same surgery, with variable visual outcomes.

Some patients seem to be unusually susceptible to cataract formation. In others, concomitant posterior synechiae, iris atrophy, iris neovascularization, or secondary glaucoma indicates a more severe degree of inflammatory damage to the anterior segment. Posterior synechiae may be etiologically related to cataract formation as localized lens opacities can occur subjacent to them. This may be on the basis of microperforation of the lens capsule. In general, severe anterior uveitis may be associated with anterior subcapsular opacities, while intermediate uveitis or persistent iridocyclitis and the use of topical and systemic steroids may be linked to posterior subcapsular cataracts (Fig. 8.1).

The presence of toxic debris and oxygen free radicals from inflammation and local ischemia induced by synechiae may damage lens fibers and epithelial cells, leading to lens opacities. The mechanism of posterior subcapsular cataract induced by corticosteroid use is not

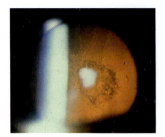

Fig. 8.1 Posterior subcapsular cataract associated with chronic steroid drops

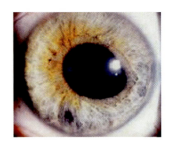

Fig. 8.2 Iris atrophy in a patient associated with anterior uveitis

well known, although it has been suggested to be related to abnormal cellular metabolism induced by electrolytic imbalance [32].

Cataract surgery in uveitic eyes remains a challenge to ophthalmologists with its intraoperative risks and the uncertainty of the postoperative course. Presentation in children and young adults, possibly uncontrolled inflammation, and associated glaucoma or hypotony often require a different surgical approach than for other types of cataracts.

There are several misconceptions about surgery in uveitic eyes, such as a uniformly poor outcome. Good visual results have been demonstrated in patients with Fuchs heterochromic iridocyclitis and in those patients with good preoperative control of intraocular inflammation [28]. Postoperative inflammation after surgery can often be controlled with medical therapy, and the incidence of phthisis bulbi and hypotony are more related to the type of uveitis than to the surgical procedure. In addition, uveitis is no longer a contraindication for the implantation of intraocular lenses.

There have been many studies of visual outcome after cataract surgery [37] implantation of posterior chamber intraocular lenses (IOLs) in patients with uveitis. While it has been a controversial subject, better lens design, better surgical techniques, and more accurate "in-the-bag" placement have resulted in intraocular lenses being used more frequently, except possibly for cases with uveitis secondary to juvenile chronic arthritis (JCA) [7, 8]. Nonetheless, complications may arise during or after surgery, such as band keratopathy, glaucoma, early capsular opacification, lens deposits, synechiae, iris atrophy (Fig. 8.2) or neovascularization, cystoid macular edema (CME), epiretinal membranes, vitreous hemorrhages, retinal detachment, and even phthisis bulbi.

For these reasons, the decision to perform cataract surgery in a uveitis patient must be carefully considered. The main indications for cataract surgery in uveitic patients are: (1) visually significant cataracts with a good prospect for improvement in acuity, (2) removal of cataracts that impair fundus assessment in patients with suspected fundus pathology or in whom a posterior segment surgical procedure is planned, and (3) removal of the lens in an eye with phacogenic uveitis. Mild cataractous changes in the early course of uveitis have little effect on visual acuity. When progressive, they may reduce visual acuity to the point where cataract extraction is necessary.

Cataract is not a reversible disease, so further visual decrease is expected if no surgery is performed. Occasionally, 20/20 visual acuity may be present in patients complaining of blurred vision, generally associated with posterior subcapsular opacities. In these cases, the patient must receive a careful explanation of the irreversibility of the cataract and the probable increase in symptoms over time, as well as the expected benefits and possible risks of surgery.

Take Home Pearls

- Cataracts are a common complication among uveitis patients, especially in persistent anterior and intermediate uveitis and form at a younger age than in the general population.
- Development of cataracts is influenced by the anatomic location, severity, and chronicity of intraocular inflammation as well as with the use of corticosteroids.
- Selection of the best surgical technique for extraction of complicated cataracts in uveitis requires background knowledge of the relationship between inflammation and cataracts.
- Misconceptions persist about surgery in uveitis; however, it is not uncommon for complications to arise during or after surgery.
- Uveitic patients may be divided into two groups: complicated cases and uncomplicated cases, according to guidelines developed by the International Ocular Inflammation Society (IOIS).

8.2 Preoperative Condition of the Patient Related to the Surgical Approach

8.2.1 Inflammation

It is of the utmost importance to achieve proper control of intraocular inflammation before, during, and after surgery. Elective surgery should be performed when inflammation has been controlled as well as possible. Phacogenic uveitis, or the need to remove the lens concomitant to other nonelective ocular procedures, is the only case in which the elimination of inflammatory signs is not necessary before surgery. It is desirable that the surgery is performed in a quiet eye in which the inflammatory reaction has been controlled for at least 3 months prior to surgery [19]. The single most important sign of inflammation is the presence or absence of inflammatory cells. Aqueous flare in anterior chronic uveitis denotes vascular incompetence of the iris and ciliary body, a consequence of vascular damage from recurrent uveitis, and should not generally be used as a guidepost for inflammatory quiescence, although it may have other significance for the eye. Inflammation in the posterior segment may be difficult to assess in patients with dense cataracts. The presence of vitreous cells does not necessarily signify active disease, because inflammatory cells clear more slowly than from the anterior chamber. The definition of optimally controlled inflammation is a patient with no cells and up to 1+ flare in the anterior chamber, no active retinal inflammation, and no CME.

Topical or periocular steroids can be used to reduce intraocular inflammation before surgery. The use of systemic steroids is seldom necessary and should be reserved for the severest cases. In severe forms of inflammation, anti-inflammatory drugs may be advisable. Topical nonsteroidal anti-inflammatory drugs (NSAIDs) may be beneficial to reduce the risk of postoperative CME via the inhibition of prostaglandin synthesis, which may be of importance, especially in eyes where the iris is manipulated, as is often the case in eyes with uveitis that have developed extensive posterior synechiae. Specific antibiotic therapy should have been completed when an infectious etiology such as tuberculosis or syphilis is suspected.

The purpose of the therapy is to reduce cellular activity in the anterior chamber to less than 1+, with a minimal vitreous infiltration by the time of surgery. Surgery must be delayed when more than 10 cells per high magnification field are detected on the anterior chamber biomicroscopy; however, in some eyes, it may be impossible to eliminate the inflammation. In those cases where the degree of inflammation behind the lens cannot be assessed, a prophylactic therapy should be prescribed for a few days before surgery and the patient managed as if an active inflammation were present.

Intraocular inflammation may be associated with high, normal, or low intraocular pressure (IOP), depending on the severity of the inflammation, deposits in the trabecular meshwork, and the damage to the ciliary body. Increased IOP may be associated with any kind of intraocular inflammation due to the chronic use of systemic or topical corticosteroids, and appear as chronic, acute, or transient. The term *uveitic glaucoma* describes high IOP associated with uveitis with optic nerve damage and visual field defects. High IOP during a short period without damage to the optic nerve can be termed *uveitis-related ocular hypertension*. Uveitic high IOP is usually associated with inflammatory damage to the trabecular meshwork and with peripheral anterior synechiae. Those eyes with posterior synechiae may eventually develop a pupillary seclusion requiring Nd:YAG laser iridotomy before cataract surgery. A specific entity characterized by high IOP during acute anterior uveitis episodes is Posner-Schlossman iridocyclitis.

The appropriate management of high IOP must include the control of the inflammation as well as the reduction of IOP. Early anti-inflammatory therapy combined with mydriatic and cycloplegic drugs should be used to reduce the formation of posterior and anterior synechiae, pupillary membranes, pupillary seclusion, and damage to the trabecular meshwork. Proper control of the IOP is recommended 2–3 weeks prior to surgery. However, medical and surgical therapy may be necessary if high IOP cannot be controlled by anti-inflammatory therapy alone. The use of cholinergic drugs should be avoided in these patients as they alter the blood–aqueous barrier (BAB) and tend to increase synechiae formation. The use of prostaglandin analogs has been associated with a higher risk of CME [36].

Low IOP may occasionally appear after severe uveitis episodes. It is generally caused by the formation of cyclitic membranes in the posterior chamber detaching the ciliary body. Occasionally, it may originate from the inflammatory destruction of the ciliary body. The appearance of a fibrinoid reaction during or immediately after surgery may be treated by the intracameral injection of 500–700 units of streptokinase or 10–25 µg of recombinant tissue plasminogen activator (rt-PA) [17].

8.2.2 Slit Lamp Evaluation

Selection of surgical procedure is influenced by the slit lamp examination. There are critical aspects of the slit lamp examination, such as anterior or posterior synechiae, presence of iridocyclitic membrane, hypotony, and shallowing of the anterior chamber without cellular inflammation but with flare in the anterior chamber. Elevated IOP (especially herpetic uveitis, lens-induced uveitis, and Posner-Schlossman syndrome) is seen, as well as iris atrophy (herpetic), posterior synechiae (especially HLA-B27 and sarcoidosis), and band keratopathy (especially JCA in younger patients and any chronic uveitis in older patients). Uveitis in a "quiet eye" should lead to consideration of juvenile idiopathic arthritis-associated uveitis, Fuchs heterochromic iridocyclitis, or masquerade syndromes (Table 8.1).

Anterior synechiae occur in the angle during chronic or acute inflammation. They may develop during low-grade chronic inflammation with only flare seen in the anterior chamber without cells noted. Significant anterior synechiae in the presence of a functioning ciliary body and compromised trabecular outflow may create severe angle-closure glaucoma despite a deep anterior chamber. Anterior synechiae more commonly are found in deeply pigmented eyes, granulomatous diseases, and traumatized eyes.

Peripheral KPs may be seen with peripheral corneal edema with herpes simplex or zoster uveitis, following acute angle-closure glaucoma, or after blunt ocular trauma. KPs must be differentiated from corneal endothelial guttae and pigment deposits. Posterior synechiae typically form during acute inflammatory episodes at the location of Koeppe nodules. Both granulomatous and nongranulomatous cases may develop posterior synechiae quite rapidly, but they usually do not appear in pars planitis. Patients with both intermediate uveitis and posterior synechiae should be evaluated thoroughly for an etiology distinct from pars planitis syndrome. Chronic anterior uveitis also frequently develops posterior synechiae, with or without gross pupillary distortion.

During vitreous examination, particularly in cases with intermediate uveitis or pars planitis (in which the sine qua non is vitreous cells), white exudative material over the inferior ora serrata and pars plana ("snowbanks"), cellular aggregates floating in the inferior vitreous ("snowballs"), or vitreous hemorrhage can be seen, especially in younger patients. Snowbanking can often be seen only with indirect ophthalmoscopy and scleral depression. Other important posterior segment signs are peripheral retinal vascular sheathing, peripheral neovascularization, mild anterior chamber inflammation, CME, posterior subcapsular cataract, secondary glaucoma, retinal gliosis, and exudative retinal detachment.

Finally, in posterior uveitis, the critical signs are cells in the anterior or posterior vitreous or both, vitreous haze, retinal or choroidal inflammatory lesions, and vasculitis (sheathing and exudates around vessels). In chronic cases, although the number of cells is considerably smaller, haze may be conspicuous.

8.2.3 Management of Associated Glaucoma

Glaucoma associated with uveitis is one of the most serious complications of intraocular inflammation. Many patients respond poorly to surgery. It is of primary importance to assess the severity of the inflammation and the etiology of the uveitis. Management includes treatment of the underlying inflammation and of the glaucoma itself (see Sect. 8.3.1.1). Special considerations should be given to the management of acute or chronic intraocular inflammation and whether corticosteroids are the cause of the high IOP. Drug therapy is the first step in the treatment of uveitic glaucoma.

When required, the outcome of glaucoma surgery in uveitic patients in general is not as good as it is in patients without uveitis [13]. The following procedures may be performed: laser iridotomy, surgical iridectomy, trabeculodialysis, trabeculectomy, trabeculectomy with wound modulation therapy, ab interno laser sclerostomy, drainage implantation, and cycloablation therapy.

Table 8.1 Slit lamp examination: most common signs

	Sign
In anterior chamber	Anterior and posterior synechiae
	Iridocyclitic membrane
	Hypotony
	Shallow anterior chamber
	Flare
	Cells
In vitreous	Vitreous cells
	Vitreous hemorrhages
	Vitreous haze
	Peripheral neovascularization
	CME
	Posterior subcapsular cataract
	Secondary glaucoma

Diode cyclophotocoagulation (TSCPC) decreases IOP more effectively than cyclocryocoagulation in children, but complications after TSCPC are more severe than after cyclocryotherapy [34]. Currently, mitomycin C is more commonly used than 5-fluorouracil to reduce bleb closure after trabeculectomy [13, 45]. Good surgical results have been reported for refractory glaucomas with the use of mitomycin C; however, the higher success rate of filtering surgery with wound healing modulation is associated with an elevated risk of hypotony, bleb leaks, and late bleb-related endophthalmitis [45].

Glaucoma drainage devices are promising in the management of progressive secondary glaucoma with uveitis. The most commonly used device is the Molteno implant [35]. Glaucoma drainage devices are uniquely suited to inflammatory glaucoma as the artificial material of the tube cannot scar. The surface of the plate forms the base of a fibrous bleb through which there is absorption of the diverted aqueous. These devices are usually reserved for refractory glaucomatous patients with uveitis who have failed to improve with other medical procedures and when recurrent inflammation is believed to be the reason for the failure of standard filter drainage procedures.

Chapters 15 and 17 discuss glaucoma surgery more thoroughly.

8.2.4 Considerations Related to Type of Uveitis

Uveitis associated with Fuchs heterochromic cyclitis (FHC) tends to be chronic and of low intensity. Posterior synechiae (Fig. 8.3) are rarely formed, and the patients are usually unaware of the problem until the first complication arises in the form of cataracts or vitreous opacities [32]. The implantation of IOLs in patients with FHC is generally satisfactory with good visual outcome. Some ophthalmologists have reported the use of heparin surface-modified lenses for all patients with FHC in whom implantation is indicated [33]. There are reports that suggest that the foldable hydrophobic acrylic IOL is the most suitable one for this type of uveitis [19].

Fuchs heterochromic cyclitis patients have few postoperative complications, although some isolated cases of vitreitis, hyphema, increased IOP, and cyclitic membrane formation have been reported [17]. Posterior capsular opacification has been described in 8–20% of patients. The problem of greatest visual significance is the development of glaucoma, which appears in approximately 10% (range 3–35%) of patients; up to 70% may require filtration surgery [32].

Some risk factors have been identified in these patients. If glaucoma is present preoperatively, it may worsen postoperatively. In cases of severe iris atrophy, the risk of postoperative uveitis appears to be higher. When rubeosis iridis is present and hemorrhage occurs during surgery, the risk of both postoperative glaucoma and uveitis is higher.

Intermediate, posterior, and panuveitis patients in which significant vitreous opacities are present can be considered for cataract surgery combined with anterior vitrectomy through a central round posterior capsulectomy created with a vitrectomy probe. In cases with severe vitreous opacification, a posterior vitrectomy via pars plana may be necessary. Most surgeons opt for conventional pars plana vitrectomy techniques in this case [23, 25]. Pars plana vitrectomy combined with lensectomy (PPV-PPL) can be the procedure of choice in cases of uveitis with vitreitis refractory to medical treatment or to free the ciliary body from posterior cyclitic membrane when there is a risk of severe ocular hypotension (Fig. 8.4). The PPV-PPL technique can also be useful in patients with JCA. The presence of vitreous opacities and peripheral retinal neovascularization with a higher risk of vitreous hemorrhage may require cataract surgery to be combined with intraoperative ablation of the fibrotic membrane new vessels by vitreous surgery.

Disadvantages of the PPV-PPL approach include the need for sulcus fixation of the posterior chamber IOL if a lens is implanted, and the potential difficulties of aspirating residual cortical debris from the posterior surface of the anterior capsule. Combined phacoemulsification and pars plana vitrectomy technique resolves these disadvantages while permitting [8, 30] the beneficial effects of pars plana vitrectomy in restoring vision, stabilizing vitreous inflammation, and reducing systemic steroid requirements in eyes with thick vitreous opacities such as those associated with sarcoidosis that is resistant to medical treatment [30]. The scleral incisions for the vitrectomy should be made first, the infusion system sutured, and upper sclerotomies occluded with scleral plugs. A small phaco incision minimizes corneal distortion and maintains closure during the vitrectomy. A capsulotomy or posterior capsulorhexis should be performed on completion of the vitrectomy because of probable rapid opacification and because it allows access of anti-inflammatory drugs to the vitreous chamber in the postoperative stage. IOL implantation can be delayed until completion of vitrectomy if desired.

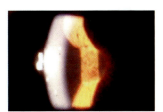

Fig. 8.3 Posterior synechiae in a patient with chronic intermediate uveitis

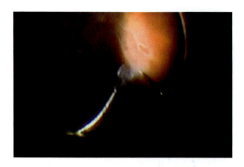

Fig. 8.4 Twenty-five-gauge instrumentation used to perform vitrectomy in a patient with vitreous opacity

This combined approach allows rapid visual rehabilitation and functional unaided vision in patients considered poor candidates for aphakic contact lens wear [10]. Although macular edema and recurrence of the inflammation may appear in up to 50% of cases of pars planitis after cataract surgery and IOL deposits in 30% of eyes, adequate control of inflammation, meticulous surgery, in-the-bag IOL implantation, and vigilant postoperative care help achieve a good visual outcome [24].

In Behçet's disease, the incidence of phthisis bulbi and hypotony in patients undergoing phacoemulsification has been reported to decrease from 25% to 2% when limited vitrectomy was performed in combination with cataract extraction [28]. It is not clear, however, whether vitrectomy combined with cataract extraction can alter the course of inflammation. Visual prognosis is significantly worse in eyes with Behçet's disease than in other types of uveitis because of the severe posterior segment complications, particularly optic atrophy [12].

Cataract extraction in patients with VKH syndrome can be safely and successfully performed if there is good preoperative and postoperative control of inflammation, careful surgical planning, and a meticulous surgical technique. The final visual outcome depends on the posterior segment complications of the syndrome [24].

Phacoemulsification and vitrectomy in multifocal chorioretinitis with panuveitis has little therapeutic benefit. When an IOL is implanted, a visual improvement of one or two lines can be expected, but visual acuity returns to preoperative values within 6 months. Multifocal chorioretinitis remains poorly understood in terms of its etiology and suitable treatment [10].

8.2.5 Preoperative Planning

As already described in this chapter, preoperative planning for complicated cataracts in uveitic patients focuses attention on the ocular examination in order to distinguish the characteristics and etiology of the disease, to assess the IOP, and to examine the vitreous and fundus. Differentiation between complicated or uncomplicated cases is according to the guidelines of the IOIS for preoperative preparation and enables selection of the best surgical technique.

The IOIS guidelines define complicated and uncomplicated cases as follows:

- Complicated patients are those in whom systemic or periocular therapy is necessary to maintain quiescent inflammation, or those in whom surgery is expected to be technically difficult.
- Uncomplicated patients are those in whom the uveitis is controlled with topical corticosteroids and in whom routine surgery is expected (Table 8.2).

8.2.6 Visual Prognosis

Visual prognosis depends on the preoperative control of inflammation and the status of the posterior pole. A minimum of 3 months of quiescence is necessary before surgery [7]. Topical, periocular, and systemic steroids and systemic immune suppressants can be used for this purpose. Etiologic diagnosis of the uveitis will be useful to determine if specific treatment can be provided. Overall, atraumatic surgery is the best anti-inflammatory. Proper management of inflammation can result in surprisingly good visual results. Potential acuity measurement (PAM) and laser interferometry may give a good estimate of the visual outcome [2]. Some authors suggest the use of color tests in the examination of patients in order to have a better idea of the posterior pole function [16].

Selection of an intraocular lens may influence visual prognosis. Intraocular lenses can be implanted in the majority of uveitic patients. Implantation of a foldable hydrophobic acrylic lens is favored by some to reduce complications [2]. The postoperative control of inflammation is extremely important in implanted patients, since the associated complications may be severe and may be a factor in a poor postoperative visual acuity. It is also important to remember that inflammation in juvenile chronic arthritis tends to worsen after cataract surgery [31]. In these patients, a careful decision regarding intraocular lens implantation must be made; otherwise the visual acuity may be suboptimal. In young children, cataract surgery will be of no value unless intensive treatment for amblyopia and correction of aphakia is performed immediately after the surgery.

Table 8.2 IOIS guidelines for patient preparation

	Guidelines
Complicated cases	Topical or periocular steroids 3 months before surgery
	NSAIDs in severe cases of inflammation
	Specific antibiotic when infective etiology is suspected
	Preoperatively: 2 days to 1 week before surgery, 1 mg/kg/day of oral prednisolone for 2 weeks plus prednisolone acetate 1% 1 drop 8 times per day and topical NSAIDs (flurbiprofen) 1 drop 4 times per day
Uncomplicated cases	Topical steroids as prescribed to maintain the inflammation as low as possible before surgery

Low-grade chronic inflammation can result in permanent damage to the optic nerve, retina, anterior chamber angle, and other structures that may preclude visual rehabilitation after cataract surgery. In the future, early surgical intervention prior to the development of permanent structural damage from inflammation or corticosteroid therapy may be shown to improve visual prognosis.

Take Home Pearls

- Prognosis depends on the control of the preoperative inflammation and the status of the posterior pole.
- Three months of quiescent inflammation is necessary before surgery.
- Intraocular lenses can be implanted in the majority of the uveitic patients.
- Iridocyclitis due to juvenile chronic arthritis tends to worsen after cataract surgery.

8.3 Surgical Planning

8.3.1 Patient Preparation

A customized approach must be established for each patient that takes into consideration the etiology of the uveitis and the cause of the vision loss, as well as the purpose of the surgery, whether to achieve vision improvement and/or to allow visualization of ocular structures. In order to avoid unrealistic expectations by the patient, it has to be established whether cataract is the main cause of vision loss or whether it is caused by optic nerve atrophy, vitreous opacification, or retinal damage. Anterior and posterior segment biomicroscopy as well as potential visual acuity measurement aid this assessment. Occasionally, B-scan examination and campimetry may be useful [43]. Similarly, the surgeon must consider whether associated surgery, such as glaucoma surgery or vitrectomy, should be performed concomitantly with phacoemulsification.

Two days to 1 week before surgery, the patient should receive a topical steroid (prednisolone acetate 1%), one drop eight times daily, and a topical NSAID such as flurbiprofen four times a day. All patients classified as complicated cases according to IOIS guidelines also receive 1 mg/kg/day of oral prednisone during the 2 weeks prior to surgery (see Sect. 8.3.1.1). Systemic steroids in children should not go beyond 3 months due to their possible side effects on growth. The use of oral NSAIDs is controversial as their efficacy as an anti-inflammatory drug is questionable in uveitis and may increase the risk of bleeding [26] (Table 8.2).

8.3.1.1 Algorithm Approach for Decision Making for Cataract in Uveitis (IOIS)

See page 92.

8.3.2 Surgical Procedure

Cataract surgery in uveitic eyes with inactive inflammation for several months can be performed similarly to that in nonuveitic eyes through a small corneal incision or via a scleral tunnel with phacoemulsification followed by the implantation of a foldable lens [32]. Good pupillary dilation is commonly difficult to achieve in uveitic eyes. Long-standing uveitis is often associated

Complicated Cases	Uncomplicated Cases
Systemic or periocular therapy needed prior to surgery Routine surgery is not anticipated	Uveitis controlled → topical steroids Routine surgery is anticipated

Topical or periocular steroids 3 months before surgery NSAIDs in severe cases of inflammation Specific antibiotics when an infective etiology (TB or syphilis) suspected High IOP associated with chronic use of topical steroids Control IOP 2–3 weeks prior to surgery	No surgery when > 10 cells per high magnification field detected in anterior chamber Only case that doesn´t need inflammatory control prior to surgery → **Phacogenic uveitis**
Uveitic glaucoma **Uveitis-related hypertension**	
Early NSAIDs + mydriatic + cycloplegic start to decrease the anterior & posterior synechiae, pupillary membrane, pupillary seclusion & damage to trabecular meshwork. (No cholinergic drugs or prostaglandin analogs) Preoperatively: 2 days to 1 week before surgery: 1 mg/kg/day of oral prednisolone for 2 weeks (in children systemic steroids should not go beyond 3 months) + prednisolone acetate 1% 1 drop 8 times per day and topical NSAIDs (flurbiprofen) 1 drop 4 times per day **A. Associated glaucoma:** Patient with 1 medication for glaucoma → medical treatment with drops prior to surgery Patient with 2 medications for glaucoma → combined surgery: filtering + phaco + mitomycin C → 0.02 mg/ml soaked sponge for 2 minutes Patient with 3 medications for glaucoma → combined surgery, but if it fails → Molteno implant In steroid-induced glaucoma → temporary immunosuppressive agents 2 weeks prior to surgery **B. Associated vitreous opacity:** Do a B-scan, PAM, campimetry or color test prior to surgery Perform combined surgery: pars plana vitrectomy + phaco or pars plana vitrectomy + lensectomy in cases of uveitis with vitreitis refractory to medical treatment. 25G → use for vitrectomy is recommended.	Phacoemulsification + IOL Prednisolone or dexamethasone 4 times per day immediately after surgery, tapering over the following 4–6 weeks
Fibrinoid reaction during or immediately after surgery → injection of 500–700 units of streptokinase or recombinant tissue plasminogen activator, 10–25 mg in anterior chamber Dexamethasone phosphate 400 mg into the anterior chamber is suggested Triamcinolone acetate injected into the vitreous chamber in combined phaco + pars plana vitrectomy. Heparin 5000 IU, 0.2 ml in 500 ml of Ringer's lactate infusion in anterior chamber is recommended	
Prednisolone or dexamethasone 4 times per day immediately after surgery tapering over the following 4–6 weeks + systemic steroids for 2 weeks with gradual tapering over 15 days In more severe cases → 1–1.5 mg/kg/day of prednisone + intensive topical steroid drops & tapered soon afterwards	

with extensive posterior synechiae and atrophy of the iris sphincter muscle.

Phacoemulsification is considered the procedure of choice in uveitic cataract surgery with better visual outcome and lower incidence of capsular opacification and postoperative inflammation than extracapsular cataract extraction. This has been attributed to smaller incision size, shorter surgical duration, and reduced surgical trauma [39].

Microincisional cataract surgery (MICS) is particularly advantageous in younger patients and patients taking high doses of corticosteroids [3]. Nuclear expression causing iris trauma is likely the most proinflammatory step in conventional extracapsular surgery [14]. Larger incision size is also significantly related to the degree of inflammation [5]. In microincisional surgery, the use of a clear corneal incision has several advantages over a scleral tunnel, such as the avoidance of postoperative hyphema, inadvertent filtering blebs, and need for cautery. This incision may be the best approach if no lens or foldable lens is implanted. If implantation of a rigid PMMA lens is planned, a limbal approach with a short scleral tunnel is preferred. Intracapsular surgery is reserved for those cases in which an important lens-induced inflammatory reaction occurred after surgery in the following eye.

Although many patients are young and surgery under general anesthesia is necessary, general anesthesia is not required for other patients, and regional anesthesia by retrobulbar or peribulbar block is preferred. Topical anesthesia is not contraindicated, but it may be risky and painful in cases in which extensive iris manipulation is expected.

8.3.3 Viscoelastics

Viscoelastic substances are commonly used to release adhesions and aid mydriasis. Dispersive viscoelastics combining hyaluronic acid and chondroitin sulfate are preferred, or a high viscosity expansive, cohesive product can be used.

More adherent posterior iris synechiae can be eliminated using an iris spatula with the viscoelastic material. In more severe cases, better mydriasis can be obtained using iris hooks placed in each quadrant through small corneal incisions, or by stretching maneuvers (Fig. 8.5) with surgical hooks under viscoelastic protection of the endothelium. In those cases in which the adherence cannot be removed or extends beyond the iris sphincter, two iridotomies can be performed at the 3 and 9 o'clock meridians. In extreme cases when the previous procedures are not successful, a superior sector iridec-

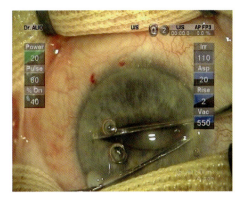

Fig. 8.5 Iris stretching maneuver in a patient with strong posterior synechiae

tomy can be performed. In some cases, a prophylactic peripheral iridectomy is recommended, as in cases of uveitis with a high tendency toward synechiae formation. Patients in whom a vitrectomy has been performed with removal of the posterior capsule do not require an iridectomy.

8.3.4 Capsulorhexis

After dilation, a capsulorhexis should be attempted. Continuous circular capsulorhexis may be difficult to perform due to the presence of secondary fibrosis of the anterior lenticular capsule. In these cases, the central part of the capsule may be cut using intraocular Vannas scissors, or a circular capsulotomy can be created using a vitrectomy probe.

Since many uveitic patients develop cataracts at an early age, the capsule is often more elastic than in older patients. This higher elasticity increases the risk of capsular rim tears. Hemorrhage during synechiolysis or capsulotomy can be dealt with by the injection of high-density viscoelastic and by raising the IOP.

The phacoemulsification procedure is accomplished by the most suitable technique for each case (Table 8.3), with chop techniques if the nucleus is very hard. The most common type of cataract is nuclear, although the lens nucleus is often relatively soft and the phacoemulsification can be easily performed [2]. Thorough cleaning of the cortex is needed to reduce the risk of postoperative inflammation and posterior capsule opacification (PCO). Cortical cleanup and aspiration of the posterior surface of the anterior capsule with low vacuum are advised in all cases. Lens epithelial cell contact with IOL will cause the cells to undergo a fibrous metaplasia and

Table 8.3 Phacoemulsification in cataract surgery (INFINITI Vision System, Alcon). Tip: microtip, 450, bottle height at 100 cm over patient's head

	Settings	
Soft cataract	Power	30% pulsed
	Vacuum	400 mmHg
	Aspiration	20 cc/min
	Burst	30 ms, on: 10, off: 30
Hard cataract	Power	100%
	Vacuum	65 mmHg
	Aspiration	20 cc/min
	Burst	30 ms, on: 5, off: 45
Fragment removal	Power	65%
	Vacuum	400 mmHg
	Aspiration	20 cc/min
	Burst	30 ms, on: 5, off: 45
Irrigation/ aspiration	Vacuum	400 mmHg
	Aspiration	30 cc/min

disrupt the BAB. Bimanual techniques give excellent results in anterior cortical cleaning.

8.3.5 Microincisional Cataract Surgery

Microincisional cataract surgery (MICS) [3] allows cataract surgery to be performed through an incision of 1.4 mm or less. A small incision correlates directly with a lower inflammatory rate postoperatively, making this technique less invasive and probably the best way to approach these patients. It seems likely that when the materials and biocompatibility of new IOLs have been improved, this will be the preferred technique. Two side-port incisions of 1.2 mm are performed at 90°. After phacoemulsification, a foldable, one-piece hydrophobic acrylic IOL is implanted into the capsular bag. Suturing the incision is advised.

8.3.6 Intraoperative Treatment

Intraocular dexamethasone phosphate (400 µg) may be instilled into the anterior chamber (intracameral) when the wound is closed [18]. Alternatively, triamcinolone acetate may be injected into the vitreous chamber at the end of combined cataract and posterior segment surgery [8]. Additionally, we use heparin 5,000 IU, 0.2 ml in 500 ml of Ringer's lactate infusion to reduce the appearance of fibrin in the anterior chamber. At the end of the surgery, an intraoperative antibiotic such as 0.1 cc of cefuroxime 1% can be injected.

8.3.7 Choice of Intraocular Lens

The decision of whether to implant an intraocular lens (IOL) in uveitic eyes remains controversial. The issues surrounding IOL placement in uveitic eyes after cataract extraction remain a key concern in the management of uveitis patients. Many features unique to a uveitic eye must be considered, such as different types of uveitis, preoperative inflammation and treatment, postoperative inflammation, and specific complications.

Presently, it seems that stringent perioperative and postoperative control of inflammation may help patients with uveitis to maintain high visual acuity over long-term follow-up [40]. There has been concern that inflammation associated with IOL implantation would increase surgical inflammation in compromised eyes. Chronic uveitis has long been considered a relative contraindication for the implantation of IOLs. The major risk factors associated with poor outcome after IOL implantation have been inflammation concentrated in the intermediate zone of the eye, such as pars planitis and panuveitis [25].

It has been shown that IOLs trigger a number of reactions, such as a foreign body inflammatory response and stimulation of the coagulation cascade. The activation of complement systems occurs through classic and alternative pathways. IOLs, especially those with prolene haptics in contact with metabolically active tissues, activate the alternative pathway [21]. There are materials such as hydrogel that do not cause any significant complement activation.

Sulcus or anterior chamber implantation are considered to be contraindicated. Several recent studies have suggested that the implantation of an IOL in the capsular bag does not increase the risk of postoperative inflammation in selected cases provided that proper antiinflammatory treatment is performed [18]. However, cellular and pigment deposits on the IOL surface (Fig. 8.6) or synechiae between the anterior surface of the IOL and the iris may develop. These lesions are often caused by a chronic latent inflammation, which may originate with the uveitis itself or be induced by the lens material. Pigment dispersion and deposition on the IOL surface seem to be multifactorial, related to surgical trauma, age of patient, and the pre-existing ocular pathology unrelated to IOL biocompatibility.

The selection of the proper type of IOL (material, design, diameter, and configuration) remains a challenge for the surgeon. The use of one-piece PMMA lenses may have some advantages in patients with uveitis as they do not activate the complement cascade, a phenomenon associated with polypropylene haptics. Surface-modified IOLs such as the heparin-coated models have been introduced and recommended for patients with uveitis as they decrease the number and severity of deposits on the surface of the IOL. Silicone lenses have induced a greater inflammatory reaction in non-uveitic patients compared with other IOL materials (PMMA, hydrogel, heparin-modified), with a higher incidence of early posterior capsule opacification, anterior chamber inflammation, and closure of the capsulorhexis. In a prospective, multinational, collaborative study sponsored by the IOIS [2], acrylic foldable lenses had a statistically significantly lower inflammatory reaction than silicone lenses within the first month after surgery, although at later visits the differences were no longer significant. Foldable acrylic showed lower inflammation than heparin surface-modified lenses in the first week after surgery, the differences disappearing later. The highest incidence of relapses has been described 1 and 6 months after surgery [2]. Both acrylic and heparin surface-modified IOLs showed the lowest incidence of relapses, while the highest was for silicone IOLs, although the differences were not significant. Posterior capsular opacification also seems to appear earlier with silicone lenses [2].

CME appeared more frequently in eyes implanted with silicone lenses than other materials, although it disappeared with adequate therapy. The deposition of pigment on the lens and pupillary membranes was higher for silicone lenses. There is also a higher incidence of small and giant cell deposition on the surface of silicone IOLs than on PMMA and acrylic lenses. Giant cells are always significant as they are a sign of foreign body reaction. Lens epithelial cells originating from the anterior capsule and migrating onto the IOL surface may cause anterior and posterior capsular opacification and phimosis of the capsulorhexis. Chapter 11 provides more information on the selection of intraocular lenses.

Take Home Pearls

- Phacoemulsification is the procedure of choice in uveitic cataract surgery.
- Microincision cataract surgery may be advantageous.
- The best anti-inflammatory is a good, atraumatic surgery.
- Clear cornea incisions are preferred over scleral tunnels.

8.4 Complications

Postoperative complications prevalent in uveitis patients are related to high IOP, corneal edema, endothelial damage, and fibrous membranes, which are described mostly in pars planitis patients [44]. Strict control of the postoperative inflammation is imperative to reduce these complications [44]. Perilenticular fibrotic membranes, described mostly in pars planitis patients, may be dense enough to resist rupture by Nd:YAG laser at high levels of energy and tend to reappear, at times associated with displacement of the lens and retinal detachment.

Decreased visual acuity is mainly caused by CME [16], epiretinal membranes [29], and glaucomatous optic nerve damage [34]. CME is the most serious, common postoperative complication in patients with chronic uveitis who undergo cataract extraction. This complication is detected in 19–35% of cases by angiography and is present in 80% of eyes with less than 20/40 postoperative visual acuity. CME can be treated with oral acetazolamide, topical NSAIDs, or topical, periocular, intravitreal, or systemic corticosteroids [8].

Posterior capsule opacification (PCO) is a form of postoperative inflammatory reaction. Its apparently higher frequency, up to 56% in the third year, seems to be related to the age of the patients [15].

Cataract surgery is regularly reported to induce exacerbation in different types of intraocular inflamma-

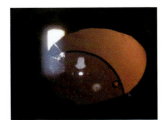

Fig. 8.6 Pigment deposits on IOL in a patient after surgery for uveitic cataract

tion. The highest incidences of relapses of inflammation appear at 1 and 6 months. A reactivation rate of 36% for ocular toxoplasmosis within 4 months of cataract surgery has been reported [7]. Prophylactic treatment with antiparasitic drugs may be considered for patients with ocular toxoplasmosis who are at risk of visual loss.

8.5 Postoperative Follow-up

Severe postoperative exacerbation of pre-existing inflammation (Fig. 8.7) should be expected. A strategy for eliminating postoperative inflammation is desirable. Topical corticosteroids are the standard of care during the immediate postoperative period to reduce ocular inflammation, prevent structural damage to the eye, and reduce patient discomfort [34]. The usual practice in uncomplicated cases is to prescribe prednisolone or dexamethasone four times daily starting immediately after surgery and then taper over the following 4–6 weeks. An acetate vehicle is the most appropriate due to its superior ocular penetration. Complicated cases may additionally receive systemic steroids started preoperatively and continuing for 2 weeks with gradual tapering over 15 days.

No strict guidelines are available for emergency cases. During the postoperative period, both topical and systemic steroids may be tapered based on the severity of ocular inflammation. In the most severe cases, moderate to high doses of oral prednisolone (1–1.5 mg/kg/day) and intensive topical corticosteroid drops should be given and tapered soon afterward.

Management may be more difficult in cases of corticosteroid-induced glaucoma, in which temporary immunosuppressive agents may be needed to control inflammation in the very early postoperative period. These drugs have to be administered prior to surgery because of variable latency periods before they become effective.

Most NSAIDs used today are cyclooxygenase inhibitors that decrease the formation of prostaglandins, which play a major role in ocular inflammation. Diclofenac drops have been shown to reduce inflammation after cataract surgery [26, 38].

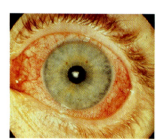

Fig. 8.7 Severe postsurgical inflammation after uveitic cataract extraction

Take Home Pearls

Topical steroids have become the standard care during the immediate postoperative period to reduce ocular inflammation.
- Uncomplicated cases: Prednisolone or dexamethasone four times daily immediately after surgery and tapering over the following 4–6 weeks
- Complicated cases: Additionally, systemic steroids started preoperatively and continuing for 2 weeks with gradual tapering over 15 days
- Most severe cases: Oral prednisolone, 1–1.5 mg/kg/day, plus intensive topical steroids tapered soon afterward.

References

1. Alio JL. Una nueva etapa en la cirugía de la catarata. Arch Soc Esp Oftalmología 2003; 78:65–66
2. Alio JL, Chipont E, BenEzza D, et al. Comparative performance of intraocular lenses in eyes with cataract and uveitis. J Cataract Refract Surg 2002; 28:2096–2108
3. Alio JL, Rodriguez-Prats JL, Galal A, editors. MICS. Panama: Highlights, 2004
4. Alio JL, Rodriguez-Prats JL, Galal A, Ramzy M. Outcomes of microincision cataract surgery versus coaxial phacoemulsification. Ophthalmology 2005; 12:1997–2003
5. Alio JL, Rodríguez-Prats JL, Galal A. Advances in microincision cataract surgery intraocular lenses. Curr Opin Ophthalmol 2006; 17:80–93
6. Amon M, Menapace R, Radax U, et al. In vivo study of cell reactions on poly(methyl methacrylate) intraocular lenses with different surface properties. J Cataract Refract Surg 1996; 22:825–829
7. Androudi S, Brazitikos P, Laccheri B, et al. Outcomes of early and late immunomodulatory treatment in patients with HLA-B27 associated chronic uveitis. Graefes Arch Clin Exp Ophthalmol 2003; 241:1000–1005
8. Androudi S, Ahmed M, Fiore T, et al. Combined pars plana vitrectomy and phacoemulsification to restore visual acuity in patients with chronic uveitis. J Cataract Refract Surg 2005; 31:472–478
9. Arellanes-García, Navarro-Lopez L, Recillas-Gispert C. Pars planitis in the Mexican Mestizo population: ocular findings, treatment, and visual outcome. Ocul Immunol Inflamm 2003; 11:53–60
10. Becker MD, Harsch N, Zierhut M, et al. Therapeutic vitrectomy in uveitis: current status and recommendations. Ophthalmologe 2003; 100:787–795

11. BenEzza D, Cohen E. Cataract surgery in children with chronic uveitis. Ophthalmology 2000; 107:1255–1260
12. Berker N, Soykan E, Elgin U, et al. Phacoemulsification cataract extraction and intraocular lens implantation in patients with Behcet´s disease. Ophthalmic Surg Lasers Imaging 2004; 35:215–218
13. Ceballos EM, Beck AD, Lynn MJ. Trabeculectomy with antiproliferative agents in uveitic glaucoma. J Glaucoma 2002; 11:189–196
14. Chee SP, Ti SE, Sivakumar M, et al. Postperative inflammation: extracapsular cataract extraction versus phacoemulsification. J Cataract Refract Surg 1999; 25:1280–1285
15. Dana MR, Chatzistefanou K, Schaumberg DA, et al. Posterior capsule opacification after cataract surgery in patients with uveitis. Ophthalmology 1997; 104:1387–1393; discussion 1393–1394
16. Durrani OM, Tehrani NN, Marr JE, et al. Degree, duration and causes of visual loss in uveitis. Br J Ophthalmol 2004; 88:1159–1162
17. Erol N. Tissue plasminogen activator in the management of anterior chamber fibrin formation. J Cataract Refract Surg 2004; 30:2254–2255
18. Foster CS, Opremcak EM. Therapeutic surgery: cornea, iris, cataract, glaucoma, vitreous, retinal. In: Foster CS, Vitale AT, editors. Diagnostic and treatment of uveitis. Philadelphia: Saunders, 2002
19. Foster CS, Rashid S. Management of coincident cataract and uveitis. Curr Opin Ophthalmol 2003; 14:1–6
20. Foster CS, Fong LP, Singh G. Cataract surgery and intraocular lens implantation in patients with uveitis. Ophthalmology 1989; 96:281–288
21. Foster CS, Stavrou P, Zafirakis P, et al. Intraocular lens removal from (corrected) patients with uveitis. Am J Ophthalmol 1999; 128:31–37
22. Foster RE, Lowder CY, Meisler DM, et al. Extracapsular cataract extraction and posterior chamber intraocular lens implantation in uveitis patients. Ophthalmology 1992; 99:1234–1241
23. Gabric N, Cupak K. Cataract surgery and uveitis. Acta Med 1991; 45:251–256
24. Gannesh SK, Babu K, Biswas J. Phacoemulsification with intraocular lens implantation in cases of pars planitis. J Cataract Refract Surg 2004; 30:2072–2076
25. Girard LJ, Rodriguez J, Mailman ML, et al. Cataract and uveitis management by pars plana lensectomy and vitrectomy by ultrasonic fragmentation. Retina 1985; 5:107–114
26. Herbort CP, Jauch A, Othemin-Girard P, et al. Diclofenac drops to treat inflammation after cataract surgery. Acta Ophthalmol Scand 2000; 78:421–424
27. Holland GN, Van Horn SD, Margolis TP. Cataract surgery with ciliary sulcus fixation of intraocular lenses in patients with uveitis. Am J Ophthalmol 1999; 128:21–30
28. Javadi MA, Jafarinasab MR, Araghi AA, et al. Outcomes of phacoemulsification and in-the-bag intraocular lens implantation in Fuchs´ heterochromic iridocyclitis. J Cataract Refract Surg 2005; 31:997–1001
29. Kaufman AH, Foster CS. Cataract extraction in patients with pars planitis. Ophthalmology 1993; 100:1210–1217
30. Koenig SB, Mieler WF, Han DP, et al. Combined phacoemulsification pars plana vitrectomy, and posterior chamber intraocular lens insertion. Arch Ophthalmol 1992; 110:1101–1104
31. Lam LA, Lowder CY, Baerveldt G, et al. Surgical management of cataracts in children with juvenile rheumatoid arthritis associated uveitis. Am J Ophthalmol 2003; 135:772–778
32. Laurell CG, Zetterstrom C, Philipson B, et al. Randomized study of the blood-aqueous barrier reaction after phacoemulsification and extracapsular cataract extraction. Acta Ophthalmol Scand 1998; 76:573–578
33. Lin CL, Wang AG, Chou JC, et al. Heparin-surface-modified intraocular lens implantation in patients with glaucoma, diabetes or uveitis. J Cataract Refract Surg 1994; 20:550–553
34. McColgin AZ, Heier JS. Control of intraocular inflammation associated with cataract surgery. Curr Opin Ophthalmol 2000; 11:3–6
35. Molteno AC, Sayawat N, Herbison P. Otago glaucoma surgery outcome study: long term results of uveitis with secondary glaucoma drained by Molteno implants. Ophthalmology 2001; 108:605–613
36. Moroi SE, Gottfredsdottir MS, Schteingart MT, et al. Cystoid macular edema associated with latanoprost therapy in a case series of patients with glaucoma and ocular hypertension. Ophthalmology 1999; 106:1024–1029
37. Okhravi N, Lightman SL, Towler HM. Assessment of visual outcome after cataract surgery in patients with uveitis. Ophthalmology 1999; 106:710–722
38. Othenin-Girard P, Tritten JJ, Pittet N, et al. Dexamethasone versus diclofenac sodium eyedrops to treat inflammation after cataract surgery. J Cataract Refract Surg 1994; 20:9–12
39. Pande MV, Spalton DJ, Kerr-Muir MG, et al. Postoperative inflammatory response to phacoemulsification and extracapsular cataract surgery: aqueous flare and cells. J Cataract Refract Surg 1996; 22:770–774
40. Rahman I, Jones NP. Long term results of cataract extraction with intraocular lens implantation in patients with uveitis. Eye 2005; 19:191–197
41. Rauz S, Stavrou P, Murray PL. Evaluation of foldable intraocular lenses in patients with uveitis. Ophthalmology 2000; 107:909–919
42. Schauersberger J, Kruger A, Abela C, et al. Course of 4 types of foldable intraocular lenses. J Cataract Refract Surg 1999; 25:1116–1120

43. Tabbara KF, Chavia PS. Cataract extraction in patients with chronic posterior uveitis. Int Ophthalmol Clin 1995; 35:121–131
44. Tessler HH, Farber MD. Intraocular lens implantation versus no intraocular lens implantation in patients with chronic iridocyclitis and pars planitis. A randomized prospective study. Ophthalmology 1993; 100:1206–1209
45. Yalvac IS, Sungur G, Turhan E, et al. Trabeculectomy with mitomycin-C in uveitic glaucoma associated with Behçet disease. J Glaucoma 2004; 13:450–453
46. Yaylali V, Ozbay D, Tatlipinar S, et al. Efficacy and safety of rimexolone 1% versus prednisolone acetate 1% in the control of postoperative inflammation following phacoemulsification cataract surgery. Int Ophthalmol 2004; 25:65–68

Perioperative Medical Management

Manfred Zierhut, Peter Szurman

Core Messages

- Preoperatively, risk factors should be analyzed, for example, type of uveitis, course of inflammation, basic diagnostic workup and complications like cystoid macular edema.
- At the time of surgery, the eye should have been completely quiet for approximately 2–3 months.
- Preoperative prophylaxis includes maintenance therapy, under which the eye remains quiet until surgery, and additional anti-inflammatory treatment beginning approximately 1–2 weeks prior to surgery, systemic or topical corticosteroids.
- Intraoperatively, intravenous methylprednisolone or intravitreal triamcinolone acetonide can be very effective in high-risk patients in preventing postoperative complications.
- Postoperative treatment should include systemic and topical corticosteroids, depending on the preoperative and intraoperative situation.

Contents

9.1	Preoperative Considerations	99	9.5	Postoperative Management	101
9.2	Timing of Surgery	99	9.6	Summary	101
9.3	Preoperative Prophylaxis	100	References		101
9.4	Intraoperative Management	100			

9.1 Preoperative Considerations

Cataract formation is a common sight-impairing complication of uveitis, occurring in up to 50% of patients depending on the type of uveitis. Cataract surgery is more complex than in nonuveitic patients and has a considerable potential for an unfavourable postoperative course. Remarkable progress has been made recently, but some general considerations should be reviewed regarding patient selection and thorough perioperative monitoring. The first step is the accurate classification of the disease entity, as a specific diagnosis will often guide the surgical strategy and determine the prognosis of cataract surgery. A standardized questionnaire is recommended for a comprehensive ocular and systemic history. This includes patient characteristics, the location of uveitis, and course and onset of intraocular inflammation. Diagnostic examinations should include an updated chest X-ray to disclose tuberculosis and sarcoidosis, Lyme disease serology, angiotensin converting enzyme and basic laboratory investigations. Thorough ophthalmic evaluation is essential to identify simultaneous ocular pathology that may also be causative for visual impairment and limit postoperative visual rehabilitation. Concomitant cystoid macular edema (CME) or glaucoma should be treated preoperatively before proceeding with cataract surgery [13]. This is even more important in cases of ocular toxoplasmosis, as cataract surgery has shown to cause exacerbation in this specific subset of patients [1].

9.2 Timing of Surgery

There is general agreement about achieving complete quiescence of intraocular inflammation for at least 2–3 months before proceeding with surgery [3]. This is usually interpreted as absence of cells in the anterior chamber, less than 2+ vitreous cells and no active chorioretinal inflammation. Patients suffering from Fuchs heterochromic cyclitis in particular will frequently fail to achieve complete quiescence even after maximal anti-inflammatory therapy, yet those patients rarely develop severe postoperative complications [12]. In contrast, other types of uveitis may respond aggressively with recurrent postoperative inflammation even with previously well-controlled disease, for example, Behçet's disease (BD), sarcoidosis and juvenile idiopathic arthritis (JIA) associated uveitis. This is due to a subclinical chronic inflammation that persists even if the eye seems to be quiescent. The history of the disease may help to evaluate the risk for an unfavourable postoperative course. It has been shown for BD that it is significantly related to the frequency of ocular attacks during the year preceding the surgery [8]. Clinical parameters may further insinuate a subclinically persistent inflammation, for example, preoperative hypotony, vitreous cells and choroidal swelling. In these cases with unfavourable prognostic factors, it has been recommended to postpone surgery until after the period of at least half a year with no ocular attacks [8].

Besides respecting a quiescent interval, supplementary anti-inflammatory treatment has been advocated by most authorities. The improved visual prognosis after cataract surgery in uveitis eyes in recent years seems to be related to the more consistent use of perioperative anti-inflammatory and immunosuppressive treatment regimens.

9.3 Preoperative Prophylaxis

The ideal preoperative prophylaxis has not been conclusively defined as yet. While some authors consider a topical prophylaxis with corticosteroid eyedrops as sufficient in most cases, other studies generally recommend systemic immunosuppression to ensure quiescence. In principle, the preoperative prophylaxis is based on three strategies.

First, the maintenance therapy has to be optimized. In cases where inflammation responds insufficiently to low-dose corticosteroid therapy, immunosuppressive treatment has to be considered or adjusted according to the course and severity of uveitis. One should take into account that most immunosuppressive drugs need several months to achieve sufficient effects. Second, after having optimized the maintenance therapy, an additional anti-inflammatory prophylaxis with topical corticosteroid eyedrops, prednisolone acetate 1% five times daily, is started 1 (and up to 2) weeks prior to surgery. Alternatively, some authors recommend dexamethasone phosphate 0.1%, but the use of phosphate-containing eyedrops could be criticized in view of potentially inducing band keratopathy.

Finally, additional systemic corticosteroid prophylaxis using prednisolone 1 mg/kg approximately 1 week prior surgery is recommended by many authors, although the prophylactic value is still under debate. Other authorities consider topical prophylaxis to be sufficient in most patients and use preoperative oral corticosteroids only in selected cases with previous or current CME, with intermediate or posterior uveitis or with known attacks of severe inflammation after previous intraocular surgery [4]. Recent studies, however, have shown that administration of preoperative oral corticosteroids results in a higher proportion of patients with a visual acuity of 20/40 or better at 3 months [10]. Alternatively, an intravenous pulse therapy using methylprednisolone or prednisolone succinate 3–5 mg/kg the day before surgery has been proposed. In contrast, non-steroidal anti-inflammatory drugs (NSAIDs) have been less favoured in recent years. Topically applied NSAID eyedrops have little effect on inflammation, while the systemic application might increase risk of intraoperative bleeding [4].

9.4 Intraoperative Management

Minimizing damage of the blood–aqueous barrier (BAB) in uveitis patients is achievable through the use of modern surgical techniques and biocompatible implants. However, uveitis patients are at higher risk for early postoperative complications like fibrin formation, synechiae and CME. Therefore, a sub-Tenon injection of dexamethasone 4 mg should be applied at the end of surgery. In high-risk patients with a history of frequent intraocular inflammation and recurrent development of CME, intravenous methylprednisolone 250 mg may be injected additionally. Alternatively, intravitreal triamcinolone acetonide 4 mg has been proposed. In a recent study, it was shown that a single injection of triamcinolone acetonide into the anterior chamber during cataract surgery was an effective prophylaxis against fibrin formation after cataract surgery in patients with juvenile idiopathic arthritis-associated uveitis. They found less fibrin formation, CME and hypotony compared to patients who received a short-term systemic steroid treatment postoperatively [7].

Another study advocates the use of heparin-sodium 10 IU/ml as an adjunct in the irrigation solution. The authors found a lower inflammatory reaction in the early postoperative period without increasing the risk of intraoperative bleeding [6].

9.5 Postoperative Management

Postoperatively, the first 3 months are most critical and notably determine the long-term outcome. It has been shown that the BAB may be compromised for several months even after uncomplicated cataract surgery in nonuveitic patients [11]. Uveitic patients are more susceptible to developing complications due to the combination of pre-existing and surgically induced breakdown of the BAB. Hence, high-dose anti-inflammatory treatment is especially important to maintain intraocular quiescence during the critical period by slowly tapering the perioperative treatment for up to 3 months [2]. Oral corticosteroids have been proven to effectively reduce the postoperative BAB damage. In most situations, the postoperative treatment of intraocular surgery of uveitic patients is handled like a recurrence, that is, treated with 1 mg/kg/day of prednisolone, and reduced by 10 mg/week, finally resulting in an individual maintenance dosage.

Meacock and colleagues found that perioperative long-term treatment (prednisolone 0.5 mg/kg/day, starting 2 weeks before surgery, reduced by 5 mg/week) was more effective than a single dose of methylprednisolone 15 mg/kg/h before surgery. However, no beneficial effect on CME incidence could be shown [9].

Postoperatively, oral corticosteroids are tapered off over a period of 8–10 weeks. The dosage depends on the severity and type of uveitis, underlying complications and the individual surgical trauma. In most cases, prednisolone 1 mg/kg/day might be a suitable dose that is reduced by 10 mg/week, finally resulting in an individual maintenance dosage.

Topical corticosteroid therapy may be reduced earlier but should be continued at a low-dose level, as this acts as an effective prophylaxis against intraocular lens deposits. One should bear in mind that visually significant giant cell deposits frequently recur as soon as corticosteroids are tapered off. Therefore, long-term maintenance of low-dose topical corticosteroids may be required. A suitable topical treatment regimen might be to start with prednisolone acetate eyedrops every 2 h, then continue five times daily for 2 weeks and taper it as required to finally achieve a maintenance dose of once a day. In patients with postoperative fibrin formation, prednisolone acetate eyedrops are given hourly, and sub-Tenon corticosteroids are injected. In cases of a persistent fibrin membrane (> 3 days), a single intracameral injection of recombinant tissue plasminogen activator (10 µg) has shown to be effective [5].

Finally, one should bear in mind that these patients are under long-term immunosuppressive treatment and consequently may have a higher risk of postsurgical bacterial infections. Therefore, a meticulous topical postoperative antibiotic prophylaxis must be considered. We found it very helpful to continue treatment with topical broad-spectrum antibiotics as long as higher dosages of topical steroids were applied.

9.6 Summary

With improvement in microsurgical techniques, biocompatible implants and consequent perioperative medical management, a successful and lasting visual recovery after cataract surgery can be achieved in most uveitic patients. Unclear at the moment is the optimal systemic steroid regimen and the role of intravitreal steroid application intraoperatively. Following preoperative precautions will lead to a high level of safety regarding postoperative inflammation.

References

1. Bosch-Driessen LH, Plaisier MB, Stilma JS, van der Lelij A, Rothova A. Reactivation of ocular toxoplasmosis after cataract extraction. Ophthalmology 2002; 109: 41–45
2. Estafanous MFG, Lowder CY, Meisler DM, Chauhan R. Phacoemulsification cataract extraction and posterior chamber lens implantation in patients with uveitis. Am J Ophthalmol 2001; 131: 620–625
3. Foster CS, Rashid S. Management of coincident cataract and uveitis. Curr Opin Ophthalmol 2003; 14: 1–6
4. Heiligenhaus A, Heinz C, Becker M. The treatment of uveitis cataract. In: Kohnen T, Koch D, editors. Cataract and Refractive Surgery. Berlin: Springer; 2005, pp. 133–152
5. Klais CM, Hattenbach LO, Steinkamp GW, Zubcov AA, Kohnen T. Intraocular recombinant tissue-plasminogen activator fibrinolysis of fibrin formation after cataract surgery in children. J Cataract Refract Surg 1999; 25: 357–362
6. Kohnen T, Dick B, Hessemer V, Koch DD, Jacobi KW. Effect of heparin in irrigating solution on inflammation following small incision cataract surgery. J Cataract Refract Surg 1998; 24: 237–243
7. Li J, Heinz C, Zurek-Imhoff B, Heiligenhaus A. Intraoperative intraocular triamcinolone injection prophylaxis for post-cataract surgery fibrin formation in uveitis associated with juvenile idiopathic arthritis. J Cataract Refract Surg 2006; 32: 1535–1539
8. Matsuo T, Takahashi M, Inoue Y, Egi K, Kuwata Y, Yamaoka A. Ocular attacks after phacoemulsification and intraocular lens implantation in patients with Behcet's disease. Ophthalmologica 2001; 215: 179–182

9. Meacock WR, Spalton DJ, Bender L, Antcliff R, Heatley C, Stanford MR, Graham EM. Steroid prophylaxis in eyes with uveitis undergoing phacoemulsification. Br J Ophthalmol 2004; 88: 1122–1124
10. Okhravi N, Lightman SL, Towler HM. Assessment of visual outcome after cataract surgery in patients with uveitis. Ophthalmology 1999; 106; 710–722
11. Sanders DR, Kraff MC, Lieberman HL, Peyman GA, Tarabishy S. Breakdown and reestablishment of blood-aqueous barrier with implant surgery. Arch Ophthalmol 1982; 100: 588–590
12. Scheilian M, Karimean F, Javadi MA, et al. Surgical management of cataract and posterior chamber intraocular lens implantation in Fuchs' heterochromic iridocyclitis. Int Ophthalmol 1997; 21: 137–141
13. Tabbara K, Chavis P. Cataract extraction in patients with chronic posterior uveitis. Int Ophthalmol Clin 1995; 35: 121–131

Lens / Chapter 10

Pars Plana Lensectomy

Emilio Dodds

Core Messages

- Pars plana vitrectomy and lensectomy (PPV-PPL) is an alternative to phacoemulsification and intraocular lens placement in some cases of uveitic cataract.
- Severe, persistent, or recurrent uveitis, especially with multiple uveitic complications and poor inflammatory control, is the usual indication for PPV-PPL.
- Visual rehabilitation with contact lenses or spectacles is possible, and improvement in visual acuity is expected in patients with visually significant cataracts.
- PPV-PPL can also be considered in eyes at risk for future complications, such as untreatable posterior capsular opacification in silicone-filled eyes.
- Retention of the anterior capsule can be considered if eventual implantation of a posterior chamber lens is anticipated.

Contents

10.1	Introduction	103	10.5	Proposed Technique 106
10.2	Cataract in Chronic and Recurrent Uveitis	103	10.6	Retinal Detachment in Viral Retinitis ... 107
			10.7	Surgical Technique in Retinal Detachment and Viral Retinitis 108
10.3	Cataract and Juvenile Idiopathic Arthritis-Associated Uveitis	105	References	108
10.4	Surgical Technique in Cataract Associated with Chronic and Recurrent Uveitis	106		

This chapter contains the following video clips on DVD: Video 5 and 6 show Pars plana lensectomy posterior approach (Surgeon: Marc de Smet) and Pars plana lensectomy anterior approach (Surgeon: Emilio Dodds).

10.1 Introduction

In patients with chronic and recurrent uveitis, cataract extraction may exacerbate inflammation not only by the effect of the surgical procedure itself, but also by inducing a reactivation of the underlying disease. In these special uveitis cases, if we perform lens extraction alone without vitrectomy, vision may be only temporarily improved, because complications may arise due to persistent inflammation and recurrences of the inflammatory condition. A complete lensectomy and vitrectomy can be the best option in some of these cases.

Another situation where we may choose pars plana lensectomy and vitrectomy as a surgical option is in those patients that require a retinal repair and a long-term tamponade with silicone oil. Good examples of this situation are seen in cases of viral retinitis such as cytomegalovirus (CMV) retinitis and acute retinal necrosis syndrome.

10.2 Cataract in Chronic and Recurrent Uveitis

Phacoemulsification can be safely performed in many cases of uveitis with well-controlled inflammation, but there are some patients in which a complete control of the inflammatory process is not possible or recurrences may appear despite aggressive systemic and local therapy.

Prior inflammatory damage to the eye may also be an impediment to performance of a phacoemulsification and placement of an intraocular lens (IOL). The best example of this situation is seen in patients with chronic uveitis like juvenile idiopathic arthritis (JIA), chronic anterior uveitis secondary to Vogt-Koyanagi-Harada (VKH) syndrome, patients with severe intermediate uveitis, and other chronic uveitides. In those cases there is still an indication for pars plana lensectomy and vitrectomy to restore vision (Figs. 10.1 and 10.2a,b). Cataract surgery in eyes with chronic uveitis entails the risk of the inflammatory process worsening, with secondary formation of pupillary membranes, glaucoma, and phthisis bulbi [1] (Fig. 10.3a,b).

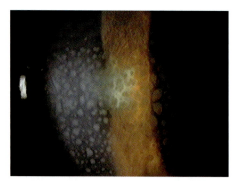

Fig. 10.1 Patient with chronic active uveitis, posterior synechiae, and cataract due to VKH. A good candidate for a combined lensectomy and vitrectomy

The use of a combined procedure with vitrectomy and lensectomy appears to have a favorable influence on the result of surgery and on the course of the inflammatory process. This technique has been described by Diamond and Kaplan, who attributed their success to the combined surgical technique itself plus the minimal amount of inflammation present in the eyes at the time of surgery after aggressive anti-inflammatory therapy. All cases that they presented had a considerable improvement in visual acuity due to removal of the cataractous lens that contributed to the visual impairment. Lensectomy/vitrectomy was performed in 25 eyes with complicated cataract and with vitreous opacities associated with uveitis. Visual acuity improved two or more lines in 24 of 25 operated eyes with a follow-up of 15 months. The effect of this therapy on the course of recurrent uveitis remains to be determined; however the authors noted a decrease in the severity of recurrent episodes in the operated eyes [2, 3]. Later Girard et al. reported on 23 consecutive eyes with chronic uveitis that also underwent a combined surgery of vitrectomy and lensectomy. The visual acuity improved in 91.3% of the eyes, and remission of the uveitis was noted in 100% of the patients with an average follow-up of 5 years. Similar results have been described by other authors with a number of patients ranging from 12 to 39 [4–7].

Pars plana lensectomy and vitrectomy appears to be the best approach to complicated cataracts with vitreous involvement because it allows a complete removal of not only the lens material but also the anterior vitreous that constitutes a scaffold along which a cyclitic membrane can develop. After this procedure, a group of patients

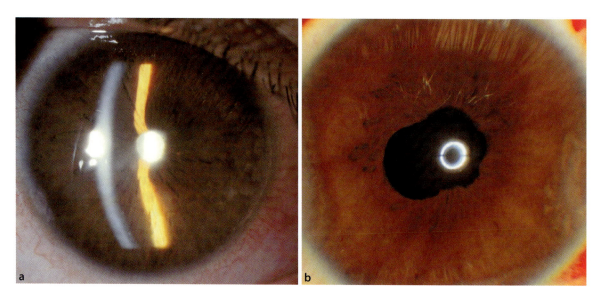

Fig. 10.2 a Patient with chronic uveitis and cataract due to JIA. b A lensectomy–vitrectomy procedure was performed

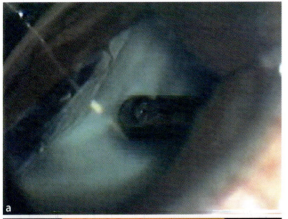

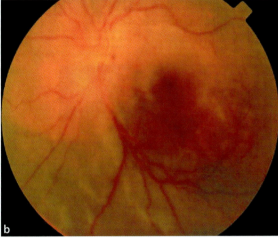

Fig. 10.3 **a** Patient with JIA with a fibrotic membrane covering the pars plana and ciliary body. **b** Patient with JIA with hypotony showing blurred disc margins and chorioretinal folds around the macula and tortuosity of the retinal vessels

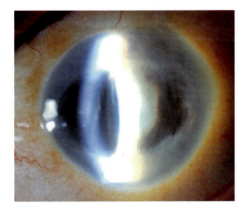

Fig. 10.4 Patient with JIA that underwent cataract surgery with IOL and ended up with phthisis bulbi

reported by Flynn et al. did not develop transpupillary or cyclitic membranes, and subjectively appear to have less inflamed eyes postoperatively [8]. Other potential advantages are that this procedure allows removal of the inflammatory debris in the vitreous to provide a clear visual access, and it also allows a better surgical access for removal of peripheral lens material in the presence of small pupils and posterior synechiae [8].

An intermediate option between phacoemulsification and pars plana lensectomy/vitrectomy in these patients with a chronic uveitis and a pathologic vitreous is to combine pars plana vitrectomy and phacoemulsification. A study was done in 36 eyes where 24 eyes had an IOL implanted while 12 were left aphakic. With this technique, visual acuity improved in 72.2% of the eyes [9].

10.3 Cataract and Juvenile Idiopathic Arthritis-Associated Uveitis

One particular situation concerning chronic uveitis and cataract arises in those patients with juvenile idiopathic arthritis. Cataract occurs in 40–60% of patients with juvenile idiopathic arthritis associated uveitis, which can be attributed not only to chronic inflammation but to corticosteroid use as well [10]. Intraocular lens implantation in those patients is controversial because several complications have been reported, including posterior synechiae, retrolental membranes, chronic inflammation, glaucoma, hypotony, phthisis, and macular edema. Most of the time, placement of intraocular lenses in these patients is contraindicated [11, 12] (Fig. 10.4).

Kanski operated on 187 eyes with lensectomy and partial vitrectomy and reported several complications, such as lens fragments dislodged into the vitreous, secondary glaucoma in 15% of the eyes, phthisis bulbi in 8%, and secondary pupillary membranes in 6% of the eyes [13]. Despite these complications, visual acuity improved in 77% of the cases, but a long-lasting cessation of uveitis was noted only in 2% of the patients [13].

Modern phacoemulsification techniques may have altered the risk–benefit ratio. Estefanous et al. showed that cataract extraction by phacoemulsification is an acceptable option for many patients with cataract and uveitis, with fewer postoperative complications due to the lesser amount of inflammation compared to extracapsular cataract extraction. Best corrected visual acuity improved in 95% of the eyes in their series [14]. When it is possible to completely control the inflammatory process in uveitic eyes, phacoemulsification and implantation of an IOL in the posterior chamber is safe, effective, and well tolerated according to another study done by Akova

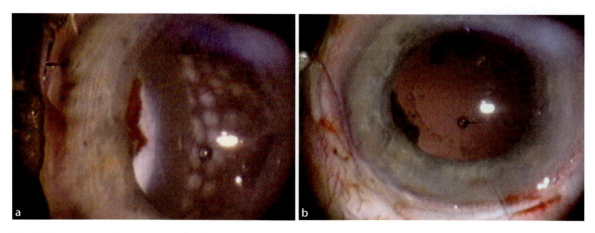

Fig. 10.5 **a** Patient with pars planitis that had a complete vitrectomy with scleral depression to remove the vitreous base. **b** Peripheral laser and lensectomy with a ring of anterior capsule left in place

et al. in 37 eyes with different types of uveitis [15]. Even in patients with juvenile idiopathic arthritis, favorable results have been reported in eight patients after phacoemulsification and posterior chamber IOL implantation by Probst and Holland, and later in five patients by Lam et al. [16, 17]. They propose that adequate long-term preoperative and postoperative control of intraocular inflammation with immunosuppressive therapy in addition to intensive topical corticosteroids is the clue to the surgical success in these patients [17].

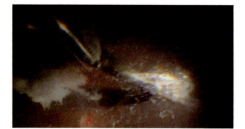

Fig. 10.6 Removal of the posterior hyaloid stained with triamcinolone

10.4 Surgical Technique in Cataract Associated with Chronic and Recurrent Uveitis

The lensectomy–vitrectomy technique reported in the literature was not the same for every patient. Diamond and Kaplan utilized a pars plana approach to completely remove the lens and capsule, and a subtotal vitrectomy was performed (central core to midperiphery) to specifically avoid the vitreous base and iris. Intravitreal dexamethasone (400 µg) was injected at the end of the procedure [2].

Girard et al. proposed the utilization of two needles, an aspirating needle and a fragmenting/aspirating needle. Both were inserted through sclerotomies at 3 mm from the limbus and into the lens in the anterior cortex. The lens was removed, and the anterior capsule was maintained with a central capsulectomy performed in order to allow a posterior chamber lens insertion at a later time [18]. Nobe et al. felt that a more complete vitrectomy was important to avoid residual vitreous opacities and recommended a pars plana approach [6].

10.5 Proposed Technique

A complete vitrectomy should include a pars plana approach to perform a central vitrectomy followed by scleral depression to remove the vitreous base, making sure that the posterior hyaloid is removed either by direct visualization or by staining the vitreous with intraocular triamcinolone (Figs. 10.5a,b and 10.6). The lens can be removed by inserting an MVR blade through the pars plana port toward the equator of the lens to allow the insertion of the vitreous cutter and remove the lens with either aspiration alone, aspiration and cut, or, if it is too hard, by utilizing the phacoemulsification tip without the sleeve and without irrigation through the same port (Figs. 10.7 and 10.8). If we can anticipate that an IOL can be inserted in the future, the anterior capsule can be maintained, and to avoid capsule opacification, a central capsulotomy can be performed, leaving an anterior capsule ring wide enough to support an IOL placed in the posterior chamber in a second procedure if possible (Fig. 10.9).

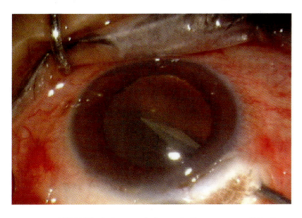

Fig. 10.7 MVR blade inserted through the equator of the lens

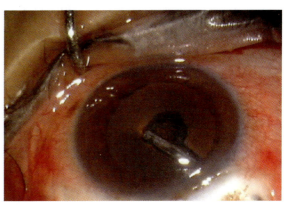

Fig. 10.8 Aspirating the lens with the vitreous cutter

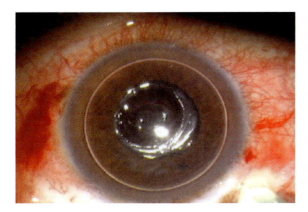

Fig. 10.9 Anterior capsule left in place for future placement of an IOL

10.6 Retinal Detachment in Viral Retinitis

Patients that require a retinal repair and a long-term silicone oil tamponade are another indication for pars plana lensectomy and vitrectomy. Good examples of this situation are seen in cases of viral retinitis, such as cytomegalovirus (CMV) retinitis, and acute retinal necrosis syndrome.

CMV retinitis is still the most common opportunistic ocular infection in patients with acquired immune deficiency syndrome, despite therapy with highly active antiretroviral therapy (HAART), because there are some patients who do not respond or cannot tolerate this therapy [19]. Retinal detachment is a well-known complication of CMV retinitis. It has been reported to occur in 33% of the eyes by 1 year after the diagnosis of the CMV retinitis [20]. Repair of these retinal detachments without the use of silicone oil was associated with high rates of redetachment. The use of silicone oil in patients with retinal detachment secondary to cytomegalovirus retinitis is associated with a high anatomical success rate [21]. Development of cataract, however, is a predictable complication in eyes that are filled with silicone oil after retinal detachment surgery, including eyes with CMV retinitis [22]. In one study, 67% of the eyes with retinal detachment due to CMV retinitis repaired with silicone oil develop a cataract in a median time of 18 months compared to 16% of the patients in the control group without surgery with silicone oil [23]. Azen et al. reported the proportion of eyes with cataract at 6 months after surgery with silicone oil tamponade was 64% among eyes with CMV retinitis and 63% in eyes without CMV retinitis, suggesting that silicone oil is the main cause of the development of cataract and not the underlying disease [24].

There are several complications that compromise the visual prognosis of these patients even after cataract surgery is performed. The final visual acuity was worse in almost all eyes after cataract surgery in one study due to complications such as redetachment, progression of retinitis, and posterior capsule opacification, a complication difficult to solve even with Nd:YAG laser capsulotomy, because the oil tamponade tends to cause adherence of the opacified capsule fragments to the posterior surface of the IOL [23].

In the era of HAART therapy, patients with AIDS have a longer life expectancy, and it is desirable to use methods to repair retinal detachments in patients with CMV retinitis that allow a better visual outcome [25]. Removal of silicone oil after repairing the detachment is an option that has been proposed in the literature with good results after 6 months in a small series of two patients [26]. According to other series, the cataractogenesis is likely to already have begun before silicone can be removed. Casswell et al. showed that 60% of the lenses that were clear at the time of oil removal developed clinically significant cataract anyway [27]. The other problem is that removal of silicone oil entails the risk of having the retina redetach. Morrison and co-workers showed that 53% of the patients redetached after a median of 4 months following oil removal and that cataract surgery performed at the time of oil removal was a statistically significant risk factor for redetachment [28]. Engstrom et al. reported favorable results with clear lens extraction by phacoemulsification with IOL placement at the time of retinal detachment repair with silicone oil tamponade. With this approach, the problem of posterior capsule opacification is still unsolved [29].

After reviewing all this issues, a good option in these cases is to perform a pars plana lensectomy at the time of retinal detachment repair. In this way, and since the expectancy of life is longer after HAART therapy for patients with AIDS, the development of a cataract and the need of another surgery to restore vision is not necessary in the short term. Visual rehabilitation can be done with either contact lenses or spectacles right after the surgical procedure is performed if the potential visual acuity is good enough. When silicone oil fills the entire vitreous cavity of the aphakic eye, the refractive correction can be expected to change by 5–9 diopters and sometimes as much as 14 diopters. Aphakic eyes become less hyperopic when filled with silicone oil. High myopia, incomplete silicone oil filling, and several other factors influence the final optical outcome [30].

10.7 Surgical Technique in Retinal Detachment and Viral Retinitis

A three-port pars plana approach is utilized to repair the retinal detachment. The lens can be removed through the pars plana as stated above for patients with chronic uveitis. A good option is to leave peripheral remnants of the anterior capsule, a capsule ring, to be able to easily place an IOL in the future. This is an option to consider after several months, only if it is possible to remove the silicone oil based on the retinal status, namely, whether it is stably attached or not. Since these eyes are going to be filled with silicone oil, an inferior iridectomy is necessary to prevent the oil from moving into the anterior chamber and contacting the corneal endothelium. It is important to make sure that the capsular remnants at 6 o'clock are also perforated to avoid blockage of the inferior iridectomy [31]. If the inferior iridectomy/capsulotomy is patent the silicone oil will be maintained in the vitreous cavity (Fig. 10.10). MacCumber and colleagues prefer to leave the entire anterior capsule, avoiding the inferior iridectomy [32]. If the visual outcomes improve with better surgical techniques, more eyes with complex retinal detachments will be candidates for secondary intraocular lens placement. Posterior chamber IOLs have fewer complications than anterior chamber IOLs or sulcus fixated lenses [33].

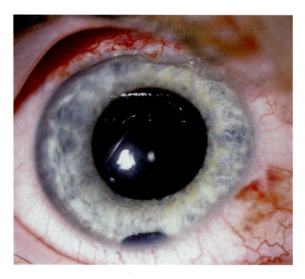

Fig. 10.10 Lensectomy and vitrectomy, inferior iridectomy, and anterior capsule ring behind the iris

The same technique can be applied to patients with acute retinal necrosis syndrome, where a long-acting tamponade is necessary to stabilize the necrotic retina that is associated with a high incidence of proliferative vitreoretinopathy [34, 35].

References

1. Hooper, P. L., N. A. Rao, et al. Cataract extraction in uveitis patients. Surv Ophthalmol 1990; 35: 120–44
2. Diamond, J. G. and H. J. Kaplan. Lensectomy and vitrectomy for complicated cataract secondary to uveitis. Arch Ophthalmol 1978; 96: 1798–1804
3. Diamond, J. G. and H. J. Kaplan. Uveitis: effect of vitrectomy combined with lensectomy. Ophthalmology 1979; 86: 1320–9
4. Girard, L. J., J. Rodriguez, et al. Cataract and uveitis management by pars plana lensectomy and vitrectomy by ultrasonic fragmentation. Retina 1985; 5: 107–14
5. Nolthenius, P. A. and A. F. Deutman. Surgical treatment of the complications of chronic uveitis. Ophthalmologica 1983; 186: 11–6

6. Nobe, J. R., N. Kokoris, et al. Lensectomy-vitrectomy in chronic uveitis. Retina 1983; 3: 71–6
7. Petrilli, A. M., R. Belfort, Jr., et al. Ultrasonic fragmentation of cataract in uveitis. Retina 1986; 6: 61–5
8. Flynn, H. W., Jr., J. L. Davis, et al. Pars plana lensectomy and vitrectomy for complicated cataracts in juvenile rheumatoid arthritis. Ophthalmology 1988; 95: 1114–9
9. Androudi, S., M. Ahmed, et al. Combined pars plana vitrectomy and phacoemulsification to restore visual acuity in patients with chronic uveitis. J Cataract Refract Surg 2005; 31: 472–8
10. Hooper, P. L., N. A. Rao, et al. Cataract extraction in uveitis patients. Surv Ophthalmol 1990; 35: 120–44
11. Foster, C. S., L. P. Fong, et al. Cataract surgery and intraocular lens implantation in patients with uveitis. Ophthalmology 1989; 96: 281–8
12. Kanski, J. J. and G. A. Shun-Shin. Systemic uveitis syndromes in childhood: an analysis of 340 cases. Ophthalmology 1984; 91: 1247–52
13. Kanski, J. J. Lensectomy for complicated cataract in juvenile chronic iridocyclitis. Br J Ophthalmol 1992; 76: 72–5
14. Estafanous M. F. G., C. Y. Lowder, D. M. Meisler, R. Chauhan. Phacoemulsification cataract extraction and posterior chamber lens implantation in patients with uveitis. Am J Ophthalmol 2001; 131: 620–625
15. Akova, Y. A., C. Kucukerdonmez, et al. Clinical results of phacoemulsification in patients with uveitis. Ophthalmic Surg Lasers Imaging 2006; 37: 204–11
16. Probst, L. E. and E. J. Holland. Intraocular lens implantation in patients with juvenile rheumatoid arthritis. Am J Ophthalmol 1996; 122: 161–70
17. Lam, L. A., C. Y. Lowder, et al. Surgical management of cataracts in children with juvenile rheumatoid arthritis-associated uveitis. Am J Ophthalmol 2003; 135: 772–8
18. Girard, L. J., J. Rodriguez, et al. Cataract and uveitis management by pars plana lensectomy and vitrectomy by ultrasonic fragmentation. Retina 1985; 5: 107–14
19. Jabs, D. A., M. L. Van Natta, et al. Characteristics of patients with cytomegalovirus retinitis in the era of highly active antiretroviral therapy. Am J Ophthalmol 2002; 133: 48–61
20. Kempen, J. H., D. A. Jabs, et al. Retinal detachment risk in cytomegalovirus retinitis related to the acquired immunodeficiency syndrome. Arch Ophthalmol 2001; 119: 33–40
21. Davis, J. L., M. S. Serfass, et al. Silicone oil in repair of retinal detachments caused by necrotizing retinitis in HIV infection. Arch Ophthalmol 1995; 113: 1401–9
22. Irvine, A. R., L. Lonn, et al. Retinal detachment in AIDS: long-term results after repair with silicone oil. Br J Ophthalmol 1997; 81: 180–3
23. Tanna, A. P., J. H. Kempen, et al. Incidence and management of cataract after retinal detachment repair with silicone oil in immune compromised patients with cytomegalovirus retinitis. Am J Ophthalmol 2003; 136: 1009–15
24. Azen, S. P., I. U. Scott, et al. Silicone oil in the repair of complex retinal detachments. A prospective observational multicenter study. Ophthalmology 1998; 105: 1587–97
25. Palella, F. J., Jr., K. M. Delaney, et al. Declining morbidity and mortality among patients with advanced human immunodeficiency virus infection. HIV Outpatient Study Investigators. N Engl J Med 1998; 338: 853–60
26. Schaller, U. C., J. C. MacDonald, et al. Removal of silicone oil with vision improvement after rhegmatogenous retinal detachment following CMV retinitis in patients with AIDS. Retina 1999; 19: 495–8
27. Casswell, A. G. and Z. J. Gregor. Silicone oil removal I. The effect on the complications of silicone oil. Br J Ophthalmol 1987; 71: 893–7
28. Morrison, V. L., L. D. Labree, et al. Results of silicone oil removal in patients with cytomegalovirus retinitis related retinal detachments. Am J Ophthalmol 2005; 140: 786–93
29. Engstrom, R. E., Jr., D. T. Goldenberg, et al. Clear lens extraction with intraocular lens implantation during retinal detachment repair in patients with Acquired Immune Deficiency Syndrome (AIDS) [correction of autoimmune deficiency syndrome] and cytomegalovirus retinitis. Ophthalmology 2002; 109: 666–73
30. Stefansson, E., M. M. Anderson, Jr., et al. Refractive changes from use of silicone oil in vitreous surgery. Retina 1988; 8: 20–3
31. Beekhuis, W. H., F. Ando, et al. Basal iridectomy at 6 o'clock in the aphakic eye treated with silicone oil: prevention of keratopathy and secondary glaucoma. Br J Ophthalmol 1987; 71: 197–200
32. MacCumber, M. W., K. H. Packo, et al. Preservation of anterior capsule during vitrectomy and lensectomy for retinal detachment with proliferative vitreoretinopathy. Ophthalmology 2002; 109: 329–33
33. Hurley C, Barry P. Combined endocapsular phacoemulsification, pars plana vitrectomy and intraocular lens implantation. J Cataract Refract Surg 1996; 22: 462–6
34. Stoffelns, B. and N. Pfeiffer. Acute retinal necrosis. Silicon oil tamponade in retinal detachment. Ophthalmologe 1997; 94: 568–72
35. Ahmadieh, H., M. Soheilian, et al. Surgical management of retinal detachment secondary to acute retinal necrosis: clinical features, surgical techniques, and long-term results. Jpn J Ophthalmol 2003; 47: 484–91

Lens / Chapter 11

Extracapsular Extraction by Phacoemulsification

Antoine P. Brézin, Dominique Monnet

Core Messages

- Uveitis consists of heterogeneous entities, and many decisions regarding cataract surgery remain empirical.
- The perioperative medical management of inflammation is as important to visual outcome as the procedure by itself.
- The surgical challenge lies mostly in obtaining a sufficient pupil dilatation.
- Visual outcome depends mostly on the state of the macula.
- Cataract surgery in Fuchs heterochromic cyclitis usually has a better visual outcome than other causes of uveitis.
- Cataract surgery in idiopathic juvenile arthritis usually has a worse visual outcome than other causes of uveitis.

Contents

11.1	Introduction 111	11.4.1.4	Intraoperative Complications 115
11.2	Preoperative Assessment 112	11.4.2	Management of Specific Etiologies 116
11.3	Timing of Cataract Surgery 113	11.4.2.1	Fuchs Heterochromic Cyclitis 116
11.4	Intraoperative Management 113	11.4.2.2	Juvenile Idiopathic Arthritis 117
11.4.1	General Considerations 113	11.4.2.3	Infectious Uveitis 117
11.4.1.1	Techniques for Pupil Dilatation 113	11.4.3	Intumescent Cataracts 117
11.4.1.2	Intraocular Lens Implantation 114	11.5	Outcome of Cataract Surgery in Patients with Uveitis 117
11.4.1.3	Intraoperative Periocular or Intraocular Injection of Corticosteroids 114	References	 118

11.1 Introduction

Cataracts are a common complication of uveitis, occurring globally in approximately 40 % of all cases of uveitis [1]. However, this frequency is highly variable according to the causes of uveitis. In many cases, particularly in posterior uveitis, the frequency of cataracts does not differ from that of the general population. At the opposite, cataracts can be observed in the majority of cases, in some etiologies of anterior uveitis, such as idiopathic juvenile arthritis [2]. Inflammation by itself may be a causal factor of cataract formation, as can corticosteroid treatment by topical, periocular, intraocular or systemic routes.

In patients with uveitis, capsular extraction by phacoemulsification is now, in standard cases, the unchallenged method of choice for cataract extraction. The intraoperative particularities of cataract extraction in patients with uveitis are usually limited to breaking iris–lens synechiae, as a first step before performing a circumlinear capsulorhexis. In most cases of cataract surgery in uveitis, the greatest challenge lies in the perioperative medical management of inflammation. Indeed, surgery in inflamed eyes or in eyes with a history of inflammation can play a triggering role in inflammatory reactions. Those reactions can be seen in the anterior segment but may also be observed in other compartments of the eye. Cystoid macular edema in particular, which is the major cause of irreversible visual loss in patients with uveitis, can be observed after cataract surgery, even in uncomplicated cases.

Preoperative assessment is critical, as factors implicating the posterior segment of the eye may participate in visual loss. Most surgeons agree that cataract surgery in uveitis should only be performed when intraocular inflammation has been controlled for more than 3 months. However, uveitis consists of very heterogeneous entities, and the levels of evidence on which decisions are made regarding cataract surgery are usually very low. Cataract surgery in patients with uveitis has benefited from the general improvement of phacoemulsification methods. Small incisions and short operative times have reduced the surgically induced breakdown of the blood–aqueous barrier. Posterior capsular rupture and the rates of other perioperative complications have become minimal. In most cases, extracapsular cataract surgery by phacoemulsification in patients with uveitis has become uneventful and can now be associated with a good prognosis.

11.2 Preoperative Assessment

In eyes with a history of intraocular inflammation, identifying the cause of uveitis should always be attempted before cataract surgery. In some cases, early cataract formation by itself may be an adjunctive item, which can help in diagnosing the cause of uveitis. For example, lens opacities are a common early finding in Fuchs cyclitis. However, in the majority of cases, the presence of a cataract does not help in identifying the cause of uveitis. Moreover, in some cases of severe panuveitis, lens opacities may mask details of fundus examination, resulting therefore in a loss of information to understand the cause of inflammation. Knowing the cause of uveitis is also helpful in making decisions regarding the perioperative medical management of uveitis (see Chaps. 8, 9, 15 and 25).

The following is a list of items that should be assessed prior to surgery:

1. Is the cause of uveitis known?
2. Do factors other than lens opacification contribute to vision loss?
   (a) Corneal opacities
   (b) Vitreous opacities
   (c) Macular lesions
      – Epiretinal membrane
      – Macular edema reversible/irreversible
      – Macular atrophy
      – Macular ischemia
      – Submacular neovascularization
      – Areas of chorioretinitis, scarred or active, involving the macula
      – Other causes of macular lesions
   (d) Optic neuropathy
3. Is ocular hypertension or glaucoma associated with lens opacification? If yes, should combined cataract and filtering surgery be considered?
4. What is the time interval since the last attack of uveitis?
5. Is a residual chronic inflammation observed?
   (a) Blood–aqueous barrier breakdown
   (b) Cells in the anterior chamber
6. Assessment of the pupil
   (a) Normal pupil dilatation
   (b) Reduced pupil dilatation, without iris–lens synechiae
   (c) Iris–lens synechiae
      – Location of synechiae
      – Risk of pupil blockage?
   (d) Postinflammatory membranes attached to the pupil
   (e) Iris atrophy
7. Assessment of anterior chamber depth
8. Cataract staging
   (a) Soft, with subcapsular opacities
   (b) Standard
   (c) Hard
   (d) White cataracts, requiring the use of dye to perform capsulorhexis
   (e) Intumescent cataract, associated with a risk of angle-closure glaucoma
9. Will fellow eye cataract surgery be also indicated in the short term?

A particularly great spectrum of situations can be seen. A soft cataract with subcapsular posterior opacities and no iris–lens synechiae may be particularly unchallenging. Conversely, a hard, white cataract, in a patient with extended iris–lens synechiae will require a long procedure, associated with a greater-than-average risk of complications.

Assessing the exact role of lens opacities in decreased visual acuity in uveitic eyes with cataracts can be difficult. Imaging of the posterior pole by angiography or by optical coherence tomography can be limited by poor pupil dilatation, by the cataract itself or by vitreous opacities (Fig. 11.1). When available, the scanning laser ophthalmoscope can be used to predict visual acuity in patients with cataracts and other factors with a potential to affect vision [3]. Even when benefits for vision are uncertain, cataract surgery may be indicated in uveitic eyes to assess the posterior segment when clinical examination has become impossible.

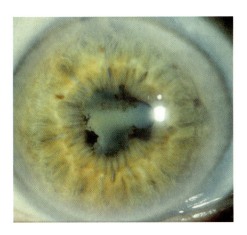

Fig. 11.1 Cataract with multiple synechiae

11.3 Timing of Cataract Surgery

Even in normal eyes, cataract surgery results in a breakdown of the blood–aqueous barrier. Numerous studies have been carried out to monitor protein levels in the anterior chamber using laser flare meter photometry [4]. Most studies have focused on the comparison of surgical techniques, such as the type of incision. Whatever the technique used, a transient increase in the blood–aqueous breakdown is observed, lasting, on average, up to 8 weeks. Because of this blood–aqueous breakdown, and perhaps because of other unknown factors, cataract surgery may trigger recurrences of intraocular inflammation in patients with a history of uveitis. However, when uveitis is effectively managed, the number and severity of relapses can actually decrease after surgery. Pivetti-Pezzi et al. studied 12 patients with anterior uveitis other than Fuchs heterochromic cyclitis, followed for 2 years after cataract surgery [5]. In their study, the number of relapses decreased from 2.74 ± 3.44 prior to surgery to 1.25 ± 1.71 after surgery.

How the base level of protein and/or cells in the anterior chamber influences the risk of exacerbation of intraocular inflammation on the occasion of cataract surgery is unknown. However, most investigators agree that the longer the time interval between the last attack of uveitis and the time when surgery is performed, the lesser the risk of a surgically induced inflammatory reaction. There is a lack of evidence-based data to quantify the relationship between the duration of the period of quiescence before surgery and the risk of recurrence of uveitis. Moreover, the risk of recurrence of uveitis according to the time interval between the last attack of uveitis and surgery is probably highly variable according to the cause of uveitis. In the study by Estafanous et al., 39 eyes with uveitis were operated by phacoemulsification and posterior chamber intraocular lens implantation [6]. The average period of quiescence before surgery was 19 months (range 0–135 months). All four eyes with mild inflammation during the immediate preoperative visit experienced recurrence of uveitis, but with no unfavorable impact on visual outcome. In the study by Alió et al. under the auspices of the International Ocular Inflammation Society Study Group of Uveitic Cataract Surgery, 140 uveitic eyes underwent phacoemulsification and posterior chamber intraocular lens implantation [7]. In this multicentric study, the object of which was to compare the performance of IOLs of various materials, the enrollment was limited to eyes with quiescent uveitis for a minimum of 3 months before surgery.

The medical management used to prepare eyes for cataract surgery is detailed elsewhere in this book (see Chaps. 8, 9 and 25). According to the cause of uveitis and to the specificities of each case, topical or systemic corticosteroids, or corticosteroids by periocular or intraocular injections, may be required to control inflammation. When flare meter measurements are available, surgery is usually only considered when values have reached a minimum plateau and when there are no remaining cells in the anterior chamber. At one end of the spectrum, some etiologies of uveitis, such as Fuchs cyclitis, usually do not require any specific preoperative management. At the other end, in severe cases of uveitis, controlling inflammation in view of cataract surgery may justify the initiation of immunosuppressive therapy.

11.4 Intraoperative Management

11.4.1 General Considerations

11.4.1.1 Techniques for Pupil Dilatation

Managing iris–lens synechiae is usually the greatest intraoperative challenge in cataract surgery of uveitic eyes. The techniques used to obtain a sufficient pupil dilatation to perform a capsulorhexis are detailed elsewhere in this book (see Chap. 13). Briefly, the methods used for pupil dilatation range from the simple breakdown of iris–lens synechiae with the cannula used to inject viscoelastic substance in the anterior chamber to the use of iris hooks inserted through multiple corneal paracentheses (Figs. 11.2 and 11.3):

1. Breakdown of synechiae with cannula during injection of viscoelastic substance
2. Pupil stretch
   (a) Bimanual stretching with Sinskey hooks or equivalent
   (b) Stretching with Beehler pupil dilator
3. Intraoperative polymethyl methacrylate (PMMA) pupil dilator ring
4. Paracenthesis with insertion of iris hooks

When appropriately performed, pupil stretching during phacoemulsification does not lead to increased complications [8]. With the use of the latest generation of phacoemulsification machines, with high vacuum levels and pressure stabilization systems, a 4–5 mm pupil dilatation may be sufficient to perform a cataract extraction.

Once a pupil dilatation has been obtained, the technique for cataract surgery in uveitic eyes does not differ from standard procedures. The complete removal of all fragments of lens cortex is a factor in the prevention of postoperative inflammatory reaction, which could be exacerbated in cases of uveitis. This removal must be performed in a masked fashion, when pupil dilatation prevents visual control of the periphery of the capsular bag. A Sinskey hook may be used to push the pupil to the periphery to check the exhaustiveness of cortical cleanup.

11.4.1.2 Intraocular Lens Implantation

The selection of intraocular lens (IOL) implantations in eyes with uveitis is detailed elsewhere in this book (see Chap. 12). A great part of the literature is based on results obtained prior to modern cataract extraction through phacoemulsification by small incisions with insertion of foldable IOLs. Most studies include heterogeneous cases of uveitis, which may limit the interpretation of the results. Moreover, when polymethyl methacrylate (PMMA) lenses are compared with foldable acrylic or silicone lenses, results should take into account the effect of the incision size on postoperative inflammation. The study by Alió et al. compared the implantation of hydrophobic acrylic, silicone, PMMA and heparin-surface-modified (HSM) PMMA IOLs, placed in the bag after phacoemulsification [7]. The acrylic group had the lowest inflammation values from one day after surgery until the 3-month follow-up.

In most studies of cataract surgery in uveitic eyes, lens placement in uncomplicated procedures is in the capsular bag. However, posterior synechiae can form between the iris and the lens capsule. To prevent that complication, some authors have intentionally placed IOLs in the ciliary sulcus of the patients with uveitis. In the study by Holland et al. of 16 eyes with uveitis, posterior synechiae which were present in 13 eyes before surgery developed in only three of these eyes postoperatively [9]. These authors argued that ciliary sulcus placement allowed the IOL to serve as a physical barrier between the iris and the lens capsule remnants.

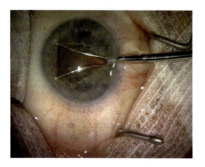

Fig. 11.2 Beehler pupil dilator

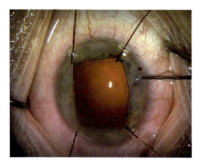

Fig. 11.3 Iris hooks

11.4.1.3 Intraoperative Periocular or Intraocular Injection of Corticosteroids

Posterior sub-Tenon injections have become widely used for the treatment of macular edema in uveitis [10, 11]. In nonuveitic eyes, intraoperative sub-Tenon's capsule triamcinolone acetonide injection has been compared to steroid drops in the treatment of ocular inflammation after cataract surgery. In double-masked controlled trials, patients were randomized prospectively into two groups treated with 1% prednisolone eyedrops or with sub-Tenon's 30 or 40 mg triamcinolone acetonide injection [12, 13]. A single intraoperative triamcinolone acetonide sub-Tenon's capsule injection demonstrated a clinically equivalent therapeutic response and ocular tolerance compared with 1% prednisolone drops in controlling postoperative inflammation after uncomplicated cataract surgery. In patients with uveitis, intraoperative sub-Tenon injections are routinely performed, in addition to systemic or topical treatment. However, its added value for the prevention of inflammatory rebounds after cataract surgery in uveitic eyes has not been evaluated yet.

Cataract surgery combined with intravitreal injection of triamcinolone acetonide has been used in patients with age-related macular degeneration, diabetic macular edema or retinal vein occlusions [14]. Intravitreal triamcinolone is now also routinely used for the treatment of uveitic cystoid macular edema [15]. As with sub-Tenon injections, intraoperative intravitreal injections are occasionally performed during cataract surgery in uveitic eyes. The standard dose for intravitreal triamcinolone is 4 mg, in 0.1 ml volume. As with sub-Tenon injection, the added value for the prevention of recurrences after cataract surgery in uveitic eyes has not been evaluated yet. Complications of sub-Tenon or intravitreal injections include increased intraocular pressure, reported in some series in more than half of patients, but mostly controlled by antiglaucoma medications [16].

Triamcinolone acetonide can also be injected in the anterior chamber at the end of cataract surgery. In a study of 22 patients with juvenile idiopathic arthritis, the injection of 4 mg of triamcinolone acetonide in the anterior chamber was compared to systemic treatment with intraoperative intravenous injection of methylprednisolone and postoperative oral prednisolone [17]. Fibrin formation was not seen after surgery in the triamcinolone group, but occurred in half of patients with systemic treatment. Additional systemic corticosteroid was not required in patients with triamcinolone acetonide anterior chamber injections.

Biodegradable systems providing sustained release of corticosteroids have been tested for the prevention of postoperative inflammatory reactions in standard cases of cataract surgery. Surodex® (Oculex Pharmaceuticals, now Allergan) contains 60 μg of dexamethasone and can be inserted in the anterior chamber or in the sulcus at the conclusion of cataract surgery. This intraocular drug delivery system was superior to eyedrops in reducing inflammatory symptoms and aqueous flare measured with the laser flare meter [18]. The use of Surodex® has not been reported in cataract surgery of uveitic eyes, but could be of interest. Other biodegradable systems providing sustained release of corticosteroids are currently in trial for the treatment of chronic uveitis. The intraoperative placement of these systems during cataract surgery in cases of uveitis could be of interest.

11.4.1.4 Intraoperative Complications

Iris Prolapse

Most of the current literature regarding intraoperative iris prolapse is based on patients treated by tamsulosin (Flomax) [19]. Intraoperative floppy-iris syndrome (IFIS) is characterized by three signs that occur during cataract extraction. The signs include a floppy iris that billows in the normal irrigation currents of the anterior chamber, a propensity for the iris to prolapse through the phacoemulsification and side-port incisions, and progressive pupil constriction during surgery. Those features, which are caused by a lack of tone of the dilator smooth muscle of the iris, are often seen in uveitic eyes.

A critical factor to prevent iris prolapse is to distance the wound from the base of the iris. In uveitic eyes with an atrophic iris, the incisions for cataract surgery should be sufficiently anterior in the cornea. Simple prolapses can be addressed by repositioning the iris with viscoelastic substance and an iris repositor. Occasionally, excess viscoelastic substance needs to be removed as it can aggravate the iris prolapse. An iridotomy at the base of the iris is often ineffective in preventing further iris trauma. A second instrument can be introduced via the paracenthesis to restrain a flaccid iris. However, in difficult cases, the most effective method to manage an iris prolapse is to apply iris hooks on each side of the primary incision [20].

Anterior Capsule Tears

In standard conditions, anterior capsule tears have been reported to occur in 0.79% of phacoemulsification surgery [21]. In uveitic eyes, the importance of an intact capsulorhexis for safe phacoemulsification and intraocular implantation can be even more critical than in standard cases. Managing a tear identified during the capsulorhexis, by redirecting the capsulorhexis to incorporate the tear, must be attempted. Obtaining a satisfactory visualization of the anterior capsule, through a sufficiently dilated pupil should always be achieved before beginning the capsulorhexis.

Rupture of the Posterior Capsule and Prolapse of the Vitreous Body

Even in nonuveitic eyes, a ruptured posterior capsule is a troublesome complication of cataract surgery which can lead to inflammatory reactions. Removing all vitreous body in the anterior chamber is necessary to minimize the risk of secondary complications. Because the vitreous body is difficult to visualize, that can be an insecure maneuver. Intracameral triamcinolone has been shown to be very helpful in this situation [22]. Approximately 0.5 ml of triamcinolone acetonide solution can be sprayed into the anterior chamber at the location where the vitreous body is likely to be. Immediately, the vitreous body appears as a white-colored gel with triamcinolone acetonide granules which can be easily removed with a vitreous cutter. This technique can be applied to complicated cataract surgery in uveitic eyes. In addition to its effect on the visualization of the vitreous, triamcinolone acetonide can also play a role in minimizing the inflammatory response that can be seen after complicated cataract surgery, with an even greater risk in eyes with a history of uveitis.

Zonular Dialysis

Weak zonules pose a difficult choice between implantation of the posterior chamber intraocular lens (PC IOL) in the capsular bag, scleral suturing of the PC IOL, or no implantation. In difficult cases, secondary IOL placement can be considered, rather than increasing the risk of inflammatory rebounds in uveitic eyes. Forcible IOL implantation enlarges zonular dialysis and causes subluxation of the IOL. Zonules should be examined after completion of phacoemulsification to decide whether an IOL may be placed in the bag or in the sulcus. Capsular tension rings are useful in the management of localized zonular dialysis, with no more than one quadrant width [23]. Various capsular stabilization devices have been designed to preserve the integrity of the lens capsule during phacoemulsification with a weak zonule [24]. However, even when cataract surgery can be safely performed with in-the-bag PC IOL placement, those systems do not preclude postoperative dislocations. The use of iris-fixated Artisan IOLs has not been reported in complicated surgery in uveitic eyes.

11.4.2 Management of Specific Etiologies

11.4.2.1 Fuchs Heterochromic Cyclitis

Many features distinguish Fuchs heterochromic cyclitis from other causes of uveitis, among which the lack of iris–lens synechiae. Discrete lens opacities are a near constant finding, and cataracts occur early in the course of the disease (Fig. 11.4). In most series, cataract surgery is performed between the age of 30 and 35 [25–27]. Fuchs heterochromic cyclitis is generally thought to have a better prognosis than other forms of chronic anterior uveitis [28]. Pre- and postoperatively, aqueous flare values in eyes with Fuchs heterochromic cyclitis are two to three times higher than in control eyes with senile cataracts [29]. Blood–aqueous barrier breakdown following phacoemulsification with posterior chamber lens implantation is relatively mild and appears to be fully reestablished to preoperative levels 6 weeks postoperatively. No complications, such as fibrin formation or synechiae, are observed, and cells on the intraocular lens optic are exceptional. Amsler's sign or hyphema occurring after ocular paracentesis is a classic feature of Fuchs heterochromic cyclitis (Fig. 11.5) [30]. Because modern phacoemulsification is performed with a positive intraocular pressure, Amsler's sign is now inconstantly observed. The outcome of phacoemulsification in eyes with Fuchs heterochromic cyclitis is summarized in Table 11.1. Even in cases with a successful anatomical outcome and good visual acuity, the patients' quality of life may be affected by the chronic perception of floaters, linked to vitreous opacities.

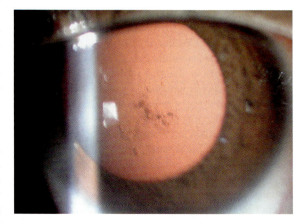

Fig. 11.4 Early lens opacities in Fuchs heterochromic cyclitis

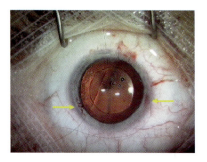

Fig. 11.5 Amsler's sign (*arrows*) during placement of a PMMA IOL in Fuchs heterochromic cyclitis

Table 11.1 Outcome of cataract surgery by phacoemulsification in Fuchs heterochromic cyclitis

	Authors		
	Ram et al.	Javadi et al.	Tejwani et al.
Year published	2002	2005	2006
Number of eyes	20	41	103
Mean age (years)	32 ± 10	35 ± 12	32 ± 12
Postoperative best corrected visual acuity	6/6 or better in 85% of eyes	20/20 in 54% of eyes	> 20/40 in 92.5% of eyes

11.4.2.2 Juvenile Idiopathic Arthritis

Lens extraction in childhood uveitis is presented in detail elsewhere in this book (see Chap. 15). Inflammatory reactions are often exacerbated, with severe breakdown of the blood–aqueous barrier. The visual outcome of cataract surgery is much less favorable than in other cases of uveitis [2]. Cataract extraction is still occasionally performed without the implantation of an intraocular lens. In young children, posterior capsulotomy and anterior vitrectomy are frequently performed intraoperatively.

11.4.2.3 Infectious Uveitis

Herpetic Uveitis

Herpetic anterior uveitis is associated with iris atrophy which is best quantified by retroillumination of the iris through the pupil [31]. When large atrophic areas are present, iris prolapse through the incisions required for phacoemulsification is a common complication (see above). Recurrences of anterior herpetic uveitis can be triggered by cataract surgery and treatment by systemic acyclovir or valacyclovir is frequently prescribed for the prevention of recurrences.

Ocular Toxoplasmosis

Cataract surgery has been suspected of triggering recurrences of active chorioretinitis in patients with a history of ocular toxoplasmosis. In a study by Bosch-Driessen et al., reactivations of ocular toxoplasmosis following cataract extraction occurred in 5 of 14 patients (5 of 15 eyes), which was higher than the incidence of recurrences in age- and sex-matched controls [32]. No additional risk factors for the development of recurrences of ocular toxoplasmosis after cataract surgery were found. Incidence of recurrences preceding surgery did not differ between patients and controls. For the authors, prophylactic treatment with antiparasitic drugs during and after the cataract surgery can be worthwhile for patients at risk of visual loss.

11.4.3 Intumescent Cataracts

Intumescent-cataracts-complicating cases of uveitis are particularly challenging. When possible, treatment of lens-induced glaucoma by a peripheral iridotomy may buy time for topical and/or systemic immunosuppression to reduce intraocular inflammation. However, in cases of severe intumescence, inflammatory phacoantigenic mechanisms may sustain intraocular inflammation. Those cases are the exception to the usual rule requiring cataract surgery to be performed only when intraocular inflammation has been managed preoperatively by medical treatment. Trypan blue staining has considerably simplified the visualization of the anterior capsule to perform a circumlinear capsulorhexis [33].

11.5 Outcome of Cataract Surgery in Patients with Uveitis

Because inflammatory rebounds may occur, postoperative monitoring in uveitic eyes requires a more frequent schedule of visits than standard modern phacoemulsifi-

Table 11.2 Outcome of cataract surgery in miscellaneous cases of uveitis

		Authors		
		Okhravi et al.	Estafanous et al.	Rahman and Jones
	Year published	1998	2000	2005
	Number of eyes	90	39	72
	Mean age (years)	50	50 ± 13	49
	Mean follow-up	10 months	20 months	7.6 years
Cataract extraction	Manual extracapsular	88 eyes (98%)		41 eyes (57%)
	Phacoemulsification	1 eye	39 eyes (100%)	31 eyes (43%)
	Visual outcome	6/12 or better in 57% of eyes	20/40 or better in 87% of eyes	6/9 or better in 74% of eyes
	Macular edema or scarring	18%	33%	24%
	Posterior capsule opacification	48%	62%	96 %

cation. The outcome of cataract surgery in uveitic eyes is highly variable, according to the cause of uveitis, the preoperative findings, the surgical procedure and mostly the long-term state of the vitreous, the macula and the optic nerve. Many large series in the literature are still based on the analysis of cases including manual extracapsular extraction [6, 34, 35]. Only very recently have a few large series been reported regarding the outcome of phacoemulsification in uveitic eyes (Table 11.2). Since uveitis is often a lifetime disease, follow-up data are still short to assess the long-term outcome of cataract surgery in uveitic eyes. Many series combine cases with a favorable prognosis, such as Fuchs heterochromic cyclitis with sight-threatening cases as in juvenile idiopathic arthritis.

References

1. Durrani OM, Tehrani NN, Marr JE, Moradi P, Stavrou P, Murray PI. Degree, duration, and causes of visual loss in uveitis. Br J Ophthalmol. 2004;88:1159–62
2. Kump LI, Castaneda RA, Androudi SN, Reed GF, Foster CS. Visual outcomes in children with juvenile idiopathic arthritis-associated uveitis. Ophthalmology. 2006;113:1874–7
3. Cuzzani OE, Ellant JP, Young PW, Gimbel HV, Rydz M. Potential acuity meter versus scanning laser ophthalmoscope to predict visual acuity in cataract patients. J Cataract Refract Surg. 1998;24:263–9
4. Ladas JG, Wheeler NC, Morhun PJ, Rimmer SO, Holland GN. Laser flare-cell photometry: methodology and clinical applications. Surv Ophthalmol. 2005;50:27–47
5. Pivetti-Pezzi P, Accorinti M, La Cava M, Abdulaziz MA, Pantaleoni FB, Long-term follow-up of anterior uveitis after cataract extraction and intraocular lens implantation. J Cataract Refract Surg. 1999;25:1521–6
6. Estafanous MF, Lowder CY, Meisler DM, Chauhan R. Phacoemulsification cataract extraction and posterior chamber lens implantation in patients with uveitis. Am J Ophthalmol. 2001;131:620–5
7. Alio JL, Chipont E, BenEzra D, Fakhry MA; International Ocular Inflammation Society, Study Group of Uveitic Cataract Surgery. Comparative performance of intraocular lenses in eyes with cataract and uveitis. J Cataract Refract Surg. 2002;28:2096–108
8. Shingleton BJ, Campbell CA, O'Donoghue MW. Effects of pupil stretch technique during phacoemulsification on postoperative vision, intraocular pressure, and inflammation. J Cataract Refract Surg. 2006;32:1142–5
9. Holland GN, Van Horn SD, Margolis TP. Cataract surgery with ciliary sulcus fixation of intraocular lenses in patients with uveitis. Am J Ophthalmol. 1999;128:21–30

10. Lafranco Dafflon M, Tran VT, Guex-Crosier Y, Herbort CP. Posterior sub-Tenon's steroid injections for the treatment of posterior ocular inflammation: indications, efficacy and side effects. Graefes Arch Clin Exp Ophthalmol. 1999;237:289–95
11. Tanner V, Kanski JJ, Frith PA. Posterior sub-Tenon's triamcinolone injections in the treatment of uveitis. Eye. 1998;12:679–85
12. Paganelli F, Cardillo JA, Melo LA Jr, Oliveira AG, Skaf M, Costa RA; Brazilian Ocular Pharmacology and Pharmaceutical Technology Research Group. A single intraoperative sub-Tenon's capsule triamcinolone acetonide injection for the treatment of post-cataract surgery inflammation. Ophthalmology. 2004;111:2102–8
13. Negi AK, Browning AC, Vernon SA. Single perioperative triamcinolone injection versus standard postoperative steroid drops after uneventful phacoemulsification surgery: randomized controlled trial. J Cataract Refract Surg. 2006;32:468–74
14. Jonas JB, Kreissig I, Budde WM, Degenring RF. Cataract surgery combined with intravitreal injection of triamcinolone acetonide. Eur J Ophthalmol. 2005;15:329–35
15. Antcliff RJ, Spalton DJ, Stanford MR, et al. Intravitreal triamcinolone for uveitic cystoid macular edema: an optical coherence tomography study. Ophthalmology. 2001;108:765–72
16. Jonas JB, Degenring RF, Kreissig I, Akkoyun I, Kampppeter BA. Intraocular pressure elevation after intravitreal triamcinolone acetonide injection. Ophthalmology. 2005;112:593–8
17. Li J, Heinz C, Zurek-Imhoff B, Heiligenhaus A. Intraoperative intraocular triamcinolone injection prophylaxis for post-cataract surgery fibrin formation in uveitis associated with juvenile idiopathic arthritis. J Cataract Refract Surg. 2006;32:1535–9
18. Tan DT, Chee SP, Lim L, Theng J, Van Ede M. Randomized clinical trial of Surodex steroid drug delivery system for cataract surgery: anterior versus posterior placement of two Surodex in the eye. Ophthalmology. 2001;108:2172–81
19. Manvikar S, Allen D. Cataract surgery management in patients taking tamsulosin staged approach. J Cataract Refract Surg. 2006;32:1611–4
20. Chan DG, Francis IC. Intraoperative management of iris prolapse using iris hooks. J Cataract Refract Surg. 2005;31:1694–6
21. Marques FF, Marques DM, Osher RH, Osher JM. Fate of anterior capsule tears during cataract surgery. J Cataract Refract Surg. 2006;32:1638–42
22. Yamakiri K, Uchino E, Kimura K, Sakamoto T. Intracameral triamcinolone helps to visualize and remove the vitreous body in anterior chamber in cataract surgery. Am J Ophthalmol. 2004;138:650–2
23. Menapace R, Findl O, Georgopoulos M, et al. The capsular tension ring: designs, applications, and techniques. J Cataract Refract Surg. 2000;26:898–912
24. Nishimura E, Yaguchi S, Nishihara H, Ayaki M, Kozawa T. Capsular stabilization device to preserve lens capsule integrity during phacoemulsification with a weak zonule. J Cataract Refract Surg. 2006;32:392–5
25. Tejwani S, Murthy S, Sangwan VS. Cataract extraction outcomes in patients with Fuchs' heterochromic cyclitis. J Cataract Refract Surg. 2006;32:1678–82
26. Javadi MA, Jafarinasab MR, Araghi AA, Mohammadpour M, Yazdani S. Outcomes of phacoemulsification and in-the-bag intraocular lens implantation in Fuchs' heterochromic iridocyclitis. J Cataract Refract Surg. 2005;31:997–1001
27. Ram J, Kaushik S, Brar GS, Gupta A, Gupta A. Phacoemulsification in patients with Fuchs' heterochromic uveitis. J Cataract Refract Surg. 2002;28:1372–8
28. Menezo V, Lightman S. The development of complications in patients with chronic anterior uveitis. Am J Ophthalmol. 2005;139:988–92
29. Nguyen NX, Kuchle M, Naumann GO. Quantification of blood–aqueous barrier breakdown after phacoemulsification in Fuchs' heterochromic uveitis. Ophthalmologica. 2005;219:21–5
30. Amsler M, Verrey F. Hétérochromie de Fuchs et fragilité vasculaire. Ophthalmologica. 1946;11:177–81
31. Van der Lelij A, Ooijman FM, Kijlstra A, Rothova A. Anterior uveitis with sectoral iris atrophy in the absence of keratitis: a distinct clinical entity among herpetic eye diseases. Ophthalmology. 2000;107:1164–70
32. Bosch-Driessen LH, Plaisier MB, Stilma JS, Van der Lelij A, Rothova A. Reactivations of ocular toxoplasmosis after cataract extraction. Ophthalmology. 2002;109:41–5
33. Jacob S, Agarwal A, Agarwal A, Agarwal S, Chowdhary S, Chowdhary R, Bagmar AA. Trypan blue as an adjunct for safe phacoemulsification in eyes with white cataract. J Cataract Refract Surg. 2002;28:1819–25
34. Okhravi N, Lightman SL, Towler HM. Assessment of visual outcome after cataract surgery in patients with uveitis. Ophthalmology. 1999;106:710–22
35. Rahman I, Jones NP. Long-term results of cataract extraction with intraocular lens implantation in patients with uveitis. Eye. 2005;19:191–7

Lens / Chapter 12

Selection of Intraocular Lenses: Materials, Contraindications, Secondary Implants

Gerd U. Auffarth

Core Messages

- Intraocular lens (IOL) selection in uveitis patients depends on the type of uveitis, expected surgical trauma and expected postoperative inflammatory reaction.
- Hydrophilic acrylic foldable IOLs and heparin surface-modified (HSM) PMMA IOLs are used most widely and tolerated in uveitis patients.
- Hydrophobic acrylic foldable IOLs may be used in cases of minimal surgical trauma and mild uveitic reactions.
- In pediatric cataract cases, heparin surface-modified PMMA IOLs may have the best long-term prognosis.
- Cataract surgery should consist of minimal invasive techniques with reduced energy application such as micro/hyperpulse technology or waterjet technology.

Contents

12.1	Introduction	121	12.9	Hydrophilic Acrylate IOLs and Uveitis	127
12.2	Development of IOL Materials	121	12.10	Hydrophobic Acrylate IOLs and Uveitis	127
12.3	Postoperative Inflammatory Reactions Following Cataract Surgery	122	12.11	Hydrophobic Silicone IOLs and Uveitis	127
12.4	Rigid PMMA IOLs	123	12.12	PMMA IOLs and Uveitis	127
12.5	Acrylate Foldable Lenses	123	12.13	Special IOLs and Uveitis	127
12.6	Silicone Foldable Lenses	124	12.14	Secondary Implants and Uveitis	127
12.7	Stability of Material	125	12.15	Contraindications for IOL Implantation in Uveitis	128
12.8	IOL Choice in Uveitic Patients	125	References		128

12.1 Introduction

Modern cataract surgery with the implantation of an intraocular lens (IOL) represents the most frequent surgical procedure in medical implantation surgery worldwide [6, 7]. The first IOLs were based on Plexiglas—polymethylmethacrylate (PMMA). Since the early to mid-1990s, foldable lenses made of silicone materials and foldable acrylate lenses with high (hydrophilic) and low (hydrophobic) water content have almost completely replaced the rigid PMMA IOLs due to further developments in cataract surgical techniques [6, 7, 11, 14, 15]. The distinction between IOL materials can be seen in their differing surface properties (Fig. 12.1). Hydrophilic IOLs (hydrophilic acrylate lenses) have an excellent biocompatibility. Therefore, they are particularly suitable for patients with uveitis, trauma, diabetes or those patients with expected vitreous surgical measures with silicone oil implantation [1, 4, 6, 14–16, 33, 34, 36]. Hydrophobic IOL materials (hydrophobic acrylate foldable lenses, silicone IOLs) are characterized by very low rates of posterior capsule opacification (PCO) if fitted with a sharp optic edge and are used with most patients for standard cataract surgery [9–11, 25–28, 30].

12.2 Development of IOL Materials

The first intraocular lenses were implanted following extracapsular cataract extraction more than 50 years

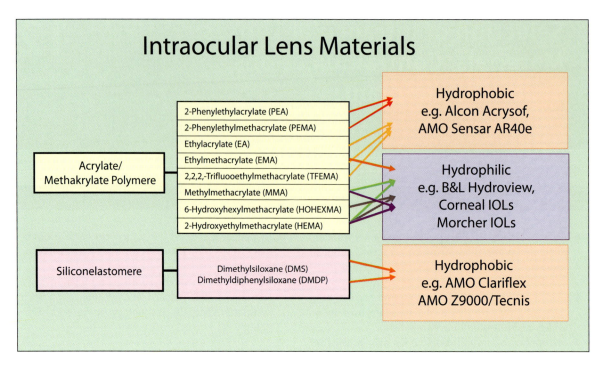

Fig. 12.1 Intraocular lens materials (modified from [14])

ago. The material, polymethylmethacrylate (PMMA), still serves as the basis for many IOLs. Until the 1990s, rigid PMMA IOLs were standard in cataract surgery. The lengthiest long-term observations and experiences of eye implants have been collected with this material [6, 8]. With the introduction of phacoemulsification and small incision surgery, foldable lenses made of silicone and different acrylates replaced rigid PMMA IOLs as standard lenses during the mid-1990s. Figure 12.1 schematically summarizes the various foldable lens materials along with their properties [6, 8]. With acrylate foldable lenses, we can distinguish between hydrophobic acrylate foldable lenses, which have a low water content (< 2%, e.g., Alcon AcrySof, AMO Sensar AR40e), and hydrophilic lenses, which have a high water content (usually > 20%, e.g., B&L Hydroview, Rayner C-flex, Corneal ACR6DE). Silicone materials are generally hydrophobic. The usually relatively thick silicone IOLs of the first generation developed into relatively thin lenses made of high refractive index silicone materials [6, 8].

12.3 Postoperative Inflammatory Reactions Following Cataract Surgery

Extracapsular cataract surgery with IOL implantation always leads to a specific inflammation reaction in the anterior segment, and generally in the entire eye [1, 4, 14, 26, 33, 34]. Figure 12.2 illustrates the sequence with which this occurs [4, 14, 26]. Initially the surgical trauma leads to a collapse of the blood–aqueous barrier. This leads to the initial postoperative inflammation reaction with Tyndall phenomenon and cells in the anterior chamber. Remaining lens epithelial cells as well as macrophages attracted by the IOL as foreign bodies synthesize transmitters (cytokines, interleukins) which maintain the inflammatory reaction and induce prostaglandin synthesis. The interaction between the IOL surface (properties of the material), immune defenses and lens epithelial cells plays an important role in this process. After 2–5 days, a second wave of delayed inflammatory reaction can occur, which can have various consequences, including fibrin formation on the IOL. In the meantime, fibrous metaplasia develops as a wound-healing reaction. With hydrophobic IOL surfaces, this can lead to an anterior capsular fibrosis. When the inflammation reaction in the anterior segment has healed, cystoid macular edema in the posterior segment can develop after several weeks due to the induction of prostaglandin synthesis [4, 6]. Hydrophilic lenses and IOL surfaces generally have a better biocompatibility, meaning that they induce the above-mentioned cascades and reactions on a smaller scale than hydrophobic IOLs [1, 4, 34]. However, through improved phacoemulsification equipment and a further minimization of trauma through a reduction of the applied ultrasound energy,

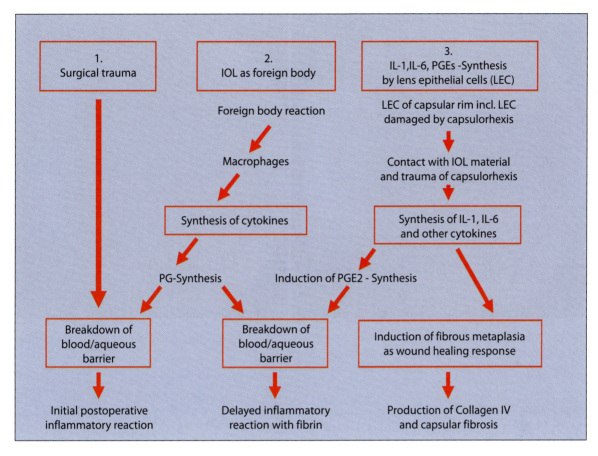

Fig. 12.2 Postoperative inflammatory reaction after cataract surgery (modified from [14])

the difference in reaction patterns of hydrophilic and hydrophobic foldable lenses is relatively small in modern surgery.

12.4 Rigid PMMA IOLs

PMMA IOLs are implanted infrequently due to the rigidity of the lenses that necessitate incisions of 5–7 mm in order to be implanted. Untreated, they have a hydrophobic surface. To improve biocompatibility, PMMA IOLs are coated with heparin. Through this process, they develop hydrophilic surface properties. Other coating materials such as polyfluorocarbon (Teflon) were also tested, although they never gained wide acceptance [6, 12, 14, 15].

At present, rigid PMMA IOLs are most often used for secondary implantation (sulcus fixated or transscleral fixated) with aphakia. A number of surgeons also prefer using the rigid material for children and adolescents because of the proven long-term compatibility. In cases of capsular bag complications, PMMA IOLs often are implanted primarily into the sulcus. HSM-PMMA IOLs also are used in patients with uveitis, trauma and congenital cataract, or in rare cases also in diabetics due to a better biocompatibility. Heparin-coated PMMA IOLs are further characterized by a smaller silicone oil adhesion compared with hydrophobic IOLs.

12.5 Acrylate Foldable Lenses

With acrylate foldable lenses, we differentiate between those with high and those with low water content (Fig. 12.1). They are offered as one-piece and three-piece IOLs. Moreover, acrylate foldable lenses can be made more hydrophilic by applying surface coatings (heparin). Today, hydrophobic acrylate foldable lenses are the most frequently implanted folding lenses. Figure 12.3 illustrates a one-piece hydrophobic acrylate foldable lens

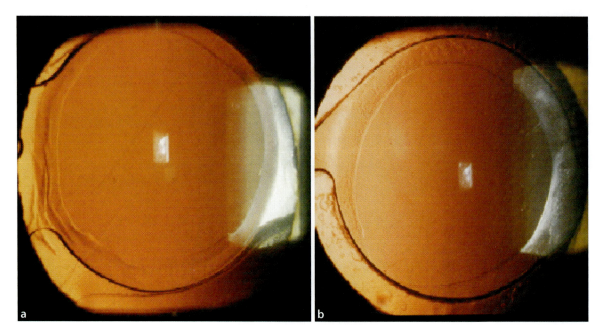

Fig. 12.3 Retroillumination photograph of a one-piece hydrophobic acrylate foldable lens on the right (Alcon AcrySof SA30AL) and a hydrophilic acrylate foldable lens on the left (Rayner Centerflex 570H)

on the right (Alcon AcrySof SA30AL) and a hydrophilic acrylate foldable lens on the left (Rayner Centerflex 570H).

Hydrophilic acrylate foldable lenses also show a very good (uveal) biocompatibility [1, 4, 14, 33, 34]. The inflammation and foreign body reaction is usually small, and the lenses are suitable for cataract surgery in cases of uveitis, trauma, diabetes and patients with high retinal detachment risk and possible silicone oil use. Hydrophilic acrylate foldable lenses are characterized by lower anterior capsule opacification than hydrophobic lenses, however PCO rates even with a sharp optic edge are higher than with hydrophobic acrylate foldable lenses [6, 9–11, 14–16, 25–28, 30, 34]. It is this last point of secondary cataract that represents the major advantage of hydrophobic acrylate foldable lenses with a sharp optic edge. In uncomplicated surgery with a centered capsulorhexis which lies completely on the optic, PCO rates of hydrophobic acrylate foldable lenses are below 5–3% over the long-term [6].

quently leading to a white opacification of the anterior capsule and a reduction of the anterior capsule opening (in extreme cases up to the anterior capsule phimosis), as well as a pronounced cellular reaction (Figs. 12.4 and 12.5) [6, 10, 13, 30]. Due to their interaction with silicone oil, these IOLs are generally not implanted in patients with diabetes or those with high myopia. As with

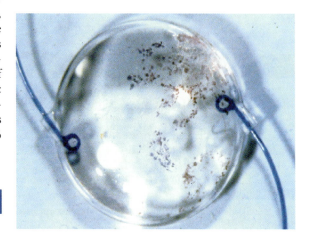

Fig. 12.4 Light microscopy photograph of a silicone IOL with cell adhesion (hematoxylin and eosin stain) explanted from a case with uveitis-glaucoma-hemorrhage (UGH) syndrome

12.6 Silicone Foldable Lenses

Today, high refractive index silicone materials are almost exclusively used. The silicone surfaces are generally referred to as hydrophobic. All silicone foldable lenses induce an anterior capsule reaction, quite fre-

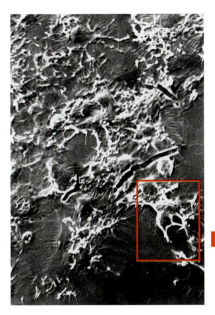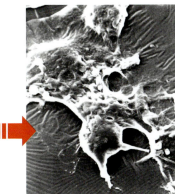

Fig. 12.5 Scanning electron microscopy of the surface of the silicone IOL in Fig. 12.4: note the accumulation of foreign body giant cells and macrophages

hydrophobic acrylate foldable lenses, silicone foldable lenses with sharp optic edges show very low PCO rates [6, 10, 13, 30].

12.7 Stability of Material

The longest experiences with IOL materials have been collected for the rigid PMMA IOLs. For these IOLs, excellent material stability was shown over several decades. However, snowflake-like opacification in the lens optic have also been described in isolated cases with PMMA IOLs (snowflake degeneration) [6, 7].

Silicone lenses have also been implanted for a long period of time (>25 years). Isolated discolorations (yellow, brown) of the lenses have been described, though these could partly be explained by production-dependent factors [6, 8].

Hydrophobic acrylate foldable lenses show similarly stable properties as compared to PMMA IOLs. However, opacification, or so-called "glistenings," were also described for these lenses. These are water-containing microvacuoles with a diameter of 5–10 µm, which were described more frequently in cases of longer implantation durations and higher IOL strength. An association to proteins and lipids in the aqueous humor and mechanical stress was also found. Several phenomena were described with hydrophilic acrylate foldable lenses [6, 22].

The SC60B-OUV model of the American manufacturer MDR achieved a sad popularity status. In this case, a complete clouding of the entire lens, including the haptics, generally resulted. Several different causes were explored. Those which were proven included calcium-phosphate-containing deposits, stability problems of the UV absorber and zinc-containing sediments on the lens surface [6, 17]. Calcium phosphate deposits were also found with the B&L Hydroview IOL [6, 14].

12.8 IOL Choice in Uveitic Patients

Modern cataract surgery does not use a single type of lens for all surgeries. The different foldable lens materials and their characteristics allow for differential application depending on the patient. Knowledge of these properties facilitates the classification of preoperative anterior segment findings and treatment methods for the ophthalmologist.

> The IOL implantation in uveitic patients depends on:
> - Type of uveitis
> - Severity of inflammation
> - Frequency of recurrent uveitis periods
> - Anterior segment status (synechiae, endothelial plaques, etc.)
> - Posterior segment status (vitrectomized eye, silicone oil filled)
> - Age
> - Density of cataract
> - Expected visual outcome
> - Type of surgical technique

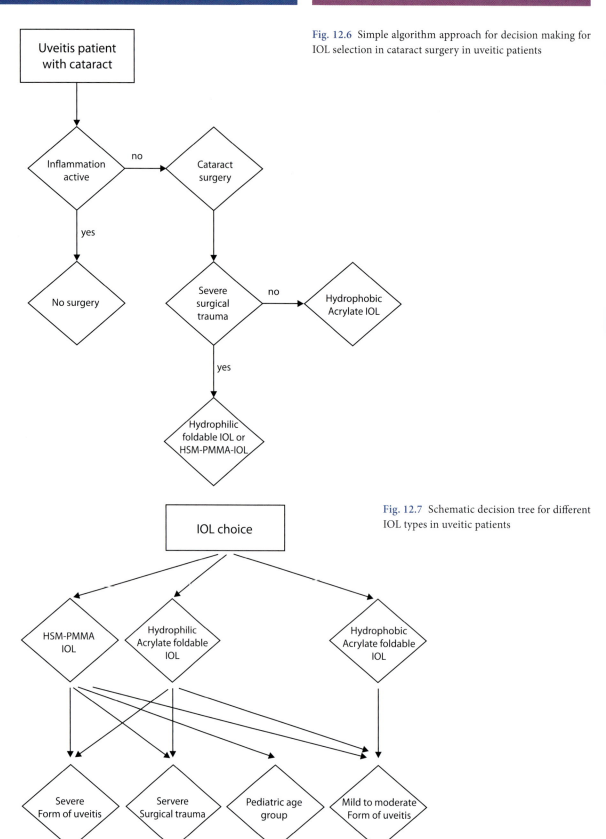

Fig. 12.6 Simple algorithm approach for decision making for IOL selection in cataract surgery in uveitic patients

Fig. 12.7 Schematic decision tree for different IOL types in uveitic patients

Cataract surgery in uveitic patients can range from minimally invasive surgical trauma in soft subcapsular cataracts without other pathologies to very traumatic cases with dense cataracts, synechiae and low endothelial cell counts. Cataract surgery can be necessary from the pediatric age group up to the "normal" age group of the elderly patient.

In general, choice of IOL type and material depends on the severity of the expected trauma and the severity of the expected reaction of the eye (Figs. 12.6 and 12.7) [2, 3, 5, 18–21, 24, 29, 31, 32, 35, 36].

12.9 Hydrophilic Acrylate IOLs and Uveitis

Hydrophilic IOLs can be used in almost every uveitis case regardless of the severity of the disease and postoperative expected inflammatory reaction. They have the best biocompatibility as described above and are used worldwide in these cases [1, 4, 6, 15, 23, 32–34]. The only exceptions may be pediatric cases, when the surgeon is unsure of the long-term tolerance of this material. In these cases, a heparin surface-modified PMMA IOL is a safe choice.

12.10 Hydrophobic Acrylate IOLs and Uveitis

There are numerous reports that implantation of hydrophobic acrylate foldable IOLs are well tolerated in uncomplicated cataract surgery in uveitic patients [2, 3, 18–21, 29, 31–32]. The advantage of reduced posterior capsule opacification in the generally younger uveitic patients is another advantage. However, cell adherence and attraction of foreign body giant cells is higher in hydrophobic acrylate IOLs. Therefore, they are only recommended in minimally invasive cases.

12.11 Hydrophobic Silicone IOLs and Uveitis

In general, hydrophobic silicone IOLs are not recommended in uveitis cataract surgery. They tend to provoke anterior capsule fibrosis, display a high degree of cell adhesion (Figs. 12.4 and 12.5) and are incompatible with silicone oil use in vitreoretinal surgery, which is also often necessary in uveitis patients [4, 6, 14, 15, 31].

12.12 PMMA IOLs and Uveitis

PMMA IOLs with heparin surface modification have been for a long time the standard IOL choice in uveitis cataract surgery. They still are a safe choice in any indication. However, the large incisions of up to 7 mm may increase the postoperative breakdown of the blood–aqueous barrier, thus resulting in a higher amount of postoperative inflammation. Nevertheless, HSM-PMMA IOLs can still be regarded as a safe alternative to hydrophilic foldable IOLs, especially in younger or pediatric patients [4, 14].

> Choice of intraocular lens includes:
> - Hydrophilic acrylic foldable IOLs and heparin surface-modified PMMA IOLs are the best-tolerated implants in uveitic patients.
> - Hydrophobic acrylic foldable IOLs may be used in cases of minimal surgical trauma and mild uveitic reactions.
> - In pediatric cataract cases, heparin surface-modified PMMA IOLs may have the best long-term prognosis.

12.13 Special IOLs and Uveitis

Special IOLs such a multifocal, blue blocking or aspherical IOLs are rarely usable in uveitic patients. These lenses are usually implanted in eyes without other pathology. Any additional ocular disease may compromise the function or advantages of these IOL types. Multifocal IOLs may result in a loss of contrast sensitivity, blue-blocking IOLs may not give any advantage to the uveitic patients who also have retinal disease and aspherical IOLs should not be used if pupil deformations or pathologies are present. As uveitis is a chronic, lifelong disease, the problems with these lenses may become even more significant over time.

12.14 Secondary Implants and Uveitis

Secondary implantation of an IOL occurs in cases where surgery was very complicated, resulting in a loss of capsular support for an IOL or in cases where an IOL was not initially implanted, such as in congenital or pediatric cataract surgery. In these cases, HSM-PMMA IOLs or hydrophilic foldable IOLs are the choice for transscleral fixation of an implant in uveitic patients. Anterior chamber IOLs or iris fixated IOLs are contraindicated as they are implanted at the site where inflammatory reactions occur [6, 8].

12.15 Contraindications for IOL Implantation in Uveitis

It is difficult to differentiate between contraindications for IOL implantation and contraindications for cataract surgery in general in uveitis. Nowadays, purely curative lens extraction without IOL implantation is a rare but possible situation. If cataract surgery is indicated to improve vision, to prevent blindness or amblyopia or to keep the patient in the work force, generally IOL implantation is possible, too.

In severe cases of Behçet's disease, or severe forms of intermediate or posterior uveitis, there might be a contraindication for cataract surgery in general, including IOL implantation.

Contraindications for cataract surgery with IOL implantation may include:
- Lens opacities not causing decreased vision
- Inflammatory choroidal effusion
- Any acute uveitis form
- Exudative retinal detachment
- Hypotony due to cyclitic membranes
- Chronic untreatable CME with macular damage
- Poor prognosis for visual improvement

Cataract surgery with IOL implantation should improve vision and quality of life in uveitic patients. A careful decision should always be based on the general situation of the patient, the stage of his disease and his expected prognosis [3–6, 14, 18–24, 31–36].

References

1. Abela-Formanek C, Amon M, Schild G, Schauersberger J, Kolodjaschna J, Barisani-Asenbaum T, Kruger A. (2002) Inflammation after implantation of hydrophilic acrylic, hydrophobic acrylic, or silicone intraocular lenses in eyes with cataract and uveitis: comparison to a control group. J Cataract Refract Surg. Jul;28(7):1153–9
2. Akova YA, Kucukerdonmez C, Gedik S. (2006) Clinical results of phacoemulsification in patients with uveitis. Ophthalmic Surg Lasers Imaging. May–Jun;37(3):204–11
3. Alio JL, Chipont E, BenEzra D, Fakhry MA. (2002) International Ocular Inflammation Society, Study Group of Uveitic Cataract Surgery. Comparative performance of intraocular lenses in eyes with cataract and uveitis. J Cataract Refract Surg. Dec;28(12):2096–108
4. Amon M. (2001) Biocompatibility of intraocular lenses. J Cataract Refract Surg. Feb;27(2):178–9
5. Androudi S, Ahmed M, Fiore T, Brazitikos P, Foster CS. (2005) Combined pars plana vitrectomy and phacoemulsification to restore visual acuity in patients with chronic uveitis. J Cataract Refract Surg. Mar;31(3):472–8
6. Apple DJ, Auffarth GU, Peng Q, Visessook N. (2000) Foldable intraocular lenses: evolution, clinicopathologic correlations and complications. SLACK Incorporated (Verlag), Thorofare, NJ, USA, ISBN 1-55642-435-3
7. Apple DJ, Peng Q, Arthur SN, Werner L, Merritt JH, Vargas LG, Hoddinott DS, Escobar-Gomez M, Schmidbauer JM. (2002) Snowflake degeneration of polymethyl methacrylate posterior chamber intraocular lens optic material: a newly described clinical condition caused by unexpected late opacification of polymethyl methacrylate. Ophthalmology. Sep;109(9):1666–75
8. Auffarth GU, Apple DJ. (2001) Zur Entwicklungsgeschichte der Intraokularlinsen. Der Ophthalmologe. 98:1017–28
9. Auffarth GU, Brezin A, Caporossi A, Mendicute J, Berdeaux G, Smith AF. (2004) Comparison of Nd:YAG capsulotomy rates following phacoemulsification with implantation of PMMA, silicone, or acrylic intra-ocular lenses in four European countries. Ophthalmic Epidemiol. Oct;11(4):319–29
10. Auffarth GU, Golescu A, Becker KA, Völcker HE. (2003) Quantification of posterior capsule opacification with round and sharp edge intraocular lenses. Ophthalmology. 110:772–780
11. Auffarth GU, Peng Q. (2000) Posterior capsule opacification: pathology, clinical evaluation and current means of prevention. Ophthalmic Practice. 18:4:172–82
12. Auffarth GU, Ries M, Tetz MR, Becker KA, Limberger IJ, Völcker HE. (2002) Posterior capsule opacification after implantation of polyfluorocarbon-coated intraocular lenses: a longterm follow-up. Dev Ophthalmol. 34:202–8
13. Auffarth GU, Wilcox M, Sims JCR, McCabe C, Wesendahl TA, Apple DJ. (1995) Analysis of 100 explanted one piece and three piece silicone intraocular lenses. Ophthalmology. 102:1144–50
14. Auffarth GU. (2005) Intraokularlinsenmaterialien. In: Kampik A, Grehn F (eds.) Augenärztliche Rehabilitation. Thieme (Publ.), Stuttgart, New York: 58–63
15. Beasley AM, Auffarth GU, Recum AV. (1996) Intraocular lens implants: a biocompatibility review. J Invest Surg. 9:399–413
16. Becker KA, Martin M, Rabsilber TM, Entz BB, Reuland AJ, Auffarth GU. (2006) Prospective, non-randomised,

long-term clinical evaluation of a foldable hydrophilic single-piece intraocular lens: results of the Centerflex FDA study. Br J Ophthalmol. Aug;90(8):971–4

17. Frohn A, Dick HB, Augustin AJ, Grus FH. (2001) Late opacification of the foldable hydrophilic acrylic lens SC60B-OUV. Ophthalmology. Nov;108(11):1999–2004

18. Ganesh SK, Babu K, Biswas J. (2004) Phacoemulsification with intraocular lens implantation in cases of pars planitis. J Cataract Refract Surg. Oct;30(10):2072–6

19. Ganesh SK, Padmaja BK, Biswas J. (2004) Cataract surgery in patients with Vogt-Koyanagi-Harada syndrome. J Cataract Refract Surg. Jan;30(1):95–100

20. Javadi MA, Jafarinasab MR, Araghi AA, Mohammadpour M, Yazdani S. (2005) Outcomes of phacoemulsification and in-the-bag intraocular lens implantation in Fuchs' heterochromic iridocyclitis. J Cataract Refract Surg. May;31(5):997–1001

21. Koura Y, Fukushima A, Nishino K, Ishida W, Nakakuki T, Sento M, Yamazoe K, Yamaguchi T, Misyoshi T, Ueno H. (2006) Inflammatory reaction following cataract surgery and implantation of acrylic intraocular lens in rabbits with endotoxin-induced uveitis. Eye. May;20(5):606–10

22. Manuchehri K, Mohamed S, Cheung D, Saeed T, Murray PI. (2004) Brown deposits in the optic of foldable intraocular lenses in patients with uveitis. Eye. Jan;18(1):54–8

23. Meacock WR, Spalton DJ, Bender L, Antcliff R, Heatley C, Stanford MR, Graham EM. (2004) Steroid prophylaxis in eyes with uveitis undergoing phacoemulsification. Br J Ophthalmol. Sep;88(9):1122–4

24. Monden Y. (2002) Intraocular lenses in patients with uveitis. Kurume Med J. 49(3):91–7

25. Nishi O, Nishi K, Akura J. (2002) Speed of capsular bend formation at the optic edge of acrylic, silicone, and poly(methyl methacrylate) lenses. J Cataract Refract Surg. Mar;28(3):431–7

26. Nishi O, Nishi K, Wada K, Ohmoto Y. (1999) Expression of transforming growth factor (TGF)-alpha, TGF-beta (2) and interleukin 8 messenger RNA in postsurgical and cultured lens epithelial cells obtained from patients with senile cataracts. Graefes Arch Clin Exp Ophthalmol. Oct;237(10):806–11

27. Nishi O, Nishi K, Wickstrom K. (2000) Preventing lens epithelial cell migration using intraocular lenses with sharp rectangular edges. J Cataract Refract Surg. Oct;26(10):1543–9

28. Nishi O. (1999) Posterior capsule opacification part 1: experimental investigations. J Cataract Refract Surg. Jan;25(1):106–17

29. Petric I, Loncar VL, Vatavuk Z, Ivekovic R, Sesar I, Mandic Z. (2005) Cataract surgery and intraocular lens implantation in children with juvenile rheumatoid arthritis associated uveitis. Coll Antropol. 29(Suppl 1):59–62

30. Rabsilber TM, Reuland AJ, Entz BB, Holzer MP, Limberger IJ, Auffarth GU. (2006) Quantitative Nachstarevaluierung von Acrylat- und Silikonintraokularlinsen mit scharfem Kantendesign. Der Ophthalmologe. Jan;103(1):25–9

31. Rahman I, Jones NP. (2005) Long-term results of cataract extraction with intraocular lens implantation in patients with uveitis. Eye. Feb;19(2):191–7

32. Ram J, Kaushik S, Brar GS, Gupta A, Gupta A. (2002) Phacoemulsification in patients with Fuchs' heterochromic uveitis. J Cataract Refract Surg. Aug;28(8):1372–8

33. Schauersberger J, Amon M, Aichinger D, Georgopoulos A. (2003) Bacterial adhesion to rigid and foldable posterior chamber intraocular lenses: in vitro study. J Cataract Refract Surg. Feb;29(2):361–6

34. Schild G, Amon M, Abela-Formanek C, Schauersberger J, Bartl G, Kruger A. (2004) Uveal and capsular biocompatibility of a single-piece, sharp-edged hydrophilic acrylic intraocular lens with collagen (Collamer): 1-year results. J Cataract Refract Surg. Jun;30(6):1254–8

35. Till JS. (2003) Collamer intraocular lens implantation with active uveitis. J Cataract Refract Surg. Dec;29(12):2439–43

36. Tognetto D, Toto L, Minutola D, Ballone E, Di Nicola M, Di Mascio R, Ravalico G. (2003) Hydrophobic acrylic versus heparin surface-modified polymethylmethacrylate intraocular lens: a biocompatibility study. Graefes Arch Clin Exp Ophthalmol. Aug;241(8):625–30

Management of Posterior Synechiae, Peripheral Anterior Synechiae, Iridocorneal Adhesions, and Iridectomy

Yosuf El-Shabrawi

Core Messages

- Surgical interventions in uveitic patients frequently produce frustrating results, due either to intraoperative complications or exuberant postoperative inflammation. The primary goal of every uveitis therapy, therefore, should be the prevention of ocular damage requiring subsequent surgery.
- Posterior synechiae are the most common ocular complications in chronic or recurrent anterior uveitis, occurring in 13–91% of affected eyes.
- Peripheral anterior synechiae are usually asymptomatic unless large areas of at least 270° are involved.
- Central iridocorneal synechiae are frequently associated with rubeotic iris vessels. Thus, due to the high frequency of intraoperative bleeding and to the high recurrence rates, a synechiolysis should rather be avoided if possible.
- Complete quiescence should be sought; however, when acute surgical interventions are required, especially in the case of iridectomies, they should not be postponed until further irreversible adverse events occur.

Contents

13.1	Introduction	132		13.3.4	Clinical Manifestation	133
13.2	Posterior Synechiae	132		13.3.4.1	Asymptomatic	133
13.2.1	Etiology	132		13.3.4.2	Symptomatic	133
13.2.2	Incidence	132		13.3.5	Procedures	133
13.2.3	Clinical Appearance	132		13.3.5.1	Medical Care	133
13.2.4	Procedures	132		13.3.5.2	Laser Care	134
13.2.4.1	Medical Treatment	132		13.3.5.3	Surgical Interventions	134
13.2.4.2	Surgical Treatment	132		13.3.5.4	Surgical Interventions for Central Iridocorneal Adhesions	134
13.2.4.3	Surgical Technique	132		13.4	Laser Iridotomy, Iridectomy	134
13.3	Peripheral Anterior Synechiae, Iridocorneal Adhesions	133		13.4.1	Laser Iridotomy	135
13.3.1	Background	133		13.4.2	Surgical Iridectomy	135
13.3.2	Etiology	133		13.5	Consecutive Medical Treatment	135
13.3.3	Incidence	133		References		136

13.1 Introduction

Uveitic eyes, even those appearing clinically quiet, tend to show unexpected intraoperative complications. Bleeding from the corneoscleral wound, the iris or detachment of Descemet's membrane following the dissection of iridocorneal adhesions may occur. Exuberant inflammation is also a dreaded postoperative complication, frequently leading to frustrating results of the ocular surgery. Hence, the main goal in treating uveitic patients should be the prevention of complications of chronic or recurrent uveitis to reduce the need for surgery in the first place [1]. If surgery is inevitable, every effort should be made to keep inflammation under control for as long as possible preoperatively, except for those situations requiring immediate surgery. In those instances, inflammatory activity should be reduced as far as possible, but surgery should not be postponed indefinitely, as this would risk additional irreversible damage [2]. Even with the most potent anti-inflammatory drugs, there may be irreversible damage to the normal ocular architecture, most commonly in the form of posterior synechiae [3–6].

13.2 Posterior Synechiae

13.2.1 Etiology

Posterior synechiae usually develop with chronic persistent or recurrent uveitis, such as HLA B27-associated uveitis, idiopathic anterior uveitis, iridocyclitis in juvenile idiopathic arthritis, sarcoidosis, intermediate uveitis, lens-induced uveitis (e.g., phacolytic, lens particle, phacoanaphylaxis) and uveitis-glaucoma-hyphema (UGH) syndrome. Infectious uveitis entities such as herpes simplex, herpes zoster, tuberculosis and syphilis may also be associated with formation of posterior synechiae. Fuchs heterochromic iridocyclitis, however, typically lacks posterior synechiae.

13.2.2 Incidence

In HLA B27-associated uveitis, posterior synechiae are described in 13–91% of cases. In patients suffering from HLA B27-negative uveitis, the numbers vary from 7% to 46% [3–6].

13.2.3 Clinical Appearance

Posterior synechiae may be present as focal adhesions, or may extend over the entire surface of the lens, if pupillary or prelental membranes are present.

13.2.4 Procedures

13.2.4.1 Medical Treatment

Newly formed synechiae should be treated with intensive local anti-inflammatory therapy in addition to short-acting mydriatics. Alternatively, mydriatic combinations (containing 0.3% cocaine hydrochloride, atropine sulfate 0.1%, adrenaline (epinephrine) 1:10,000.03) [7] can be injected subconjunctivally into the inferior fornix. Subconjunctival mydriatic combinations should, however, be used with care, since adverse cardiac events may occur.

13.2.4.2 Surgical Treatment

Posterior synechiae surgery is usually combined with cataract surgery or to ensure optimal visualization for vitrectomy. Local, circumscribed adhesions can easily be lysed with a blunt spatula or by injection of high molecular weight ophthalmic viscoelastic devices (OVD). Sharp dissections of posterior synechiae should be avoided.

13.2.4.3 Surgical Technique

Depending on the surgeon's experience, the extent of the posterior synechiae, the patient, as well as additional surgical steps planned, such as vitrectomy, the procedure can be done under general, retrobulbar, peribulbar as well as topical anesthesia. After a corneal incision, attempts can be made to hydrodissect the posterior synechiae using a 27-gauge cannula attached to a 2 ml syringe filled with a mydriatic agent such as adrenaline 1:10,000. Alternatively, circumscribed synechiae are usually easily lysed with an iris spatula. In instances of pupils of less than 3 mm, large prelental membranes should be expected. In these eyes, the dissection of posterior synechiae should be attempted only in the presence of intracameral high molecular weight OVD, to maintain constant intraocular pressure as otherwise bleeding from iris vessels can be expected.

The high molecular OVDs may be applied either directly into the anterior chamber or, after performing an iridectomy, beneath the iris onto the anterior lens capsule, thus lifting the iris from the lens capsule or prelental membrane; this disrupts the iris adhesions, coming from the periphery toward the sphincter of the pupil. If this proves to be inefficient, a small, sharp dissection of adhesions at the sphincter may be performed, using either Vannas scissors, or alternatively, a 23-gauge needle. This is then followed by a blunt dissection for 360° using an iris spatula. In addition, rubeotic iris vessels should be carefully cauterized prior to the dissection from the anterior lens capsule, again to prevent or at least lower the risk of bleeding.

13.3 Peripheral Anterior Synechiae, Iridocorneal Adhesions

13.3.1 Background

In the presence of chronic anterior or intermediate uveitis, a membrane may form between the iris and the trabecular meshwork. If this membrane contracts, an anterior pulling mechanism will result in an angle-closure glaucoma. In rare instances, cyclitic membranes may also grow, coming from the angle over the entire surface of the iris and the peripheral cornea. The anterior pulling mechanisms of such a membrane lead to an irreversible destruction of the ciliary body, followed by ciliary body failure, hypotony and ultimately resulting in a phthisical eye. To evaluate the full extent of the presence of peripheral anterior synechiae, imaging studies using ultrasound biomicroscopy (UBM) or corneal specular microscopy may be required.

13.3.2 Etiology

As already described for posterior synechiae, peripheral anterior synechiae (PAS) as well as central anterior iridocorneal adhesions usually develop with chronic persistent or recurrent forms of uveitis, including JIA-associated iridocyclitis, interstitial keratitis, lens-related uveitis, sarcoidosis and intermediate uveitis, as well as UGH syndrome. Infective causes include herpes simplex, herpes zoster, tuberculosis and syphilis. Anterior synechiae are typically not found in Fuchs heterochromic iridocyclitis.

13.3.3 Incidence

Peripheral anterior synechiae are rare.

13.3.4 Clinical Manifestation

13.3.4.1 Asymptomatic

Unless large areas of at least 270° are involved, PAS are usually asymptomatic. The morbidity of PAS lies in the occlusion of the angle followed by angle-closure glaucoma.

13.3.4.2 Symptomatic

1. Acute angle closure: Produces the classic symptoms of acute angle-closure glaucoma, such as ocular pain, headaches, nausea, blurred vision and halos.
2. Subacute: History of multiple transient attacks, which consist of mild ocular pain, reduced vision and halos.
3. Chronic with vision loss due to glaucomatous optic neuropathy.

13.3.5 Procedures

13.3.5.1 Medical Care

Treatment of PAS should only be considered when there is an increase in intraocular pressure or progressive narrowing of the angle, as no specific medical management is available. Anti-glaucoma treatments that may be administered when there is increased IOP include topical beta-blockers, topical alpha-agonists, topical carbonic anhydrase inhibitors, as well as topical prostaglandin analogs. Miotics and epinephrine should be avoided in uveitic patients, as they can increase inflammation and may lead to posterior synechiae. Short-acting cycloplegics should be used to prevent posterior synechiae. But again, the main focus should always be control of inflammation. Thus, depending on the activity of the uveitis, topical corticosteroids or immune modulatory treatment should be administered to minimize inflammation and, subsequently, the formation of additional PAS.

13.3.5.2 Laser Care

Since persistent inflammation usually produces significant scarring in the trabecular meshwork (TM) within 6 months, a surgical intervention should be considered at an early stage of the disease. Afterward, the angle can still be opened, but the TM will not function normally due to scarring.

1. As a primary step, anterior chamber (AC) compression with a Zeiss gonioprism may be successful in breaking a pupillary block or early posterior synechiae.
2. Nd:YAG/argon laser iridotomy: Due to the high incidence of secondary closure of more than 50% after an average of 85 days, YAG/argon laser iridotomy usually proves to be a frustrating choice.
3. Argon laser peripheral iridoplasty: When PAS continue to form after an iridotomy, laser iridoplasty might be tried. By creating burns in the peripheral iris that cause the iris to contract, the iris is pulled away from the TM, rupturing PAS. It may even be used to prevent an acute angle-closure attack and/or break up posterior synechiae by enlarging the pupil.
4. Nd:YAG peripheral synechiolysis can be attempted in early synechial closure but may not be effective if the synechiae are firm. Laser synechiolysis should be attempted before surgical goniosynechiolysis.

13.3.5.3 Surgical Interventions

1. Viscodissection after anterior chamber (AC) paracenthesis with subsequent injection of a viscoelastic device into the AC.
2. Surgical goniosynechiolysis: Using a smooth-tipped irrigating cyclodialysis spatula, the iris can be separated from the TM, rupturing the PAS. This is not recommended unless synechial closure is 270° or more.
3. Surgical iridectomy is performed when an iridotomy is indicated but is not feasible.
4. If significant glaucomatous cupping associated with visual field loss is present, a filtering operation would be preferred to goniosynechiolysis.

13.3.5.4 Surgical Interventions for Central Iridocorneal Adhesions

Since anterior synechiae have a very high recurrence rate after surgery, in addition to the fact that surgical dissection of the membranes from the cornea may be challenging, due to local detachment of Descemet's membrane, or bleeding, they should be left in place and untouched if at all possible. Only in the rare instances in which large cyclitic membranes grow onto the anterior surface of both the iris and the corneal endothelium should an early intervention be attempted. In these patients, after intracameral instillation of a high molecular OVD, blunt dissection of the membrane from both the iris surface as well as the cornea should be attempted. This should be followed by an extensive vitrectomy, whereby special care has to be taken that the ciliary body is freed from the membrane as extensively as possible. If cyclitic membranes growing onto the iris surface are seen, surgery should be planned as soon as possible, as otherwise the dissection of the membrane, due to its large extension, proves highly difficult. In addition, frequently the development of an ocular hypotony may occur, caused by ciliary body failure because of a long-standing cyclitic membrane.

13.4 Laser Iridotomy, Iridectomy

Patients with larger posterior synechiae may develop secondary glaucoma due to pupillary block and subsequent angle closure. In contrast to laser iridotomies in individuals without intraocular inflammatory diseases, there is a high early failure rate of YAG iridotomy in patients with angle-closure glaucoma secondary to pupillary block from uveitis. Patients with intraocular inflammatory diseases show a tendency toward secondary closure. A study by Spencer et al. [8] comparing iridotomies in uveitic patients with those in "normal" glaucoma patients very clearly demonstrated this tendency toward a higher incidence of failure. In the study group of 11 uveitic patients, 28 iridotomies were performed on 15 eyes; of these 28 iridotomies, 17 failed. Using Kaplan–Meier survival analysis, the median time to failure was 85 days. In the control group of 65 "normal" glaucoma patients, 66 iridotomies were performed on 66 eyes. None of the iridotomies in the control group failed.

13.4.1 Laser Iridotomy

The yttrium aluminum garnet (YAG) laser may be applied directly in the superior peripheral iris. In heavily pigmented irises, which are usually thicker, a prior treatment with approximately 20 spots of an argon laser at 200 mW, 0.1 s duration, and 50 µm spot size [1] may be recommended, as it leads to thinning of the iris and so reduces intraoperative bleeding. This pretreatment is then followed by a YAG laser in the center of the areas previously prepared with the argon laser. If bleeding does occur, pressure should be applied on the globe be pressing with the contact lens. Due to the tendency toward secondary closure of the iridotomies, at least two drains should be applied.

13.4.2 Surgical Iridectomy

A 2–3-mm-wide circumferential corneal incision close to the limbus is created. In some instances, this may be preceded by a one-clock-hour limbal peritomy. This corneal incision should reach only to the level of Descemet's membrane at first and not yet perforate the anterior chamber. Then with one continuous cut, Descemet's membrane should be incised to collapse the anterior chamber. This is usually followed by prolapse of the iris. The iris can then be excised easily using Vannas scissors. If the iris does not prolapse spontaneously, mild pressure onto the sclera may make it do so. If this again is not effective, iris tissue may be grasped with forceps.

Due to frequent closures of small iridectomies, sector iridectomies should be performed with 360° posterior synechiae. Special care should be taken that a full thickness iridectomy is performed; this must include the pigmented epithelium. In addition, in pseudophakic eyes of uveitic patients, care has to be taken that the iridectomy is functional, since often, after inadequately performed cataract surgery, residual lens material may occlude drainage. In these instances, the iridectomy should be irrigated with a 27-gauge cannula, but care has to be taken not to disrupt the vitreous anterior hyaloid face and so cause a spontaneous vitreous prolapse.

After a successful iridectomy has been performed, a mild massage of the wound to the central cornea will result in spontaneous regression of the iris back into the eye, followed by tight closure of the corneal wound using 10-0 nylon sutures. After surgery, subconjunctival steroid injections in addition to local antibiotics should be given.

13.5 Consecutive Medical Treatment

For both surgical interventions in posterior synechiae as well as iridectomies, the perioperative medical treatment should include 1 mg/kg/day of systemic corticosteroids, especially in patients who required systemic corticosteroid therapy for previous uveitis episodes. We usually give topical nonsteroidal drugs four times a day for about a week preoperatively, to reduce intraoperative miosis as well as postoperative inflammation. In addition, a subconjunctival corticosteroid injection (betamethasone, 2–4 mg, or methylprednisolone, 15 mg in 0.5 ml) is given at the time of surgery. The surgeon should be cautious and expect, even in a previously relatively quiet eye, the development of delayed inflammation a few days after surgery following the intensive preoperative anti-inflammatory treatment. Patients should be checked at short intervals, if possible even daily for the first week.

> **Take Home Pearls**
>
> - Surgical treatment of posterior synechiae includes blunt hydrodissection, synechiolysis with high molecular weight ophthalmic viscoelastic devices (OVD) or small, sharp incisions of the adhesion sites followed by further blunt dissection.
> - Local, circumscribed posterior synechiae are usually lysed by either hydrodissection in conjunction with a mydriatic agent or a blunt iris spatula.
> - Sharp dissections should be minimized.
> - With small pupils of less than 3 mm, large prelental membranes should be expected.
> - Peripheral anterior synechiae are frequently clinically asymptomatic unless more than 270° are involved. They may be treated using either viscodissection or surgical goniosynechiolysis, using a smooth-tipped irrigating cyclodialysis spatula. This is, however not recommended unless synechial closure is 270° or more.
> - Due to the high failure rate of YAG iridotomy in instances of angle-closure glaucoma in uveitic patients, an iridectomy should be performed instead.
> - Due to frequent closures of small iridectomies, sector iridectomies should be performed with 360° posterior synechiae.

References

1. Foster CS, Vitale AT. Diagnosis and treatment of uveitis. Philadelphia: Saunders; 2002
2. Nussenblatt RB, Palestine AG, Whitecup SM. Uveitis: fundamentals in clinical practice. Saint Louis: Mosby; 2003
3. Chang JH, McCluskey PJ, Wakefield D. Acute anterior uveitis and HLA-B27. Surv Ophthalmol 2005;50(4):364–88
4. Linssen A, Meenken C. Outcomes of HLA-B27-positive and HLA-B27-negative acute anterior uveitis. Am J Ophthalmol 1995;120(3):351–61
5. Monnet D, Breban M, Hudry C, et al. Ophthalmic findings and frequency of extraocular manifestations in patients with HLA-B27 uveitis: a study of 175 cases. Ophthalmology 2004;111(4):802–9
6. Power WJ, Rodriguez A, Pedroza-Seres M, Foster CS. Outcomes in anterior uveitis associated with the HLA-B27 haplotype. Ophthalmology 1998;105(9):1646–51
7. Heiligenhaus A, Heinz C, Becker MD. Treatment of uveitis cataract. In: Krieglstein GK, Weinreb RN, editors. Cataract and refractive surgery—essentials in ophthalmology. Heidelberg: Springer; 2004
8. Spencer NA, Hall AJ, Stawell RJ. Nd:YAG laser iridotomy in uveitic glaucoma. Clin Experiment Ophthalmol 2001;29(4):217–9

Lens / Chapter 14

Complications Post Cataract Surgery in the Uveitic Eye

Marie-José Tassignon, Dimitrios Sakellaris

Core Messages

- The pathogenesis of the postoperative inflammatory reaction in uveitic eyes is breakdown of the blood–aqueous barrier (BAB).
- The postoperative inflammatory reaction consists of a uveal response and a capsular response.
- Both types of inflammatory response also appear in normal eyes after cataract surgery, but the reaction in uveitic eyes is more pronounced and prolonged.
- The degree of the postoperative uveal and capsular response depends on the type of uveitis, the type of the IOL biomaterial and the perioperative medication strategy.
- The perioperative medical and surgical plan for uveitis patients should be decided on an individual basis.
- The uveitic cataract patient should be warned that pre- and postoperative care will be more demanding.

Contents

14.1	Introduction	137	14.4	Postoperative Ocular Hypertension, Glaucoma and Hypotony	141
14.2	Postoperative Inflammation	138	14.5	Cystoid Macular Edema and Retinal Detachment	141
14.2.1	Uveal Response	138			
14.2.2	Capsular Response	139	14.6	Hyphema and Rubeosis	141
14.3	Clinical Features of Capsular Response	139	14.7	The Bag-in-the-Lens Surgical Technique as a New Surgical Approach	142
14.3.1	Posterior Capsule Opacification	139			
14.3.2	Postoperative Synechiae	140	References		142
14.3.3	Capsular Contraction and IOL Dislocation	140			

This chapter contains the following video clips on DVD: Video 7 shows Bimanual capsular peeling, Video 8 shows Anterior capsulorhexis with the use of the ring caliper, Video 9 shows Implantation of the bag-in-the-lens and Video 10 shows Posterior capsulorhexis and injection of viscoelastic in the space of Berger (Surgeon: Marie Jose Tassignon).

14.1 Introduction

Uveitis may affect children, young adults, adults or the elderly, commonly giving rise to early- or late-onset cataract in relation to the type, location and intensity of inflammation and corticosteroid use [4, 13]. Inflammation can be preferentially located in the anterior segment, the ciliary body, or the posterior segment of the eye or can affect all eye compartments. Patients suffering from anterior and/or intermediate uveitis are more prone to develop cataract than patients with posterior uveitis only [19]. Inflammation can be mild, moderate or severe and as a consequence may jeopardize visual outcome after cataract surgery due to associated glaucoma, vitreoretinal or choroidal pathology. The blood–aqueous barrier (BAB) of the eye is usually impaired.

Furthermore, cataracts in uveitic patients are often associated with small pupils, posterior synechiae, pupillary membranes, decreased corneal transparency and fragile iris vessels, which make cataract surgery more difficult for the surgeon and increase the surgical risk. Primary posterior chamber intraocular lens (IOL) implantations have been controversial because the foreign body reaction exacerbates the uveal BAB due to surgery. However, recent studies have reported favorable results from cataract surgery with IOL implantation in patients with various types of uveal inflammation [1–4, 12]. Some types of uveitis give particularly good results, for example, Fuchs heterochromic iridocyclitis, in which cataract surgery and IOL implantation can be performed without hesitation [9, 20]. In other types of uveitis, such as juvenile idiopathic arthritis (JIA) associated uveitis and phacoanaphylactic uveitis, IOL implantation remains controversial.

Cataract surgery in uveitic patients should only be performed after extensive evaluation of all ocular and systemic factors that might influence inflammation. Even a so-called burned-out uveitis case may present severe postoperative inflammation after uneventful cataract surgery.

Perioperative medication plays a major role in postoperative outcomes. Except for Fuchs heterochromic iridocyclitis, each uveitic eye undergoing cataract surgery should be prepared carefully before surgery, either with anti-inflammatory drugs or systemic anti-inflammatory or immunosuppressive medication, depending on the preoperative ocular and systemic condition. It is generally accepted that one step higher of topical, local or systemic medication should be prescribed preoperatively than the medication under which uveitis control has been achieved. A standard operating procedure is not applicable for the uveitic patient undergoing cataract surgery. On the contrary, a case-by-case approach is advised.

14.2 Postoperative Inflammation

Posterior chamber IOL implantation, and more specifically the intracapsular implantation or lens-in-the-bag (LIB) implantation technique, is currently the most common surgical technique used, including in uveitic patients. This procedure consists of implanting a J- or C-looped IOL in the capsular bag as illustrated in Fig. 14.1a. With this implantation technique, contact of the biomaterial with the capsule occurs along the posterior surface of the optic, the haptics and partially along the anterior surface of the optic.

The inflammatory reaction induced by surgery and the implantation of an IOL has been studied extensively by Abela-Formanek et al. [1–3]. Because the IOL prosthesis that replaces the natural crystalline lens is manufactured from a foreign biomaterial, recognition and acceptance need to occur. In uveitis, alteration in the immune system and chronic BAB breakdown in the uvea can be exacerbated by surgical stress. This reaction is called the uveal response, and it influences foreign

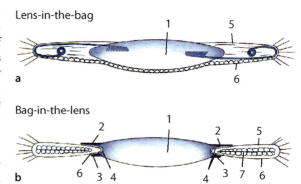

Fig. 14.1 Schematic drawing of the lens-in-the-bag (**a**) and the bag-in-the-lens (**b**) IOL positioning. IOL in place (*1*), anterior haptic (*2*), posterior haptic (*3*), lens groove in which the anterior and the posterior capsule rims are inserted (*4*), anterior capsule (*5*), posterior capsule (*6*), lens epithelial cells (*7*)

body acceptance in the early postoperative period and long term, depending on the biomaterial used. It is characterized by cellular deposition of small cells, large epitheloid and giant cells on the surface of the IOL. Activation of complement and inflammatory mediators (FGF, VGF, interleukins, etc.) [5] triggers lens epithelial cell (LEC) outgrowth and transformation, causing the well-known clinical features of anterior capsule opacification (ACO), posterior capsule opacification (PCO) and capsular contraction. This has been called the capsular response and is inherent to the surgical technique used (LIB). The foreign body reaction is facilitated because of the easy access of the inflammation mediators into the capsular bag through the anterior capsulorhexis.

14.2.1 Uveal Response

Small cellular deposits originate from monocytes that are released in the aqueous of the anterior chamber due to the breakdown of the BAB [29]. They appear the first postoperative day and peak at days 3 to 7, depending on the IOL biomaterial [1]. Their number decreases gradually 3–6 months postoperatively.

Epitheloid cells originate from macrophages and when merged, form giant cells [28, 29]. These cells are most commonly found in prolonged inflammatory reactions and peak 3 months postoperatively. They may last for months or even years and may reappear even after surgical cleansing or Nd:YAG laser IOL polishing [2]. Both small and large cells and even giant cell deposits are found in normal eyes after cataract surgery,

Table 14.1 Summary of uveal and capsular response of different IOL materials. **a** Uveal response. **b** Capsular response

a	Hydrophobic acrylic	Hydrophilic acrylic	Silicone
Small cell deposits	++	++	++
Giant cell deposits	++++	++	++

b	Hydrophobic acrylic	Hydrophilic acrylic	Silicone
ACR	+++	+++	+++
ACO	++	++	++
PCO in 3-mm zone	+	++	+
PCO in 3–6-mm zone	+	++	+

Intensity of reaction: + small, ++ mild, +++ moderate, ++++ severe
ACR anterior capsule rim opacification, *ACO* anterior capsule opacification, *PCO* posterior capsule opacification

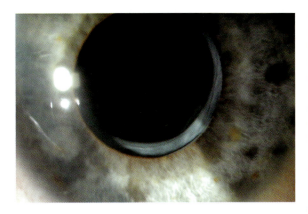

Fig. 14.2 Anterior capsule opacification and cellular IOL deposits: late uveal and capsular response

though their presence is usually more pronounced and prolonged in uveitic eyes (Fig. 14.2). The uveal response may account for differences among biomaterials, with less good results for the hydrophobic IOLs, as summarized in Table 14.1a [1].

14.2.2 Capsular Response

After cataract surgery, residual LECs at the capsular equator, and to a lesser degree along the anterior capsule, can grow and migrate, causing Elschnig pearl formation. Transformation and differentiation of the LECs into myofibroblasts can cause wrinkles and opacification of the lens capsule [8]. LEC outgrowth is decreased in the presence of inflammatory cytokines, which are released in higher concentrations and for a longer period in uveitis. The balance in cases of uveitis will thus be tipped toward LEC transformation and differentiation rather than LEC outgrowth [18]. LEC outgrowth and transformation are also present in normal eyes, but are more pronounced in the uveitic eye. The IOL biomaterial may also influence the capsular response, with less good results for the hydrophilic acrylic IOLs as summarized in Table 14.1b [1, 3].

14.3 Clinical Features of Capsular Response

14.3.1 Posterior Capsule Opacification

Posterior capsule opacification (PCO) is the most common complication after cataract surgery but has been reduced drastically the last decade thanks to improvement in surgical techniques, the use of hydrophobic IOL materials, square-edged IOL designs, and other innovations [7, 27]. Nd:YAG laser surgery remains the treatment of choice for an estimated 16% of normal eyes at 4 years postoperatively [7]. In uveitic patients and children, the incidence of PCO and Nd:YAG laser capsulotomy is much higher [23, 24]. Because of the lack of large-scale studies, exact numbers are unavailable, but 62% PCO and 31% Nd:YAG laser capsulotomy after an average follow-up of 20 months was reported in one study [12]. In an international study population, including the most benign cases of uveitis, 34.2% PCO was found after a 1-year follow-up [4].

Primary posterior capsulorhexis (PCCC) has been proposed but found to be unsuccessful in preventing PCO [30]. Iris capture is an option that has been studied in children and showed to be effective but not frequently used in uveitic patients [15]. PCCC is often, but incorrectly, considered damaging to the aqueous–vitreous barrier. Using fluorophotometry, this hypothesis has been refuted [10].

14.3.2 Postoperative Synechiae

Posterior synechiae are often present preoperatively in uveitic eyes (Fig. 14.3). Numbers on the order of 80% of cases have been proposed [16]. Their presence influences the surgical procedure. Iris manipulation during cataract surgery may exacerbate the uveal inflammatory reaction. Newly formed postoperative posterior synechiae are located between the anterior capsular rim and the papillary margin [17]. It is therefore advisable to use short-acting mydriatics and avoid miotics postoperatively. The entire margin may adhere to the capsular rim, giving rise to iris bombé in the absence of peripheral iridectomy. In severe cases, the entire posterior surface of the iris may react with the anterior capsule. Close postoperative monitoring is mandatory in order to titrate topical anti-inflammatory medication and mydriatics. Nd:YAG laser iridotomy can resolve iris bombé in the absence of peripheral iridectomy. Chronic inflammation may reclose the iridotomy, justifying a surgical approach as a primary or secondary step.

Tissue plasminogen injection in the anterior chamber, and more recently triamcinolone injections, have been proposed, although no long-term follow-up is available [6]. A surgical approach is not recommended since it may trigger inflammation. Nd:YAG laser synechiolysis has been proposed in mild cases in order to restore pupillary integrity. Pupillary membrane formation is uncommon but can be found in the early postoperative period in severely inflamed eyes. The first approach is medical by increasing the anti-inflammatory medication. The pupillary membrane will shrink as soon as the inflammation is under control. Nd:YAG laser is a good option to clear the visual axis, provided the eye is quiet.

Recurrences of synechiae are possible with time and are a sign of low-grade chronic uveal reaction. Postoperative anterior synechiae may cause ocular hypertension. Surgical detachment of anterior synechiae should be considered with care since bleeding and choroidal effusion may be induced. Dissection with high viscosity hyaluronic acid may be an option provided they are completely removed postoperatively in order to avoid severe hypertension.

14.3.3 Capsular Contraction and IOL Dislocation

The most severe stage of capsular response is capsular contraction syndrome (Fig. 14.4), a postoperative condition that is also found in nonuveitic patients [25]. Generally, it is not treated, but a surgical approach with capsular peeling to restore capsular integrity and refractive outcome is a new therapeutic option for this annoying postoperative condition. Capsular contraction may lead to capsular dislocation (Fig. 14.5), which is a late to very late (> 15 years) complication after cataract surgery [14]. Capsular dislocation is due to weakening of the zonular fibers with time. It is not specifically related to uveitis since this complication has also been described in myopia, pseudoexfoliation and in other conditions associated with fragile zonular fibers like Marfan's syndrome and homocystinuria. In most of the cases, these eyes do not present signs of clinical ocular inflammation. Treatment may vary between repositioning of the capsular bag using Cionni rings or other devices [14], or extraction of the capsular bag–IOL complex and implantation of an IOL fixated at the level of the iris. It is important to avoid IOLs positioned at the level of the iridocorneal angle in uveitis for obvious reasons, such as increased risk of peripheral anterior synechiae.

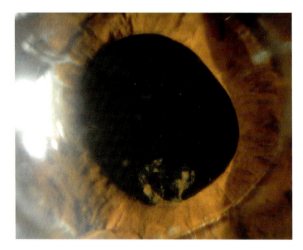

Fig. 14.3 Postoperative posterior synechiae on the primary IOL after an iris-claw toric IOL implantation to correct astigmatism after penetrating keratoplasty

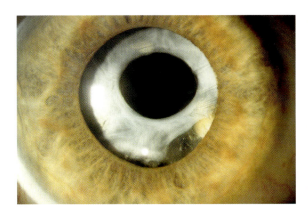

Fig. 14.4 Capsule contraction syndrome in sarcoidosis

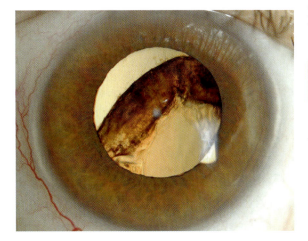

Fig. 14.5 Inferonasal IOL dislocation 15 years after surgery

14.4 Postoperative Ocular Hypertension, Glaucoma and Hypotony

Early postoperative hypotony is due to tractional ciliary body detachment or decreased secretion of the ciliary body due to ciliary body edema. Edema of the ciliary body will resolve in most of the cases. Ciliary detachment, however, will need a surgical approach by vitrectomy since the vitreous is a fundamental cause of the complication. The eye may be filled with expansile gas or silicone depending on the clinical severity.

Prolonged or late postoperative hypotony is an uncommon and severe complication in uveitis and is a consequence of ciliary body destruction due to inflammation. It is a severe complication because treatment is often unsuccessful and the eye ends up in most of the cases in phthisis. Vitrectomy and silicone filling of the eye can be proposed, but often with poor results [22]. High-frequency echography will help making the differential diagnosis between ciliary body edema and detachment [16].

Postoperative hypertension is a common complication after routine cataract surgery. Since it may be due to swelling of the trabecular meshwork, obstruction from cellular deposits, anterior synechiae or neovascularization, and because these conditions are more often seen in uveitic patients, it is to be expected that postoperative hypertension will be more frequent in uveitic eyes. Postoperative monitoring is again strongly recommended. Treatment is most often medical by topical or systemic antiglaucomatous medication. Glaucoma may be a preoperative condition, and in that case may influence postoperative outcome. Preexisting glaucoma will need closer postoperative monitoring to avoid postoperative hypertony.

14.5 Cystoid Macular Edema and Retinal Detachment

Cystoid macular edema (CME) has been for a long time the most feared complication of cataract surgery in uveitic eyes. An incidence of 50% has been found [23]. It is not proven, however, whether the incidence of CME is increased by IOL implantation [4]. Using optical coherence tomography (OCT), it has been possible to better monitor this posterior segment complication. A certain degree of CME is present in normal eyes after cataract extraction, and a higher amount would be expected in uveitic eyes after cataract surgery. In recent studies, triamcinolone injections have been proposed for the treatment of postoperative CME [6]. No large studies are available in uveitic patients using this drug. It is not known whether retinal detachment (RD) is more common in uveitic patients, but when it occurs, a greater risk of proliferative vitreoretinopathy may exist.

14.6 Hyphema and Rubeosis

Hemorrhages are frequently encountered during cataract surgery in Fuchs heterochromia (Amsler's sign) but resolve rapidly and will seldom cause postoperative hyphema. However, in vasculitis-associated uveitis, hyphema may be a common complication after cataract surgery.

Rubeosis may be present preoperatively and worsen postoperatively or may appear postoperatively in ischemic retinal conditions. Ischemia of the retina and retinal neovascularization should be assessed preoperatively. Panretinal photocoagulation, cryocoagulation and intravitreal or intracameral injection of bevacizumab (Avastin®) to reduce VEGF levels may be an option in addition to appropriate anti-inflammatory medication [26].

14.7 The Bag-in-the-Lens Surgical Technique as a New Surgical Approach

The surgical approach of this new concept of IOL implantation is illustrated in Fig. 14.1b. In the drawing, it can be observed that contact of the IOL biomaterial with the capsular bag is reduced to a small rim at the level of the groove present at the periphery of the lens optic and defined by both lens haptics. Anterior capsulorhexis is performed with the use of a ring calliper for optimal centration of the IOL, and PCCC is also performed. Because the anterior and posterior lens capsules are inserted into this groove, a tight and sealed capsular space is created in which the LECs, left behind after cataract surgery, are captured. These residual LECs do not come in contact with complements, interleukins or growth factors, triggering the LEC outgrowth and transformation. This IOL modification nullifies the capsular inflammatory response after cataract surgery. In addition, this IOL is manufactured with hydrophilic acrylic, which lessens the uveal inflammatory response. This IOL should theoretically reduce PCO and postoperative foreign body reaction.

Implantation of this IOL began in late 1999. Clinical experience has since been published showing that this IOL was well tolerated and that no PCO did occur in 100 normal patients followed for 1–4 years [21]. In addition, the IOL completely controlled PCO in children operated for congenital cataract [31]. Clinical experience with more than 650 cases, including some uveitic eyes and many diabetic eyes, shows no PCO and no unexpected postoperative inflammation or vitreous reaction despite the routinely performed PCCC. On theoretical and clinical basis, this IOL implantation technique should give excellent results in uveitic eyes (Fig. 14.6). However, more uveitis cases have to be performed before drawing final conclusions.

Take Home Pearls

- IOL implantation should be the standard procedure in all uveitic eyes, with possibly JIA-associated uveitis as the only exception.
- Using the standard lens-in-the-bag technique of implantation, hydrophobic acrylic IOL results in the lowest capsular response but the highest uveal response.
- The bag-in-the-lens procedure is a new surgical technique that resolves the problem of posterior capsule opacification. Since the lens is hydrophilic acrylic, uveal response is very low.
- Most postoperative complications are treated medically rather than surgically.
- Postoperative hypotony is most often found in JIA-related uveitis and needs a surgical approach in case of detachment of the ciliary body.
- Capsular contraction syndrome can be operated by capsular peeling, restoring the capsular bag and the postoperative refractive outcome.

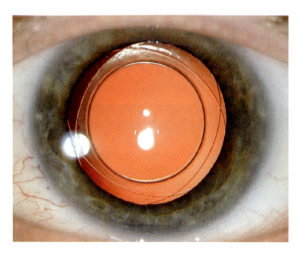

Fig. 14.6 Postoperative aspect of a Fuchs heterochromic uveitic eye implanted with a BIL: 6-month follow-up

References

1. Abela-Formanek C, Amon M, Schauersberger J, et al. (2002) Results of hydrophilic acrylic, hydrophobic acrylic, and silicone intraocular lenses in uveitic eyes with cataract. Comparison to a control group. J Cataract Refract Surg 28:1141–1152
2. Abela-Formanek C, Amon M, Schauersberger J, et al. (2002) Uveal and capsular biocompatibility of 2 foldable acrylic and intraocular lenses in patients with uveitis or pseudoexfoliation syndrome. Comparison to a control group. J Cataract Refract Surg 28:1160–1172

3. Abela-Formanek C, Amon M, Schild G, et al. (2002) Inflammation after implantation of hydrophilic acrylic, hydrophobic acrylic, or silicone intraocular lenses in eyes with cataract and uveitis. Comparison to a control group. J Cataract Refract Surg 28:1153–1159
4. Alió JL, Chipont E, BenEzra D, Fakhry MA (2002) International Ocular Inflammation Society Study Group of Uveitic Cataract Surgery. Comparative performance of intraocular lenses in eyes with cataract and uveitis. J Cataract Refract Surg 28:2096–2108
5. Andersson J, Ekdahl KN, Lambris JD, Nilsson B (2005) Binding of C3 fragments on top of adsorbed plasma proteins during complement activation on a model biomaterial surface. Biomaterials 26:1477–1485
6. Antcliff RJ, Spalton DJ, Stanford MR, et al. (2001) Intravitreal triamcinolone for uveitic cystoid macular edema: an optical coherence tomography study. Ophthalmology 108:765–72
7. Apple DJ, Peng Q, Visessok N, et al. (2001) Eradication of posterior capsule opacification. Documentation of a marked decrease in Nd:YAG posterior capsulotomy rates noted in an analysis of 5416 pseudophakic human eyes obtained post-mortem. Ophthalmology 108:505–518
8. Aslam TM, Aspinall P, Dhillon B (2003) Posterior capsule morphology determinants of visual function. Graefes Arch Clin Exp Ophthalmol 241:208–212
9. Avramidis S, Sakkias G, Traianidis P (1997) Cataract surgery in Fuchs' heterochromic iridocyclitis. Eur J Ophthalmol 7:149–151
10. De Groot V, Hubert M, Van Best JA, et al. (2003) Lack of fluorophotometric evidence of aqueous–vitreous barrier disruption after posterior capsulorhexis. J Cataract Refract Surg 29:2330–2338
11. De Groot V, Tassignon MJ, Vrensen GFJM (2005) 'Bag-in-the-lens' implantation effectively prevents posterior capsule opacification: in vitro study on human eyes and in vivo study in rabbits. J Cataract Refract Surg 31:398–405
12. Estafanous MF, Lowder CY, Meisler DM, Chauhan R (2001) Phacoemulsification cataract extraction and posterior chamber lens implantation in patients with uveitis. Am J Ophthalmol 131:620–625
13. Foster CS, Fong LP, Singh G (1989) Cataract surgery and intraocular lens implantation in patient with uveitis. Ophthalmology 96:281–287
14. Gimbel HV, Condon GP, Kohnen T, et al. (2005) Late in-the-bag intraocular lens dislocation: incidence, prevention and management. J Cataract Refract Surg 31:2193–2204
15. Guell JL, Barrera A, Manero F (2004) A review of suturing techniques for posterior chamber lenses. Cataract surgery and lens implantation. Curr Opin Ophthalmol 15:44–50
16. Heiligenhaus A, Heinz C, Becker M (2005) The treatment of uveitic cataract. In: Kohnen T, Koch DD (eds) Cataract and refractive surgery. Springer, Berlin
17. Holland GN, Van Horn SD, Margolis TP (1999) Cataract surgery with ciliary sulcus fixation of intraocular lenses in patients with uveitis. Am J Ophthalmol 128:21–30
18. Hollick EJ, Spalton DJ, Ursell PG, Pande MV (1998) Biocompatibility of poly(methylmethacrylate), silicone, and AcrySof intraocular lenses: randomised comparison of the cellular reaction on the anterior lens surface. J Cataract Refract Surg 24:361–366
19. Hooper PL, Rao NA, Smith RE (1990) Cataract extraction in uveitis patients. Surv Ophthalmol 35:120–144
20. Javadi MA, Jafarinasab MR, Araghi SAA, et al. (2005) Outcomes of phacoemulsification and in-the-bag intraocular lens implantation in Fuchs' heterochromic iridocyclitis. J Cataract Refract Surg 31:997–1001
21. Leysen I, Coeckelbergh T, Gobin L, et al. (2006) Cumulative neodymium:YAG laser rates after bag-in-the-lens and lens-in-the-bag intraocular implantation: comparative study. J Cataract Refract Surg 32:2085–2090
22. Morse LS, McCuen BW (1991) The use of silicone oil in uveitis and hypotony. Retina 11:399–404
23. Okhravi N, Lighrman SL, Towler HM (1999) Assessment of visual outcome after cataract surgery in patients with uveitis. Ophthalmology 106:710–722
24. Rauz S, Stavrou P, Murray PI (2000) Evaluation of foldable intraocular lenses in patients with uveitis. Ophthalmology 107:909–919
25. Reyntjens B, Tassignon MJ, Van Marck E (2004) Capsular peeling in anterior capsule contraction syndrome: surgical approach and histopathological aspects. J Cataract Refract Surg 30:908–912
26. Rosenfeld PJ (2006) Intravitreal Avastin: the low cost alternative to Lucentis. Am J Ophthalmol 142:141–143
27. Saika S (2004) Relationship between posterior capsule opacification and intraocular lens biocompatibility. Progr Ret Eye Res 23:283–305
28. Samuelson TW, Chu YR, Kreiger RA (2000) Evaluation of giant-cell deposits on foldable intraocular lenses after combined cataract and glaucoma surgery. J Cataract Refract Surg 26:817–823
29. Shah SM, Spalton DJ (1995) Natural history of cellular deposits on the anterior intraocular lens surface. J Cataract Refract Surg 21:466–471
30. Tassignon MJ, De Groot V, Vervecken F, Van Tenten Y (1998) Secondary closure of posterior continuous curvilinear capsulorhexis in normal eyes and eyes at risk of postoperative inflammation. J Cataract Refract Surg 24:1333–1338
31. Tassignon MJ, De Groot V, Vrensen GFJM F (2002) Bag-in-the-lens implantation of intraocular lens. J Cataract Refract Surg 28:1182–1188

Lens / Chapter 15

Cataract Surgery in Childhood Uveitis

Arnd Heiligenhaus, Carsten Heinz, Bahram Bodaghi

Core Messages

- Cataract formation is a frequent complication in childhood uveitis.
- Management of cataract in childhood uveitis is particularly difficult.
- Patient selection is important for successful surgery.
- Steroid-sparing immunosuppression may decrease the incidence of cataract.
- Preoperative evaluation is required in order to specify the course and etiology of uveitis.
- Complete quiescence of inflammation must be obtained before surgery.
- Surgical trauma should be minimized.
- IOL implantation may be proposed in selected patients with well-controlled JIA-associated uveitis.
- Postoperatively, the anti-inflammatory medication must be increased and continued for 8–12 weeks.

Contents

15.1	Spectrum of Cataract Formation 146	15.14.1	General Concerns 153
15.2	Pathophysiology 146	15.14.2	Indications and Contraindications for IOL Implantation 153
15.3	Basic Considerations for IOL Implantation 146	15.14.3	Published Reports of IOL Implantation in Children with Uveitis 154
15.3.1	Uveal Biocompatibility 147	15.14.4	Placement of the Intraocular Lenses 155
15.3.2	Capsular Biocompatibility 147	15.14.5	IOL Material 155
15.4	Indications for Cataract Surgery in Childhood Uveitis 148	15.14.6	IOL Design 155
15.5	Amblyopia 148	15.14.7	Secondary IOL Implantation 155
15.6	Contraindications to Cataract Surgery .. 149	15.14.8	IOL Explantation 156
15.7	Preoperative Examination 149	15.15	Management of Intraoperative Complications 156
15.7.1	Etiology of Uveitis 150	15.15.1	Band Keratopathy 156
15.7.2	Visual Acuity and Amblyopia 150	15.15.2	Synechiae 156
15.7.3	IOL Calculation 150	15.15.3	Miosis 156
15.8	Timing of Surgery 150	15.15.4	Hyphema 157
15.9	Preoperative Anti-Inflammatory Medication 151	15.16	How to Avoid and Manage Typical Postoperative Complications ... 157
15.10	Intraoperative Medication 151	15.16.1	Postoperative Inflammatory Reactions .. 157
15.11	Phacoemulsification 151	15.16.1.1	Topical Medication 157
15.11.1	Incisions 151	15.16.1.2	Systemic Medication 158
15.11.2	Continuous Curvilinear Capsulorhexis .. 151	15.16.1.3	Intraocular Injection of Triamcinolone .. 158
15.11.3	Hydrodissection 152	15.16.2	Capsule Opacification 158
15.11.4	Removal of the Nucleus and Cortex 152	15.16.2.1	Posterior Capsule Opacification 158
15.12	Lensectomy and Anterior Vitrectomy via Limbal Incision 152	15.16.2.2	Anterior Capsule Opacification 159
15.13	PPV and Cataract Removal 153	15.16.2.3	The Situation in Children: Techniques to Reduce PCO 159
15.14	IOL Implantation 153		

15.16.3	Ocular Hypertension and Glaucoma	159
15.16.4	Ocular Hypotony	160
15.16.5	Synechiae	160
15.16.6	Hyphema and Rubeosis	161
15.16.7	Cellular Deposits on the IOL	161
15.16.8	Cystoid Macular Edema	161
15.16.9	Amblyopia	161
15.17	Visual Outcome After Cataract Surgery in Patients with Uveitis	162
References		162

This chapter contains the following video clip on DVD: Video 11 shows Cataract surgery in JIA-associated uveitis (Surgeon: Matthias Becker).

15.1 Spectrum of Cataract Formation

In childhood uveitis, cataract is a frequent complication and may lead to severe visual disturbances. It is more common in childhood uveitis than in the adult form. In our tertiary referral center, cataract was seen in 317 of 1,506 (21%) adult uveitis patients but in 128 of 446 (37%) children with this condition.

While cataract formation is rare in posterior uveitis, it commonly develops in anterior (up to 50%) and intermediate uveitis [1–3]. Additional risk factors are a noninfectious, chronic course of uveitis, fibrin formation, long-term and high-dose corticosteroid treatment, and previous pars plana vitrectomy (PPV) [4]. Cataract occurs particularly frequently in Fuchs heterochromic iridocyclitis (FHC) and in patients with uveitis that is associated with juvenile idiopathic arthritis (JIA). Notably, 20–35% of patients present with cataract at the time of uveitis diagnosis [5, 6].

Cataract surgery in childhood uveitis, especially in juvenile idiopathic arthritis patients [7], is associated with a high rate of complications, including postoperative fibrin formation, development of posterior synechiae, ocular hypotony after cataract, giant cell deposition on intraocular lenses (IOL), and decentration of IOLs. However, the final outcome can be good if the surgical technique, pre- and postoperative medication, and monitoring of the patient are chosen properly [8].

Take Home Pearls

- Cataract formation is a frequent complication of childhood uveitis with severe visual disturbances.
- Cataract surgery in childhood uveitis is associated with a high complication rate.

15.2 Pathophysiology

The typical cataract seen in children with uveitis is posterior subcapsular cataract. Posterior synechiae are often present, with focal areas of anterior capsule necrosis and underlying lens opacities. Fibrinous pupillary membranes overlying the lens are often accompanied by opacification under the anterior capsule.

Cataract formation at the posterior pole of the lens can be explained by the missing epithelial barrier and because this is the thinnest part of the lens capsule. Inflammatory stimuli or degeneration might induce proliferation of abnormal lens epithelial cells (LEC). These abnormal cells produce extracellular basal membrane material and extracellular matrices before they degenerate along with surrounding lens fibers [9].

Careful control of inflammation and limited use of systemic and topical corticosteroids and more aggressive use of steroid-sparing immunosuppression may decrease the incidence of cataract by avoiding inflammatory relapses [7, 10].

15.3 Basic Considerations for IOL Implantation

The surgical treatment of cataract in children with uveitis poses a challenge. Surgery was previously performed without implanting an intraocular lens. The three main surgical procedures used included (1) lensectomy with vitrectomy, (2) phacoemulsification through a limbal incision followed by PPV, and (3) standard phacoemulsification associated with posterior capsulorhexis and anterior vitrectomy with IOL implantation in selected patients.

Pediatric cataract surgery and correction of aphakia have changed dramatically in the past few years [11–14]. However, even without uveitis, postoperative ocular inflammation occurs in a high percentage of children [15].

Visual rehabilitation is poor if aphakic contact lenses are not tolerated. This causes amblyopia, especially in unilateral forms of uveitis. PPV and lensectomy with complete excision of the posterior capsule may constrain the patient to a lifelong dependence on aphakic correction. In the last decade, several studies showed that IOL implantation is also an option for children with uveitis. Of all issues related to surgical technique, IOL implantation is probably the most controversial. Unfortunately, small case series, short follow-up, and the absence of controlled studies prevent drawing clear conclusions.

The outcome of cataract extraction with IOL implantation in uveitis patients depends in part on the biocompatibility of the lens material used. Indeed, any implanted material acts as an artificial surface that can trigger a foreign body reaction. Reactions on the lens surfaces are considered a marker for the degree of biocompatibility of the implanted lens material. Uveal biocompatibility describes the relationship to the vascular tissue of the eye, and capsular biocompatibility to the contact with the remaining LEC [16]. Uveal and capsular biocompatibility may differ, with one excellent and one poor, according to which parameter is investigated.

15.3.1 Uveal Biocompatibility

The breakdown of the blood–aqueous barrier (BAB) is a striking event that occurs immediately after surgical incisions. The average time required to re-establish the BAB is 3 months [17]. The increase in cells and cytokines in the anterior chamber (AC) influences the degree of both uveal and capsular biocompatibility. Activation of the complement cascade (primarily the alternative pathway) initiates an inflammatory response to the artificial material. Fragments of C3 bind to the surface of the implant, and C5 is released into the aqueous humor [18]. Chemotactic C5-derived peptides support polymorphonuclear leukocyte (PMN) influx into the AC. The PMN adhere to the surface-bound C3 fragments and amplify adhesion and aggregation of additional cells [19].

In children of 18 months or younger with cataract in the absence of uveitis, immaturity of the immune system may explain the relative absence of a significant postoperative inflammation. Serum from normal young children is deficient in total complement, and the ability to stimulate alternate pathway mechanisms is diminished. In a newborn child, leukocytes have a decreased ability for phagocytosis. Both B and T lymphocytes are functionally immature. However, this is not true for older children and for uveitis patients of any age and may explain the more aggressive inflammatory reaction that is noted after cataract surgery in the majority of older children with uveitis.

The lens capsule is permeable to low-molecular-weight crystallins [20]. However, the nature of these proteins differs with age. Turnover of existing crystallins is very high early in life [21], but the immune deviation that confers tolerance may be altered after cataract surgery, and the release of lens antigens can overwhelm the tolerance mechanism.

Some degree of foreign body reaction occurs in all eyes after cataract surgery in order to clear debris from the IOL surface. The first cells noted on the surface are small and spindle-shaped macrophages. Epithelioid or giant cells, resembling uni- or multinucleated macrophages, are found at the end of the first week. While most of these cells usually disappear, some cells can be found on IOLs years later. An early giant cell reaction with few cells occurs within the first month in many patients, but they clear after some weeks without having any clinical impact. The late reaction is regarded as a foreign-body reaction to the IOL. Groups of multinucleated cells appear usually after the first month and are often located at the pupillary border. Cells most probably originate from the anterior segment vessels or from synechiae.

Macrophages are abundant in the aqueous humor from uveitis patients after cataract surgery. While the expression of the typical macrophage cytokines IL-1 and IL-12 is low or absent, respectively, a shift towards a T helper cell type 1 cytokine expression (IL-2 and IFN-γ) is found. These data suggest that long-standing immunosuppressive therapy or chronic uveitis modifies macrophage function [22]. It has been speculated that the alteration of macrophage functions and the modified cytokines in the aqueous humor of uveitis patients may delay the clearing of cells from the AC.

Other studies have shown that the surface of foreign bodies adsorbs proteins within seconds or minutes after AC implantation. These include fibrinogen, albumin, γ-globulin, and small amounts of fibronectin and coagulation factors [23]. The consistence of this initial layer appears to differ with the IOL material and may, therefore, explain why uveal and capsular biocompatibility depends on the lens material [23].

15.3.2 Capsular Biocompatibility

The capsular bag grows exponentially with globe size and is approximately 7.6 mm at 9 months [24]. The average size of an adult lens is 12 mm. The use of large IOLs may decrease capsular retraction in uveitic eyes but can also stretch the capsular bag and cause glaucoma [25]. The haptics of many modern IOLs are flexible so that tissue erosion and distortion can be avoided.

Capsular biocompatibility is determined by lens epithelial cell (LEC) migration, by anterior capsule opacification (ACO), and posterior capsule opacification (PCO). These parameters are associated with BAB breakdown and protein adsorption of the IOL. In uveitis, the BAB is severely damaged in the eyes, and cytokine levels are modified, which has a significant influence on the capsular biocompatibility. Adsorption patterns differ considerably among IOL materials. Linnola and coauthors [23] showed that fibronectin is responsible for the IOL attachment to the capsular bag. This bioactive bond between lens and capsule may inhibit migration of LEC and reduce the PCO rate.

> **Take Home Pearls**
>
> - Any IOL material induces a foreign body reaction.
> - Uveal biocompatibility influences the degree of cell deposits on the IOL.
> - Capsular biocompatibility influences "after cataract."

15.4 Indications for Cataract Surgery in Childhood Uveitis

The major reason for surgery is poor vision. However, the contribution of cataract to visual deterioration must be distinguished from other factors, such as vitreous opacities, cystoid macular edema (CME), or amblyopia. Additionally, dense fibrin membranes that occlude the optical axis in the absence of cataract are frequently observed in patients with JIA-associated uveitis.

Indications for cataract surgery in children with uveitis:
- Poor vision (≤ 20/70) due to lens opacity
- Presence or development of amblyopia
- Opacity obscuring fundus view through undilated pupil
- Dense uni- or bilateral lens opacity
- Moderate unilateral lens opacity
- Progressive moderate lens opacity
- Lack of improvement in vision with occlusion therapy in partial lens opacity
- Young patient age (especially ≤ 2 years)
- Lens opacity located at posterior pole
- Desire to increase peripheral visual field in dense lens opacity
- Leakage of lens proteins causing phacoantigenic uveitis
- Inability to judge posterior pole due to dense lens opacity
- Inability to safely perform vitreous or macular surgery due to dense lens opacity

Surgery is indicated when a cataract is extensive or when partial opacities are present and vision does not improve with occlusion therapy. Due to the increased risk of amblyopia, surgery may be required earlier when unilateral cataract has formed than when bilateral cataract is present. Surgery is indicated when vision is less than 20/70 due to lens opacification or loss of central fixation or if visual deprivation has produced strabismus.

In partial lens opacification (< 1.5–2 mm) with partial visual obstruction, occlusion therapy can be attempted in conjunction with optimal correction or dilation of the pupil to provide a clear visual axis. Not all cataracts are progressive. Therefore, frequent monitoring of visual acuity and pupil size is mandatory. Unfortunately, cataract formation in uveitis is generally located in a central position at the posterior pole, which greatly affects visual acuity. Even in irreversible visual deprivation amblyopia, an increase in peripheral visual field may be desirable.

Cataract surgery for phacoantigenic uveitis may be required immediately if lens protein is leaking and causing inflammation. Removal of a dense cataract may be necessary to improve the assessment of abnormalities that are critical for developing a treatment plan, e.g., CME, neovascularization of retinal vessels, choroidal neovascularization, retinal detachment, or uveal effusion. In addition, dense cataract may prevent vitreous or macular surgery from being safely performed.

> **Take Home Pearls**
>
> - The contribution of cataract to visual deterioration must be distinguished from other factors, such as vitreous opacities, CME, or amblyopia.

15.5 Amblyopia

Amblyopia is caused by abnormal structural and functional evolution of the lateral geniculate nucleus and striate cortex as a result of abnormal visual stimulation during the sensitive period of visual development. Whether amblyopia can be reversed depends on the stage of maturity of the visual system at the time vision became abnormal, the duration of deprived vision, and the age at which therapy was instituted. The most critical period is in the first 2 years. The sensitivity to amblyopia gradually decreases up to the age of 6 or 7 years, when visual maturation is complete. Thus, early treatment of dense cataract is essential.

The development of amblyopia depends on the size, location, and density of the cataract. When opacities are large enough to obscure the fundus viewed through an undilated pupil, amblyopia may develop. However, when retinal structures can be visualized, conservative treatment may be considered. Children must be closely monitored when partial cataract is treated conservatively. Occlusion therapy is required in unilateral amblyopia, and clinical evaluation should also assess the visual behavior, including monocular and binocular fixation patterns.

Take Home Pearls

- Early recognition and treatment of amblyopia is required to obtain a good outcome for vision.

15.6 Contraindications to Cataract Surgery

Active inflammation, except phacoantigenic uveitis, represents a contraindication to surgery (Fig. 15.1). Relatively good vision and the advantages of accommodation must be considered. Loss of accommodation after surgery is one of the major disadvantages, and spectacles, often bifocals, are required.

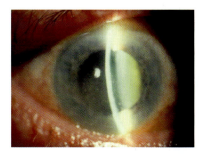

Fig. 15.1 Contraindication to cataract surgery: active uveitis with keratoprecipitates and anterior chamber cells

Take Home Pearls

- Surgery is contraindicated in active inflammation.
- Cataract extraction leads to loss of accommodation.

15.7 Preoperative Examination

It is important to plan cataract surgery on a case-by-case basis, considering age, complications, etiology, and ease with which long-term control of inflammation is achieved. The issues of surgical technique, IOL implantation, and perioperative medications differ profoundly among uveitis patients.

At preoperative evaluation, the etiology of uveitis should be specified. The ophthalmological examination should always include best corrected visual acuity tests, screening for amblyopia, slit-lamp evaluation, tonometry, and ophthalmoscopy. Additional tests may be indicated, such as interferometry, ultrasonography, fluorescein angiography, visual field assessment, or electrophysiological tests. Laser flare photometry is a valuable tool for evaluating anterior chamber inflammation. It has direct implications for postoperative medical care and drug tapering, especially in complicated conditions, such as JIA-associated uveitis.

Content of preoperative evaluation for cataract surgery in children with uveitis:
- Required:
  - Ophthalmology:
    - Visual acuity
    - Slit-lamp evaluation with mydriasis
    - Tonometry
    - Ophthalmoscopy with mydriasis
    - Screening for amblyopia
    - IOL calculation
  - Comprehensive review of systems
  - Consultation at pediatric rheumatology
  - Laboratory investigation
  - Radiological investigation
- Facultative:
  - Interferometry
  - Laser flare photometry
  - Ultrasound (e.g., impaired visualization of posterior pole)
  - Optical coherent tomography (e.g., macular edema)

- Fluorescein angiography (e.g., macular edema, manifestation at posterior pole)
- Visual field (e.g., glaucoma, manifestation at optic disc or posterior pole)
- Electrophysiological tests (e.g., chloroquine treatment)

15.7.1 Etiology of Uveitis

The management of uveitic cataract depends in principle on the underlying etiology and anatomic type of uveitis. In each individual, a comprehensive review of systems, consultation with a pediatric rheumatologist, and laboratory and radiological investigations are required.

15.7.2 Visual Acuity and Amblyopia

Surgery is required if visual acuity decreases. Most children who are 4 years or older can be tested monocularly with letter optotypes. Furthermore, amblyopia may develop. If a child has unilateral cataract, or if cataract formation is significantly more advanced in one eye, which is generally the case in children with uveitis, occlusion therapy may be indicated. In rare situations, both eyes may be operated during the same surgical intervention; however, the second operation can be postponed for 1–2 months.

In patients under 2 years with unilateral cataract, implantation of an IOL may improve amblyopia, "after cataract," and probably also the surgical management of secondary glaucoma. Deprivation amblyopia is by far the greatest concern, and in this age group, the aim of surgery is to establish emmetropia. Although the refraction will change considerably in the subsequent years and the eye may become myopic, it may be possible to prevent amblyopia. When the desired refractive error is not achieved with the IOL, a supplementary contact lens may be used. However, intractable postoperative inflammation represents the greatest treatment challenge, especially in children with JIA.

In bilateral cataract, the best solution is probably to try to establish emmetropia when the child becomes an adult. The amount of the intended hyperopia differs according to the age at surgery. It is important to inform the parents and patients before the surgery that the child will probably need bifocal glasses lifelong.

15.7.3 IOL Calculation

Before surgery, keratometric and axial length measurements are performed to calculate the IOL power. In uncooperative children, these examinations are carried out under general anesthesia directly before surgery. The preferred technique is optical measurement with the IOLMaster (Carl Zeiss Meditec AG, Jena, Germany). However, for technical reasons, it may not be possible to acquire correct measurements, e.g., if the opacity is dense in the posterior capsule, which is typical in children with uveitis. Then, IOL is calculated acoustically.

> **Take Home Pearls**
>
> - Patient selection is important for the success of surgery.
> - Preoperative evaluation is mandatory in order to specify the etiology and course of uveitis.
> - Amblyopia must be considered.
> - IOL calculation depends on age and whether surgery is needed in one or both eyes.

15.8 Timing of Surgery

The immature visual system of a young child is sensitive to opacities that interfere with the focusing of light on the retina. If the retina is not stimulated with focused images, amblyopia develops as a result.

Inflammation must be in complete remission, e.g., 10 cells or less in the slit-lamp high-power field in the anterior chamber (1+, according to previously published classification [26]), or the flare value obtained with laser photometry under maximal topical and/or systemic therapy must be at the minimum before cataract surgery can be planned. Indeed, at least 8 weeks of remission of inflammation before surgery are usually recommended [4, 27]. Surgery should be deferred if inflammation persists or frequently recurs. The experience of ocular attacks during the previous year may indicate the postoperative course, as has been observed in Behçet's disease [28], sarcoidosis, and also in JIA-associated uveitis. In these patients, appropriate anti-inflammatory medication must be adjusted first before proceeding with surgery. It has been noted repeatedly that low intraocular pressure, cells in the vitreous body, and thickening of the choroid may also represent signs of inflammation.

> **Take Home Pearls**
>
> ■ Complete quiescence of inflammation for at least 8 weeks before surgery is recommended.

15.9 Preoperative Anti-Inflammatory Medication

Anti-inflammatory medication is generally started before surgery. Application of topical corticosteroids, such as prednisolone-acetate 1% five times daily for 1 week in addition to the ongoing individual treatment regimen is often sufficient.

Patients suffering from an endogenous uveitis with a devastating chronic course and vision-threatening complications should receive immunosuppressants in advance. Most of these drugs must be given 1–3 months before they achieve sufficient anti-inflammatory effects.

> **Take Home Pearls**
>
> ■ The frequency and intensity of uveitic recurrences prior to surgery help predict the likely postoperative course.
> ■ Additional perioperative topical steroids are often sufficient in mild or episodic uveitis.
> ■ Immunosuppression in advance of surgery should be considered in severe or chronic uveitis.

15.10 Intraoperative Medication

Directly before surgery, mydriatic and nonsteroidal eyedrops are instilled to improve intraoperative pupil dilation. At the end of surgery, a transseptal injection of 4 mg dexamethasone or 40 mg triamcinolone acetonide may be given. In children in whom there is a risk that a fibrin membrane will form or CME will develop postoperatively, an intravenous injection of methylprednisolone 250 mg or an intraocular injection of triamcinolone 2–4 mg may be considered. If the intraocular pressure is greater than 35 mmHg, intravenous acetazolamide is injected 30 minutes before surgery.

15.11 Phacoemulsification

In children, general anesthesia is used. The surgical trauma should be minimized: if the duration of surgery is short, there is less inflammation. The optimal procedure depends on the etiology and course of uveitis and on the preference of the surgeon and the individual situation of the eye. Phacoemulsification with in-the-bag intraocular lens (IOL) implantation is the preferred surgical technique for the majority of uveitis patients [27, 29, 30].

15.11.1 Incisions

For the majority of children, a scleral incision is recommended [27]. Small incisions (2.5–3 mm) are preferred, as they induce less inflammation. Although the 12 o'clock position that is protected by the upper lid is safe in children, temporal or corneal incisions are preferred in patients who may require filtrating glaucoma surgery. The incisions should be secured with absorbable 10-0 polyglactin sutures.

15.11.2 Continuous Curvilinear Capsulorhexis

Compared to the can-opener technique, the risk of long-term malposition and decentration of the IOL and PCO rate is greatly reduced with continuous curvilinear capsulorhexis (CCC). Leaving a peripheral ring of anterior and posterior capsules and their zonular attachments intact guarantees stable in-the-bag fixation of the IOL haptics.

Complete CCC without tears is important when attempting to implant the IOL. Fibrous capsular bands can be excised with a cutter or fine scissors. For the central opening of the posterior capsule, forceps, a cutter, or fine intraocular scissors may be used.

An intact, well-centered CCC that overlaps the optic edge is required for the procedure. A larger opening (> 5 mm) reduces more of the LECs and reduces the development of capsule contraction syndrome, which occurs more frequently in children with uveitis [31].

CCC may be particularly difficult in children. As the capsule is thin and elastic, the risk of tearing it when moving to the periphery is high. Therefore, the use of a viscoelastic substance is highly recommended as it creates space for safe instrumentation in the anterior chamber and pushes back the anterior capsule posterior in small eyes with a high vitreous pressure. While performing the CCC clockwise, the capsule must be continuously regrasped with the forceps. A cystotome/bent needle may be used instead. Alternatively, the capsule is punctured at 12 o'clock and then grasped with forceps inferiorly toward the 6 o'clock position. The rhexis is then completed by pulling the flap to the 12 o'clock position.

A vitrectomy cutter can also be used to open the anterior capsule with low risk of anterior capsular tears, especially in children less than 6 years old [82].

15.11.3 Hydrodissection

Although hydrodissection generally has many advantages, it is rarely necessary in children with uveitis as the inner nucleus is usually soft. The capsule is thin and fragile in these patients, and therefore hydrodissection should be performed with caution in order to avoid tears of the posterior capsule and lose lens cortex into the vitreous body.

15.11.4 Removal of the Nucleus and Cortex

In children, it is almost always possible to remove the nucleus with irrigation and aspiration. Otherwise, phacoemulsification is currently the preferred technique. The chip-and-flip technique is most useful for soft nuclei. Initially, a central bowl is sculpted in the nucleus until a thin central plate remains. With a second instrument introduced through the side-port incision, the nucleus is pushed to the center of the capsular bag. Under rotation, the rim is carefully emulsified clockwise as the nucleus is rotated. Then, the edge of the central chip is elevated and the remaining nucleus flipped and removed by irrigation and aspiration. The calcified fragments that are more frequently found at the equator of the lens in chronic iridocyclitis are removed by phacoemulsification.

Compared with cataract in the elderly, dense cataract formation is rare in uveitis in childhood. Then, either phacochop, divide and conquer, or phacofracture techniques are used. The remaining cortex is completely removed by irrigation and aspiration in order to minimize postoperative inflammation, capsule shrinkage, and fibrosis (Fig. 15.2).

> **Take Home Pearls**
>
> - For children, general anesthesia is used.
> - Small scleral incisions are preferred.
> - CCC is difficult in children due to elasticity of the capsule. Vitrectorhexis is an alternative in children younger than 6 years.
> - In childhood, the nucleus and cortex can often be removed by irrigation and aspiration.
> - Phacoemulsification is preferred in dense and calcified cataract.

15.12 Lensectomy and Anterior Vitrectomy via Limbal Incision

The intact anterior hyaloid membrane and vitreous body increase the risk of cyclitic membrane formation with subsequent development of hypotony and phthisis. Inflammatory membranes that commonly develop after surgery in JIA uveitis patients may be very dense, leading to complete IOL coverage ("cocoon"), iris capture, and iris bombé. In selected cases of chronic inflammation and dense infiltration of the anterior vitreous, complete removal of the lens, capsule, and anterior vitreous body is recommended [32]. Briefly, a peritomy and a small scleral incision are prepared. Then the nucleus and the cortex are removed and large diameter capsulotomies of the anterior and posterior lens capsule and anterior vitrectomy are performed. Generally, no IOL is implanted in these patients [32, 33].

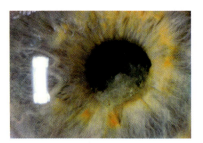

Fig. 15.2 Elschnig pearls in a patient with remaining cortex after cataract surgery

> **Take Home Pearls**
>
> - Intact anterior hyaloid membrane and vitreous body increase the risk of cyclitic membrane formation.
> - Lensectomy with anterior vitrectomy is preferred in children with JIA-associated iridocyclitis when intraocular implantation is not performed.

15.13 PPV and Cataract Removal

When vitreous opacification or another vitreoretinal complication exists, PPV combined with phacoemulsification is the procedure of choice. The visual outcome is better and the phthisis rate lower than with PPV combined with lensectomy [34].

Indications for vitrectomy include persistent, dense vitreous opacities, vitreous hemorrhage, traction retinal detachment, and epiretinal membrane formation. CME refractory to medical therapy may be a relative indication, especially in the presence of other coexisting vitreoretinal complications. The visual outcome in patients who undergo PPV with or without lensectomy can be excellent [35]. The principal limiting factor for visual recovery is the macular pathology and amblyopia.

Take Home Pearls

- Pars plana vitrectomy is combined with cataract surgery for vitreous opacification or vitreoretinal complications.

15.14 IOL Implantation

15.14.1 General Concerns

Optical correction of aphakia in children represents a challenge [36]. Aphakic glasses are a poor solution because they restrict the visual field and induce prismatic effects. Contact lenses are useful but associated with a nonnegligible risk of infection or poor compliance. Epikeratophakia is also limited for this indication because of increased cost, epithelial healing problems, interface scarring, and nonavailability of lenticles.

The best available means of achieving visual rehabilitation after cataract surgery is IOL implantation. In general, the rate of complications associated with the implantation of an IOL has been low in the adult population. However, children with JIA uveitis commonly have severe chronic inflammation, and long-term follow-up clinical trials are still needed. The issue of whether IOL implantation in uveitis patients can be recommended is controversial.

Irrespective of uveitis, the optical rehabilitation strategies, including glasses, contact lenses, or implantation of intraocular lenses, differ with respect to surgical intervention, age, unilateral/bilateral disease, and ongoing costs (Table 15.1).

15.14.2 Indications and Contraindications for IOL Implantation

An IOL can be implanted in uveitis under the following conditions: burned-out uveitis of any etiology, intermediate uveitis, sarcoidosis, Fuchs uveitis syndrome, inactive infectious uveitis (e.g., toxoplasmosis, herpetic uveitis, tuberculosis, borreliosis), and endogenous posterior uveitis without active iridocyclitis. In contrast, IOL implantation is not recommended in patients under 2 years of age or in patients with active uveitis of any etiology, an aggressive course of inflammation despite immunosuppression, or an uncertain course of uveitis.

Phacoemulsification with IOL implantation, no IOL implantation, or combined pars plana vitrectomy in children with uveitis:
- Phacoemulsification with IOL implantation is recommended in cases of:
  - Burned-out uveitis
  - Intermediate uveitis
  - Sarcoidosis
  - Fuchs uveitis syndrome
  - Inactive infectious uveitis
  - Endogenous posterior uveitis without active iridocyclitis
  - Selected patients with JIA uveitis
- IOL implantation is not recommended in cases of:
  - Patients ≤2 years of age
  - Active iridocyclitis
  - Aggressive course of uveitis while on high-dose immunosuppression
  - Uncertain uveitis course
- Combined pars plana vitrectomy is recommended in cases of:
  - Visually significant dense vitreous opacities
  - Vitreous hemorrhage
  - Visually significant epiretinal membrane
  - Rhegmatogenous or tractional retinal detachment
  - CME with vitreomacular traction

Table 15.1 Considerations for different means of optical rehabilitation in aphakia

	Glasses	Contact lenses	IOL
Surgical Procedure	No	No	Yes
Age	> 6 months	Any	> 12 months
Unilateral/bilateral	Bilateral	Either	Either
Ongoing costs	Yes	Yes	No
Recovery time	Immediately	1 week	4 weeks
Optical quality	Fairly good	Fairly good	Good
Power modification	Yes	Yes	Glasses/CL
Eyedrops possible	Yes	Restricted	Yes
Band keratopathy	Irrelevant	Relevant	Irrelevant

CL contact lens, *IOL* intraocular lens

15.14.3 Published Reports of IOL Implantation in Children with Uveitis

There is general agreement that IOLs should not be routinely implanted in patients with JIA-associated uveitis. Care must be taken, and IOLs should only be placed in patients in whom inflammation can be controlled for an extended period of time before surgery [37].

Binkhorst states that IOL implants in children require an exceptional amount of experience and good judgment, not only in surgical skill, but also in patient evaluation during the postoperative period, even if patient cooperation is poor [38].

It has been suggested in the past that implantation of IOL aggravates inflammation and encourages the formation of membranes in the anterior chamber. There is no doubt that concerns regarding IOL implantation in inflamed eyes are justified. However, recent studies have shown that results can be highly satisfactory after cataract surgery and IOL implantation in patients with certain uveitis types. When patients with chronic uveitis were randomly assigned for cataract extraction with or without IOL implantation, no significant differences in the final vision and complications were found between the two groups [39].

Another study reported a series of seven children with JIA-associated uveitis. Five patients were adults and two patients were younger than 10 years of age. Postoperative complications were significantly more common in children than in adults [40].

In 2000, Lundwall and Zetterström described seven children (10 eyes) with uveitis that underwent IOL implantation with posterior capsulotomy. The mean follow-up after surgery was 28 months. Postoperative vision reached 20/50 to 20/20 in all but two eyes. Opacities or membranes requiring reoperation developed in seven eyes, and glaucoma developed in another three. Complications were reported in 70% of the operated eyes. Only one child, who did not receive systemic immunosuppressive therapy, lost vision [41].

Lam et al. described IOL implantation in six eyes of five patients with JIA who were 12 years or younger. This retrospective study showed good results with longer periods of follow-up than previous series. The authors attributed their results to the aggressive anti-inflammatory treatment used for the meticulous control of ocular inflammation [42].

More recently, BenEzra and Cohen reported visual outcome of cataract surgery in children with chronic uveitis. Twenty eyes of 17 children with a preoperative VA of 6/120 or less were studied and followed up for 5 years. IOL implantation was performed in 10 eyes of 10 children, and the pars plana approach was used in another 10 eyes of seven children. Monocular surgery in younger children was associated with poor tolerance of contact lenses, leading to amblyopia and strabismus on longer follow-up. Importantly, children with JIA-associated uveitis were younger and had more severe and sustained complications. However, other than corticosteroids, no additional immunosuppression was used [43].

We have recently reported on the long-term visual outcome of 22 eyes in 16 children with uveitis who underwent cataract surgery. Posterior capsulorhexis and IOL implantation were performed in 16 eyes. In this group, cataract was due to JIA-associated uveitis in nine children. A final postoperative logMAR visual acuity of 0.3 or better was achieved in all cases. However, corticosteroids and/or immunosuppressive regimens were required in 50% of the patients for the control of inflammation. Long-term postoperative complications included posterior capsular opacification (18%) requiring Nd:YAG capsulotomy in two patients, Elschnig pearls (27%), glaucoma (25%), and cystoid macular edema (19%). The observations suggested that pre-, peri-, and postoperative control of ocular inflammation, including immunosuppressive medication, is mandatory in children with uveitis undergoing cataract surgery and IOL implantation [44].

15.14.4 Placement of the Intraocular Lenses

In uveitis patients, in-the-bag fixation of IOLs should be anticipated. When rapid PCO is expected, optic capture through a primary posterior CCC may be chosen [45]. However, sulcus fixation may be required if the capsule ruptures, and the degree of inflammation is slightly higher when IOL haptics are placed into the sulcus and not in the bag.

Contact between the IOL haptic and the iris is inadvisable. As permanent rubbing of the haptic against the uveal tissue may increase inflammation, iris-claw IOLs are contraindicated in uveitis patients. Angle-supported IOLs should also be avoided because of the risk of uveitis, glaucoma, and hyphema (UGH) syndrome. The safety of transsclerally sutured IOLs in uveitis has not been proven as yet.

15.14.5 IOL Material

Chronic postoperative inflammation may also result from the IOL material. The biocompatibility of the IOLs can be assessed by the degree of postoperative aqueous cells and flare and cell and pigment deposits on the lens surface.

Lower laser-flare levels and cellular deposits on the IOLs were observed with heparin surface-modified (HSM) PMMA IOLs than with unmodified PMMA IOLs [46, 47]. Compared to the other IOL materials, reduced PCO rates and postoperative inflammation were seen with acrylic IOLs [27]. Fewer uveitis relapses occurred after implanting an HSM-PMMA lens than after unmodified PMMA IOL implantation. Silicone IOLs were associated with increased inflammation and PCO and the highest incidence of relapses [27, 48].

Previously, Wilson and colleagues [24, 49] investigated the biomaterial, sizing, and design of IOLs in children. A one-piece, all PMMA, C-loop, capsular IOL that was both flexible and that showed favorable re-expansion characteristics was recommended. More recently, the authors have reported a good biocompatibility of the hydrophobic acrylic AcrySof® lens. This IOL can be inserted into a small incision, and its squared edge may result in delayed PCO. In 2001, Wilson et al. reported a series of 110 eyes implanted with an AcrySof (MA-60) lens as compared with 120 eyes implanted with a PMMA lens. IOL cell deposits were seen in 6.4% of AcrySof lenses and 19.2% of PMMA lenses. The YAG laser capsulotomy rate was similar in the two groups [50]. The use of heparin surface-modified PMMA lenses decreases the rate of giant cell deposition.

For the acrylic material of the AcrySof® IOL, there was firm contact between the IOL and posterior capsule as a result of adhesion to collagen IV, laminin, and fibronectin, which probably prevents migration of the LEC; acrylic IOLs also had the lowest grade of cell deposits [27, 51]. PCO was more severe in hydrophilic acrylic IOL than in hydrophobic acrylic IOLs. However, the greater the inflammation, the less the biocompatibility of the acrylic material [31].

15.14.6 IOL Design

It has been shown recently that a sharp, square optic edge of the posterior chamber (PC) IOL is capable of reducing migration of LEC to the posterior capsule [52]. The sharp-edge design delayed PCO development in uveitic eyes [31]. In order to reduce the risk of IOL distortion and dislocation, IOLs with large optical zones, e.g., 6 mm or more, are preferred.

15.14.7 Secondary IOL Implantation

If patients request secondary IOL implantation, implantation of a large-optic IOL into the ciliary sulcus may be considered. Sharma et al. have suggested secondary capsule-supported intraocular lens implantation in children [53]. Their retrospective study was performed in a series of 27 children (35 eyes) not satisfied with aphakic glasses or who did not tolerate contact lenses. Postoperative complications included uveitis (five eyes) that followed extensive synechiolysis, peripheral anterior synechiae (two eyes), and retinal detachment (one eye).

Bilateral uveitis (possibly sympathetic ophthalmia) resulting in blindness in a child after secondary IOL implantation for unilateral congenital cataract has been reported [54]. In children with uveitis, secondary IOL implantation may not be proposed if uveitis has not been under control for a long period of time. As inflammation may recur after secondary implantation even when uveitis is under control, we do not recommend this procedure during infancy until more controlled studies have been conducted.

15.14.8 IOL Explantation

Even under perioperative control of inflammation and careful patient selection and by intensifying the anti-inflammatory medication, some patients do not tolerate IOLs. This is the consequence of the prolonged breakdown of the blood–aqueous barrier or the sustained activity of the underlying inflammation. Patients with systemic diseases characterized by chronic inflammation (sarcoidosis and JIA) are at higher risk for this complication [55]. Deposits of giant cells, fibrin, and debris on the IOLs have also been observed in clinically silent eyes.

The IOL may have to be removed because of chronic uveitis that does not respond to inflammatory treatment, perilenticular membrane formation, or cyclitic membrane formation with progressive hypotony [55]. Attempts to stabilize the condition include capsulectomy, membranectomy, and vitrectomy. After IOL removal, the uveitis was brought under control and vision improved in 74% of the patients [55].

> **Take Home Pearls**
>
> - The best available means for visual rehabilitation after cataract surgery is IOL implantation.
> - IOL may be implanted in burned-out uveitis, intermediate uveitis, Fuchs uveitis, inactive infectious uveitis, and endogenous posterior uveitis.
> - IOLs may be implanted in selected patients with well-controlled JIA-associated uveitis, often requiring immunosuppressive therapy.
> - In-the-bag fixation of IOLs should be planned.
> - Acrylic and HSM-IOL material reduce PCO rate, postoperative inflammation, and cell deposits.
> - The sharp-edge design delays PCO development in uveitic eyes.

15.15 Management of Intraoperative Complications

15.15.1 Band Keratopathy

Band keratopathy is a frequent complication in chronic anterior uveitis, particularly when associated with JIA. Dense opacities may require chelation with EDTA before or in conjunction with cataract surgery. Phototherapeutic keratectomy may be used to treat recurrences (Fig. 15.3).

15.15.2 Synechiae

Posterior synechiae are present in up to 80% of uveitis patients. Circumscribed posterior synechiae can easily be lysed by injecting high-molecular-weight viscoelastic material or applying it with a spatula. The firmly fixed adhesions may be dissected with fine scissors.

Thin pupillary membranes are often present. The lens may be completely obscured by a thick fibrin membrane that may also contract the pupil margins and fix the iris to the anterior lens capsule. Typically, these membranes are difficult to peel from the anterior surface of the capsule or from the pupil margin. After making an incision in the center of the membrane with a 27-gauge needle and injecting viscoelastics between the membrane and the capsule, the membrane can be grasped with forceps and bluntly dissected with intraocular scissors or a cutter.

15.15.3 Miosis

Miosis is a very common finding in patients with uveitis (Fig. 15.4). The pupil can be sufficiently dilated after synechiae are lysed or after injecting adrenergic solution (epinephrine 1:1,000). To reduce the risk of bleeding from iris vessels, postoperative inflammation, and fibrin formation, the pupil margin can be gently dilated using a hook. However, sclerosis of the dilator muscle, circular membranes or diffuse adhesion of the posterior iris to the lens capsule may preclude sufficient dilation of the pupil. Then, the surgeon may have to use iris hooks and gently stretch the iris sphincter with both hands to obtain a sufficient pupil size. Some of the fibrovascular membranes can be gently pulled off the pupil margin. Others need to be disrupted by two or more incisions. Several 0.5-mm radial marginal iridotomies of the sphincter muscle may be required to obtain a symmetrically dilated pupil (Fig. 15.5). Rarely, iris retractors are used for this procedure.

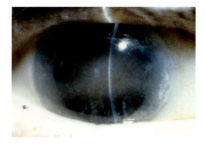

Fig. 15.3 Recurrent band keratopathy in a child with uveitis and juvenile idiopathic arthritis

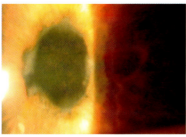

Fig. 15.4 Posterior synechiae and miosis in a patient with chronic anterior uveitis

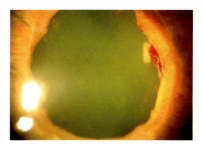

Fig. 15.5 Same patient as shown in Fig. 15.4. Several 0.5-mm radial marginal iridotomies of the sphincter muscle were performed to obtain a dilated pupil

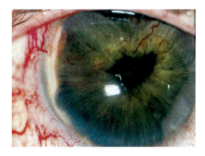

Fig. 15.6 Massive rubeotic vessels with high risk to intraoperative hyphema during cataract surgery

15.15.4 Hyphema

Intraoperative hyphema may be caused by accidentally disrupting the iris during phacoemulsification, when dissecting synechiae or fibrous membranes from the pupil margin or iridotomies, or from rubeotic vessels located at the pupil margin (Fig. 15.6), from the scleral tunnel incision, or in the anterior chamber angle (e.g., in Fuchs uveitis). This complication is managed by injecting viscoelastics, by increasing the IOP by raising the infusion bottle, or by compressing the bleeding vessel with forceps. Rarely, wet-field cauterization is required.

Take Home Pearls

- Cataract surgery in uveitis patients may be particularly challenging due to band keratopathy, synechiae, miosis, and fibrovascular membranes.
- Careful planning of an atraumatic operative approach is required.

15.16 How to Avoid and Manage Typical Postoperative Complications

15.16.1 Postoperative Inflammatory Reactions

Postoperative treatment of uveitis patients must be adjusted to the surgical procedure and the degree of inflammation and cannot be standardized. While inflammation frequently occurs in the early postoperative period in children with anterior endogenous uveitis, it is rare in infectious posterior uveitis [30, 37]. Generally, corticosteroid dosages are increased after surgery, and this augmented treatment should be continued for 8–12 weeks [27, 31]. When the dosages are tapered off too early, hypotony, CME, posterior synechiae, and IOL cell deposits may result.

15.16.1.1 Topical Medication

Many patients with anterior uveitis need only topical corticosteroids. During the first week, up to hourly applications may be necessary. Frequent application of topical eyedrops (e.g., hourly) might be impaired by patient compliance in young children. The dosage can be subsequently tapered off, while maintaining the grade of cells in the anterior chamber at 1+ or less. Additional transseptal injections of dexamethasone may be useful in patients with a high degree of inflammation, and especially when a fibrin membrane has formed.

15.16.1.2 Systemic Medication

Many patients, and in particular those with intermediate or posterior uveitis, are treated with systemic corticosteroids before surgery. All patients who required systemic corticosteroids in the past or who are at high risk of developing CME should be treated with systemic corticosteroids. Oral therapy may be started with 1–2 mg/kg, which can usually be tapered off within 6 weeks.

High intraocular corticosteroid levels can also be obtained by an intraoperative intravenous methylprednisolone injection. However, most recent observations suggest that oral steroids continued for several weeks after surgery may be more effective to reduce inflammation after cataract surgery [56]. As many JIA patients suffer side effects from long-term systemic steroid treatment for their arthritis, the higher postoperative dosages might be particularly disadvantageous [57], and immunosuppressive treatment or combined drug regimens may be indicated.

15.16.1.3 Intraocular Injection of Triamcinolone

We recently described our experience with intraoperative intraocular injection of triamcinolone acetonide in 12 JIA patients with uveitis in whom cataract surgery was performed using the lensectomy–vitrectomy technique. The observations were compared with another group of 10 patients who received intraoperative high-dose methylprednisolone and postoperative oral steroids. The groups did not differ with respect to the uveitis complications, visual acuity, and systemic immunosuppression.

At approximately 1 year after surgery, VA had improved in all patients and did not differ between the groups. In the triamcinolone group, fibrin formation and hypotony were not detected during the entire postoperative follow-up period. In the systemic treatment group, however, fibrin had formed in five patients, and they required high, frequent steroid eyedrops and subconjunctival dexamethasone injections. Postoperative hypotony developed in four patients in the systemic treatment group, and CME was noted for the first time in another patient. In addition, the number of anterior chamber (AC) cells at days 2 and 14 after surgery was lower in the TA group than in the systemic treatment group. Triamcinolone crystals were found on the surface of the iris and in the vitreous body up to day 14, but they were absent on day 30 after surgery. No significant postoperative complications related to intraocular TA were found.

Triamcinolone acetonide is a crystalline form and is hydrophobic. When injected under Tenon's capsule or intraocularly, it appears to provide a prolonged therapeutic effect with few systemic side effects [58–63]. After a single intravitreal injection of triamcinolone, the half-life is 18.6 days, and measurable concentrations lasted for approximately 3 months if vitrectomy had not been performed previously [64]. There have only been a few reports on its use in the anterior chamber [65].

Our observations suggest that a single intraoperative intraocular injection of triamcinolone in combination with postoperative low-dose topical steroid applications is effective in preventing fibrin formation after cataract surgery in JIA children with uveitis and obviates the necessity for additional postoperative systemic steroids or prolonged frequent topical applications. In this regard, TA injection was more effective than intraoperative methylprednisolone and a short postoperative course of oral prednisolone.

> **Take Home Pearls**
>
> - Corticosteroid dosages are increased after surgery, and treatment should be continued for 8–12 weeks.
> - Many patients with anterior uveitis need only supplemental topical corticosteroids.
> - A single intraoperative intraocular injection of triamcinolone in combination with postoperative low-dose topical corticosteroids is effective in preventing fibrin formation after cataract surgery.

15.16.2 Capsule Opacification

15.16.2.1 Posterior Capsule Opacification

Posterior capsule opacification (PCO), also termed "after cataract," is a consequence of the proliferation of LEC on the posterior capsule. The development of peripheral PCO depends on the quality and thoroughness of surgical cortical removal. The incidence of central PCO is lower when IOLs are fixated in the bag and is higher when one or both haptics are out of the bag. Regardless of the surgical aspects, PCO develops more frequently in uveitis; capsule opacification has been observed in up to 80% of the uveitis patients [4, 66]. The high PCO rate in distinct uveitis types, particularly in chronic inflammation and in the youngest children, must be considered when deciding on the appropriate surgical method. In children with chronically active uveitis, lensectomy may be more suitable than phacoemulsification.

Primary posterior capsule opening in children is suggested as a routine procedure, and IOL optic capture may be performed. Even when a posterior capsulorhexis has been carried out, LEC may grow on the vitreous surface of the back of the IOL optic and can be found some months after surgery. Posterior rhexis and anterior vitrectomy seem to be one way to further decrease PCO rates.

Many uveitis patients require multiple Nd:YAG laser capsulotomy treatments. In chronically active uveitis, the fibrotic membranes may need to be surgically disrupted with the use of a Sato knife or cutter. Through a small limbal incision, high-viscosity viscoelastics are injected into the anterior chamber to stabilize it during the procedure. An incision is made in the pars plana and a sharp thin knife inserted behind the iris and IOL to divide the membrane. For anterior vitrectomy, both the LEC growing in the pupil and the anterior part of the vitreous are removed. However, this does not necessarily prevent later formation of retrolenticular membranes in children with uveitis.

15.16.2.2 Anterior Capsule Opacification

Anterior capsule opacification (ACO) is caused by residual anterior LEC located on the anterior capsular leaf after rhexis. LEC may transdifferentiate to myofibroblasts when traumatized during rhexis or aspiration or when in contact with IOL. This may cause shrinkage and whitening of the anterior capsule, capsular fibrosis, and phimosis. As LEC have some potential to migrate, cell growth may be seen on the IOL.

15.16.2.3 The Situation in Children: Techniques to Reduce PCO

High proliferation rates and confluence times are typical for LECs in children [67]. LEC proliferation can open up the capsular sealing line. Polishing the posterior capsule may reduce PCO.

Primary posterior capsulorhexis (PPCCC) should be performed in all children. Even after this procedure, the capsular opening may be subsequently closed by proliferating LECs using the anterior hyaloid surface as a scaffold. Therefore, anterior vitrectomy can also be performed to reduce the risk of after cataract [68]. Additional posterior optic capture may also further reduce the PCO rate [69]. There is controversy regarding the efficacy of PPCCC with posterior IOL optic capture when performed without anterior vitrectomy [45].

The sharp posterior optic edge IOL design reduces the PCO rate [70]. Capsular fusion of the anterior and posterior capsule and LEC transformation into myofibroblasts and collagen deposit along the optic rim can create a strong and permanent capsular sealing line. Theoretically, complete removal of the LECs during the cataract surgery is the most effective measure to reduce after cataract. As removal of LECs at the equator cannot be controlled and is incomplete, this cannot be achieved clinically; application of chemicals or immunotoxins selectively targeting LECs may represent a future strategy, but this is not feasible yet [71].

Interestingly, the results of prospective studies regarding polishing the anterior capsule are unfavorable. The procedure was effective in preventing fibrosis, but ineffective in reducing regenerative after cataract. As capsular fibrosis is an important factor for capsular sealing, it may be compromised with removal of the anterior LECs [72].

Previously, capsular bending rings were introduced to reduce after cataract. They provide a capsular bend at the equator and maintain the anterior capsule at a pronounced distance from the posterior capsule. In randomized studies, the PCO score was significantly reduced [73, 74].

> **Take Home Pearls**
>
> - High rates of lens epithelial cell proliferation are typical for children.
> - Primary posterior CCC should always be performed.
> - The combination of posterior rhexis with anterior vitrectomy is suggested.
> - Posterior IOL capture may be performed to reduce capsule opacification.
> - A capsular bending ring may be considered.
> - Polishing of the anterior capsule cannot be recommended.

15.16.3 Ocular Hypertension and Glaucoma

Secondary open-angle glaucoma is a frequent finding in uveitis and is more common in anterior than in posterior uveitis. The immediate postoperative increase in intraocular pressure may be caused by swelling or obstruction of the trabecular meshwork by inflammatory cells or red blood cells. Major causes of a long-term increase in intraocular pressure are neovascularization and peripheral anterior synechiae. Secondary glaucoma is also a common complication in pediatric cataract surgery. Whereas it is uncommon in the first postoperative weeks, it develops frequently thereafter.

Glaucoma medication should be optimized preoperatively. As postoperatively elevated IOP in uveitis patients often normalizes after inflammation subsides, the anti-inflammatory regimen should also be adjusted carefully. The glaucoma medication is given as single or combination drug treatment, as required. Drugs that can be recommended for uveitis patients include primarily dorzolamide, brinzolamide, beta-blocking agents, and brimonidine. For short-term therapy, systemic administration of acetazolamide can be instituted.

Angle-closure glaucoma after cataract surgery in uveitis patients mostly results from circular posterior synechiae with subsequent iris bombé and pupillary block. YAG laser is the preferred treatment approach. Since small iridotomies often subsequently occlude in chronically active uveitis, surgical peripheral iridectomy may be preferred. Interestingly, implantation of an IOL into the capsular bag reduces the development of glaucoma [75].

preoperative hypotony is present [32], this is not an absolute contraindication to cataract surgery. Preoperative use of ultrasound biomicroscopy can identify ciliary body traction syndrome and detachment.

Surgical removal of the membranes is technically very difficult and carries a high complication rate, such as postoperative bleeding, retinal detachment, uveal effusion, and phthisis. However, surgery may be the only therapeutic option to prevent loss of vision. Permanent silicone oil tamponade to reattach the ciliary body is occasionally helpful to prevent phthisis or improve vision [76].

Take Home Pearls

- Early hypotony is typically noted immediately after surgery.
- It must be managed promptly in order to avoid secondary vision-threatening complications.

Take Home Pearls

- Glaucoma medication should be optimized preoperatively.

15.16.4 Ocular Hypotony

Early hypotony is typically noted within the first few postoperative weeks after cataract surgery. This may be the result of ciliary body detachment with and without uveal effusion, remaining ciliary traction membranes, or reduced secretion that is caused by active cyclitis. It must be managed promptly to avoid secondary complications, such as CME, serous macular detachment, choroidal folds, and phthisis.

Management includes a course of high doses of topical, transseptal, or systemic corticosteroids, and immunosuppressive treatment must be adjusted individually in patients with persisting inflammation. In addition, wound leakage must be excluded as it occurs more frequently in children.

In some patients, ocular hypotony persists after quiescence of inflammation has been achieved. The probability of phthisis ensuing is particularly high when the ciliary body begins to atrophize. Although persistent hypotony has been seen more often in eyes in which

15.16.5 Synechiae

Synechiae between the iris and IOL or lens capsule are often associated with persistent or recurrent inflammation. Iris bombé and angle-closure glaucoma may eventually result. In patients with chronically active uveitis (e.g., JIA-associated uveitis), pupillary capture of the iris that pushes the IOL forward into the anterior chamber can develop. Consequently, uveitis relapses cannot be prevented and the use of short-acting mydriatics is required.

Newly formed synechiae should be treated immediately with high doses of topical and transseptal corticosteroids; intraocular injection of triamcinolone may be helpful. Furthermore, the use of topical lytic cocktails (atropine, neosynephrine, and phenylephrine) may be indicated. The injection of tissue plasminogen activator (TPA) into the anterior chamber within the first few weeks after surgery may prevent synechiae from forming [77].

Take Home Pearls

- Postoperative synechiae and pupillary capture may be prevented with short-acting mydriatics.

- Newly formed synechiae are treated with topical or intraocular corticosteroids, lytic cocktails, or tissue plasminogen activator injection.

15.16.6 Hyphema and Rubeosis

Patients with Fuchs uveitis, herpes iridocyclitis, or vasculitis have an increased risk of developing postoperative hyphema. Inflammation must then be treated with topical corticosteroids; short-lasting mydriatics are given to prevent additional synechiae from forming. The elevated IOP is treated with glaucoma medication. Intraocular injections of triamcinolone or bevacizumab can be used to achieve regression of rubeosis and avoid re-bleeding.

The incidence of neovascularization is increased after lensectomies. Proliferation can be inhibited by administering anti-inflammatory medication, intraocular bevacizumab, or by systemic interferon-α or β. Panretinal photocoagulation, peripheral retinal cryocoagulation, or PPV may be required.

15.16.7 Cellular Deposits on the IOL

While a few cells can be found on the surface of IOLs in the majority of otherwise healthy patients, cell deposits are found more frequently in patients with uveitis. Higher numbers of cells impair visual acuity and fundus visualization.

In a recent study [51], IOLs in these patients were compared to those in individuals with no history of uveitis. The cell deposits were found more frequently on silicone than on PMMA IOLs. Acrylic IOLs had the lowest number of cell deposits. In uveitis patients, a lower incidence of giant cells was found on HSM-PMMA IOLs than on unmodified PMMA IOLs [27]. The highest degree of cell deposition was found on silicone IOLs [27].

It is not wise to implant an IOL in patients with selected types of uveitis that are known for their increased risk for dense cell deposition, e.g., in patients with chronically persistent disease, such as JIA uveitis. In order to prevent or minimize cell deposition in uveitis patients, high doses of topical corticosteroids should be given for 8–12 weeks postoperatively.

Cell deposits can be easily removed from the IOL surface by YAG laser polishing. A major drawback of this method is that giant cells frequently adhere to the IOL within a few weeks as soon as corticosteroids are tapered off [31]. As a consequence, long-term maintenance of topical corticosteroids may be required. Topical nonsteroidal anti-inflammatory agents may also be helpful.

Take Home Pearls

- Long-term maintenance of topical steroidal and nonsteroidal anti-inflammatories may be required to reduce the IOL cell deposits.

15.16.8 Cystoid Macular Edema

Cystoid macular edema (CME) is a serious complication after cataract surgery in patients with uveitis. While it has been noted in up to 50% of total patients, the incidence in uveitis in childhood is unknown. Generally it is noted within the first weeks after surgery [4, 30]. In previous studies, CME has represented the limiting factor in up to 80% of the patients with postoperative vision of 20/40 or less.

CME can be treated with high doses of topical or systemic corticosteroids and with systemic acetazolamide [78, 79]. Topical nonsteroidal anti-inflammatory agents may also be helpful.

Intravitreal triamcinolone [57] or intravitreal bevacizumab, or systemic TNF-alpha inhibitors might be used in therapy-refractive cases. Treatment response is measured primarily by visual acuity and optical coherence tomography (OCT) because Amsler tests and fluorescein angiography usually cannot be performed in the youngest children.

Take Home Pearls

- CME often occurs within the first postoperative weeks after cataract surgery in uveitis patients and must be treated aggressively.

15.16.9 Amblyopia

Clinical evaluation is continued postoperatively whereby visual behavior is assessed, including fixation tests. Occlusion therapy is adjusted to the visual development in each individual.

In many patients, aphakia can be visually rehabilitated well with rigid gas-permeable contact lenses. Contact lens fitting and patching should be initiated early after surgery. Poor compliance and intolerance can hinder visual rehabilitation in children with aphakia. Although contact lenses allow topical therapy to be continued, this increases the risk of infections. In the presence of band keratopathy, unpreserved lubricants or EDTA treatment should be used.

15.17 Visual Outcome After Cataract Surgery in Patients with Uveitis

While complications in the postoperative course are common, the functional results are generally encouraging. It is difficult to compare previous studies because different uveitis types have been investigated [4, 8, 27, 37, 66].

In one previous report, 57% of the patients had a visual acuity of 6/12 or better and 90% had improved vision [36]. Another study showed that 73.3% had visual acuity of 20/30 or better and 56.6% had significantly improved vision [66]. In a further retrospective study, visual acuity improved in 95%, and 87% attained a vision of 20/40 or better [29]. A recently published prospective study has noted that 88.6% showed improvement in vision and 46.3% had visual acuity of 20/40 or better 1 year after surgery. It appeared that acrylic and PMMA lenses provided better vision than silicone lenses [27].

In most of the studies, the predominant reasons for limited vision were preoperative macular pathologies, glaucoma, phthisis, unilateral cataract, age of 3 years or younger, and amblyopia [1, 7, 10, 30, 32, 80, 81]. It is surprising that the postoperative complications, such as CME, synechiae, pupillary membranes, and cellular deposits on the IOL, were ultimately less commonly responsible for poor vision.

Causes of poor visual outcome after cataract surgery in children with JIA-associated uveitis:
- Severe uveitis recurrences (fibrin formation, synechiae) before age 5 years
- Cataract development with visual deterioration at an early age (≤3 years)
- Glaucoma
- Phthisis
- Unilateral moderate or dense cataract
- Preoperative long-term visual deterioration due to cataract
- Preoperative presence of strabismus or amblyopia
- Preoperative presence of cystoid macula edema
- Preoperative presence of macular pucker or RPE atrophy
- Chronically active uveitis despite immunosuppression therapy

The final outcomes differed markedly between the diverse uveitis etiologies. Visual results were generally the best in Fuchs uveitis syndrome patients. Outcome was mostly poor in those JIA patients that already demonstrated vision-threatening complications at the initial presentation. Compared to the patients with anterior uveitis, those with intermediate or posterior uveitis had, in general, poor visual outcome after cataract surgery because of other visual limitations [4].

Take Home Pearls

- The predominant reasons for limited vision were macular pathology, glaucoma, phthisis, unilateral cataract, age of 3 years or younger, and amblyopia.
- Outcome was poor in JIA patients who already demonstrated vision-threatening complications at initial presentation.

References

1. Hooper PL, Rao NA, Smith RE (1990) Cataract extraction in uveitis patients. Surv Ophthalmol 35:120–144
2. Rosenberg KD, Feuer WJ, Davis JL (2005) Ocular complications of pediatric uveitis. Ophthalmology 111:2299–2306
3. Mingels A, Hudde T, Heinz C, et al. (2005) Vision-threatening complications in childhood uveitis. Ophthalmologe 102:477–484
4. Okhravi N, Lightman SL, Towler HMA (1999) Assessment of visual outcome after cataract surgery in patients with uveitis. Ophthalmology 106:710–722
5. Kanski JJ (1977) Anterior uveitis in juvenile rheumatoid arthritis. Arch Ophthalmol 95:1794–1797
6. Kotaniemi K, Kautiainen H, Karma A, et al. (2001) Occurrence of uveitis in recently diagnosed juvenile chronic arthritis. A prospective study. Ophthalmology 108:2071–2075

7. Foster CS, Barrett F (1993) Cataract development and cataract surgery in patients with juvenile rheumatoid arthritis-associated iridocyclitis. Ophthalmology 100:809–817
8. Heger H, Drolsum L, Haaskjold E (1994) Cataract surgery with implantation of IOL in patients with uveitis. Acta Ophthalmol (Copenh) 72:478–482
9. Scott JD (1982) Lens epithelial proliferation in retinal detachment. Trans Ophthalmol Soc U K 102:385–389
10. Kaufman AH, Foster CS (1993) Cataract extraction in patients with pars planitis. Ophthalmology 100:1210–1217
11. Knight-Nanan D, O'Keefe M, Bowell R (1996) Outcome and complications of intraocular lenses in children with cataract. J Cataract Refract Surg 22:730–736
12. Malukiewicz-Wisniewska G, Kaluzny J, Lesiewska-Junk H, et al. (1999) Intraocular lens implantation in children and youth. J Pediatr Ophthalmol Strabismus 36:129–133
13. Menezo JL, Taboada JF, Ferrer E (1985) Complications of intraocular lenses in children. Trans Ophthalmol Soc U K 104:546–552
14. Morgan KS (1995) Pediatric cataract and lens implantation. Curr Opin Ophthalmol 6:9–13
15. Brady KM, Atkinson CS, Kilty LA, et al. (1995) Cataract surgery and intraocular lens implantation in children. Am J Ophthalmol 120:1–9
16. Amon M (2001) Biocompatibility of intraocular lenses. J Cataract Refract Surg 27:178–179
17. Sanders DR, Kraff MC, Lieberman HL, et al. (1982) Breakdown and reestablishment of blood–aqueous barrier with implant surgery. Arch Ophthalmol 100:588–590
18. Kazatchkine MD, Carreno MP (1988) Activation of the complement system at the interface between blood and artificial surfaces. Biomaterials 9:30–35
19. Mondino BJ, Rao H (1983) Hemolytic complement activity in aqueous humor. Arch Ophthalmol 101:465–468
20. Sandberg HO, Closs O (1979) The alpha and gamma crystallin content in aqueous humor of eyes with clear lenses and with cataracts. Exp Eye Res 28:601–610
21. Voorter CE, De Haard-Hoekman WA, Hermans MM (1990) Differential synthesis of crystallins in the developing rat eye lens. Exp Eye Res 50:429–437
22. Murray PI, Clay CD, Mappin C, et al. (1999) Molecular analysis of resolving immune responses in uveitis. Clin Exp Immunol 117:455–461
23. Linnola RJ, Werner L, Pandey SK, et al. (2000) Adhesion of fibronectin, vitronectin, laminin, and collagen type IV to intraocular lens materials in pseudophakic human autopsy eyes. Part 1: histological sections. J Cataract Refract Surg 26:1792–1806
24. Wilson ME, Apple PPJ, Bluestein EC, et al. (1994) Intraocular lenses for pediatric implantation: biomaterials, designs, and sizing. J Cataract Refract Surg 20:584–591
25. Dahan E, Drusedau MU (1997) Choice of lens and dioptric power in pediatric pseudophakia. J Cataract Refract Surg 23:618–623
26. Jabs DA, Nussenblatt RB, Rosenbaum JT (2005) Standardization of Uveitis Nomenclature (SUN) Working Group. Standardization of uveitis nomenclature for reporting clinical data. Results of the First International Workshop. Am J Ophthalmol 140:509–516
27. Alio JL, Chipont EC, BenEzra D, et al. (2002) Comparative performance of intraocular lenses in eyes with cataract and uveitis. J Cataract Refract Surg 28:2096–2108
28. Matsuo T, Takahashi M, Inoue Y, et al. (2001) Ocular attacks after phacoemulsification and intraocular lens implantation in patients with Behçet disease. Ophthalmologica 215:179–182
29. Estafanous MFG, Lowder CY, Meisler DM, et al. (2001) Phacoemulsification cataract extraction and posterior chamber lens implantation in patients with uveitis. Am J Ophthalmol 131:620–625
30. Foster RE, Lowder CY, Meisler DM, et al. (1992) Extracapsular cataract extraction and posterior chamber intraocular lens implantation in uveitis patients. Ophthalmology 99:1234–1241
31. Abela-Formanek C, Amon M, Schauersberger J, et al. (2002) Uveal and capsular biocompatibility of 2 foldable acrylic lenses in patients with uveitis or pseudoexfoliation syndrome. Comparison to a control group. J Cataract Refract Surg 28:1160–1172
32. Kanski JJ (1992) Lensectomy for complicated cataract in juvenile chronic iridocyclitis. Br J Ophthalmol 76:72–75
33. Holland GN (1996) Intraocular lens implantation in patients with juvenile rheumatoid arthritis-associated uveitis: an unsolved management issue. Am J Ophthalmol 122:255–257
34. Tabbara KF, Chavis PS (1995) Cataract extraction in patients with chronic posterior uveitis. Int Ophthalmol Clin 35:121–131
35. Mieler WF, Will BR, Lewis H, et al. (1988) Vitrectomy in the management of peripheral uveitis. Ophthalmology 95:859–864
36. Dharmaraj S, Azar N (2005) Controversies of implanting intraocular lenses in infancy. Int Ophthalmol Clin 45:61–81
37. Foster CS, Fong LP, Singh G (1989) Cataract surgery and intraocular lens implantation in patients with uveitis. Ophthalmology 96:281–288
38. Binkhorst CD, Gobin MH, Leonard PA (1969) Post-traumatic artificial lens implants (pseudophakoi) in children. Br J Ophthalmol 53:518–529
39. Tessler AH, Farber MD (1992) Intraocular lens implantation versus no intraocular lens implantation in patients with chronic iridocyclitis and pars planitis. Ophthalmology 100:1206–1209
40. Probst LE, Holland EJ (1996) Intraocular lens implantation in patients with juvenile rheumatoid arthritis. Am J Ophthalmol 122:161–170

41. Lundvall A, Zetterstrom C (2000) Cataract extraction and intraocular lens implantation in children with uveitis. Br J Ophthalmol 84:791–793
42. Lam DS, Law RW, Wong AK (1998) Phacoemulsification, primary posterior capsulorhexis, and capsular intraocular lens implantation for uveitic cataract. J Cataract Refract Surg 24:1111–1118
43. BenEzra D, Cohen E (2000) Cataract surgery in children with chronic uveitis. Ophthalmology 107:1255–1260
44. Terrada C, Bodaghi B, Burtin T, et al. (2005) Implantation of intraocular lens in children with uveitis: long-term visual outcome and prognosis. American Academy of Ophthalmology. Chicago
45. Vasavada AR, Trivedi RH, Singh R (2001) Necessity of vitrectomy when optic capture is performed in children older than 5 years. J Cataract Refract Surg 27:1185–1193
46. Borgioli M, Coster DJ, Fan FT, et al. (1992) Effect of heparin surface modification of polymethylmethacrylate intraocular lenses on signs of postoperative inflammation after extracapsular cataract extraction. Ophthalmology 99:1248–1255
47. Lin CL, Wang AG, Chou JCK, et al. (1994) Heparin-surface-modified intraocular lens implantation in patients with glaucoma, diabetes, or uveitis. J Cataract Refract Surg 20:550–553
48. Schauersberger J, Kruger A, Abela C, et al. (1999) Course of postoperative inflammation after implantation of 4 types of foldable intraocular lenses. J Cataract Refract Surg 25:1116–1120
49. Wilson ME, Bluestein EC, Wang XH (1994) Current trends in the use of intraocular lenses in children. J Cataract Refract Surg 20:579–583
50. Wilson ME, Elliott L, Johnson B, et al. (2001) AcrySof acrylic intraocular lens implantation in children: clinical indications of biocompatibility. J AAPOS 5:377–380
51. Hollick EJ, Spalton DJ, Ursell PG, et al. (1998) Biocompatibility of poly (methyl methacrylate), silicone, and AcrySof intraocular lenses: randomized comparison of the cellular reaction on the anterior lens surface. J Cataract Refract Surg 24:361–366
52. Nishi O, Nishi K, Sakanishi K (1998) Inhibition of migrating lens epithelial cells at the capsular bend created by the rectangular optic edge of a posterior chamber intraocular lens. Ophthalmic Surg Lasers 29:587–594
53. Sharma A, Basti S, Gupta S (1997) Secondary capsule-supported intraocular lens implantation in children. J Cataract Refract Surg 23:675–680
54. Wilson-Holt N, Hing S, Taylor DS (1991) Bilateral blinding uveitis in a child after secondary intraocular lens implantation for unilateral congenital cataract. J Pediatr Ophthalmol Strabismus 28:116–118
55. Foster CS, Havrou P, Zafirakis P, et al. (1999) Intraocular lens-explantation in patients with uveitis. Am J Ophthalmol 128:31–37
56. Meacock WR, Spalton DJ, Bender L, et al. (2004) Steroid prophylaxis in eyes with uveitis undergoing phacoemulsification. Br J Ophthalmol 88:1122–1124
57. Antcliff RJ, Spalton DJ, Stanford MR, et al. (2001) Intravitreal triamcinolone for uveitic cystoid macular edema: an optical coherence tomography study. Ophthalmology 108:765–772
58. Paganelli F, Cardillo JA, Melo LAS, et al. (2004) A single intraoperative sub-tenon's capsule triamcinolone acetonide injection for the treatment of post-cataract surgery inflammation. Ophthalmology 111:2102–2108
59. Jonas JB (2002) Concentration of intravitreally injected triamcinolone acetonide in aqueous humour. Br J Ophthalmol 86:1450–1451
60. Jonas JB, Hayler JK, Panda-Jonas S (2000) Intravitreal injection of crystalline cortisone as adjunctive treatment of proliferative vitreoretinopathy. Br J Ophthalmol 84:1064–1067
61. Young S, Larkin G, Branley M, et al. (2001) Safety and efficacy of intravitreal triamcinolone for cystoid macular oedema in uveitis. Clin Experiment Ophthalmol 29:23–26
62. Sonoda KH, Enaida H, Ueno A, et al. (2003) Pars plana vitrectomy assisted by triamcinolone acetonide for refractory uveitis: a case series study. Br J Ophthalmol 87:1010–1014
63. Wadood AC, Armbrecht AM, Aspinall PA, et al. (2004) Safety and efficacy of a dexamethasone anterior segment drug delivery system in patients after phacoemulsification. J Cataract Refract Surg 30:761–768
64. Beer PM, Bakri SJ, Singh RJ, et al. (2003) Intraocular concentrations and pharmacokinetics of triamcinolone acetonice after a single intravitreal injection. Ophthalmology 110:681–686
65. Yamakiri K, Uchino E, Kimura K, et al. (2004) Intracameral triamcinolone helps to visualize and remove the vitreous body in anterior chamber in cataract surgery. Am J Ophthalmol 138:650–652
66. Rauz S, Stavrou P, Murray PI (2000) Evaluation of foldable intraocular lenses in patients with uveitis. Ophthalmology 107:909–919
67. El-Osta AA, Spalton DJ, Marshall J (2003) In vitro model for the study of human posterior capsule opacification. J Cataract Refract Surg 29:1593–1600
68. Koch DD, Kohnen T (1997) Retrospective comparison of techniques to prevent secondary cataract formation after posterior chamber intraocular lens implantation in infants and children. J Cataract Refract Surg 23:657–663
69. Kugelberg M, Zetterstrom C (2002) Pediatric cataract surgery with or without anterior vitrectomy. J Cataract Refract Surg 28:1770–1773
70. Buehl W, Findle O, Menapace R (2002) Effect of an acrylic intraocular lens with a sharp posterior optic edge on posterior capsule opacification. J Cataract Refract Surg 28:1105–1111

71. Meacock WR, Spalton DJ, Hollick EJ (2000) Double masked prospective ocular safety study of a lens epithelial cell antibody to prevent posterior capsule opacification. J Cataract Refract Surg 26:716–721
72. Menapace R, Wirtitsch M, Findl O, et al. (2005) Effect of anterior capsule polishing on posterior capsule opacification and neodym:YAG capsulotomy rates: three-year randomized trial. J Cataract Refract Surg 31:2067–2075
73. Menapace R, Findl O, Georgopoulos M (2000) The capsular tension ring: designs, applications, and techniques. J Cataract Refract Surg 26:898–912
74. Nishi O, Nishi K, Menapace R, et al. (2001) Capsular bending ring to prevent posterior capsule opacification: 2 year follow-up. J Cataract Refract Surg 27:1359–1365
75. Asrani S, Freedman S, Hasselblad V, et al. (2000) Does primary intraocular lens implantation prevent "aphacic" glaucoma in children? J AAPOS 4:33–39
76. Morse LS, McCuen BW (1991) The use of silicone oil in uveitis and hypotony. Retina 11:399–404
77. Heiligenhaus A, Steinmetz B, Lapuente R, et al. (1998) Recombinant tissue plasminogen activator in cases with fibrin formation after cataract surgery: a prospective randomized multicentre study. Br J Ophthalmol 82:810–815
78. Cox SN, Hay E, Bird AC (1988) Treatment of macular edema with acetazolamide. Arch Ophthalmol 106:1190–1195
79. Schilling H, Heiligenhaus A, Laube T, et al. (2005) Long-term effect of acetazolamide of patients with uveitic chronic cystoid macular edema is limited by persisting inflammation. Retina 25:182–188
80. Paikos P, Fotopoulou M, Papathanassiou M, et al. (2001) Cataract surgery in children with uveitis. J Pediatr Ophthalmol Strabismus 38:16–20
81. Moorthy RS, Rajeev B, Smith RE, et al. (1994) Incidence and management of cataracts in Vogt-Koyanagi-Harada syndrome. Am J Ophthalmol 118:197–204
82. Wilson ME Jr, Trivedi RH, Bartholomew LR, Pershing S (2007) Comparison of anterior vitrectorhexis and continuous curvilinear capsulorhexis in pediatric cataract and intraocular lens implantation surgery: a 10-year analysis. J AAPOS 11:443–446

Glaucoma / Chapter 16

Surgical Management of Uveitis-Induced Angle-Closure Glaucoma

Kaweh Mansouri, Tarek Shaarawy

Core Messages

- Angle-closure glaucoma in uveitis can be caused mechanically by iris bombé associated with posterior synechiae or by anterior rotation of the ciliary body and is often acute.
- Angle-closure glaucoma can also result from incremental angle damage and peripheral anterior synechiae related to inflammation, pigment release or neovascularization.
- Iridotomy or iridectomy may resolve iris bombé. The role of goniosynechiolysis in resolving peripheral anterior synechiae is unclear.
- Indications for surgery are similar to those for any glaucoma that is not controlled medically; however, pre- and postoperative control of inflammation is essential.
- Indications for particular types of surgery in uveitic angle-closure glaucoma are limited. Success has been reported in small series with multiple techniques.

Contents

16.1	Introduction	167
16.1.1	Pupillary Block Secondary to Posterior Synechiae	168
16.1.2	Peripheral Anterior Synechiae	168
16.1.3	Forward Rotation of the Ciliary Body	168
16.1.4	Ultrasound Biomicroscopy	168
16.2	General Approach and Surgical Management	168
16.2.1	Laser Peripheral Iridotomy	168
16.2.2	Iridectomy	169
16.2.3	Filtering Surgery	169
16.3	Trabeculectomy	169
16.4	Nonpenetrating Glaucoma Surgery	169
16.5	Cataract Surgery	170
16.6	Drainage Devices	170
16.6.1	Molteno Implant	170
16.6.2	Ahmed Glaucoma Valve	170
16.6.3	Goniosynechiolysis	170
16.6.4	Cyclodestruction	170
16.6.5	Cyclocryotherapy	170
16.6.6	Goniotomy	171
16.7	Special Considerations	171
References		171

16.1 Introduction

Secondary glaucoma is a serious complication of intraocular inflammation with potentially devastating outcomes. It poses a challenging management problem, and medical therapy often fails to reach a desirable intraocular pressure (IOP). The onset of definite chronic glaucoma is commonly preceded by periods in which the ocular pressure rises with even minimal signs of inflammation in the eye [1].

Any cellular or biochemical modification of aqueous humor can lead to morphological changes of the iridocorneal angle. The angle can be closed (completely or partially) or open. This chapter discusses the former.

Secondary angle closure can occur in inflammatory glaucomas through various mechanisms. Usually, the glaucoma associated with uveitis is the result of more than one of these. These are crucial to identify on gonioscopic examination.

16.1.1 Pupillary Block Secondary to Posterior Synechiae

Posterior synechiae appear more commonly in granulomatous uveitis. In anterior uveitis, inflammatory cells, cellular debris and proteins present in the aqueous humor stimulate the development of posterior synechiae between the posterior surface of the iris and the anterior capsule of the lens. The more extensive they are, the more restricted pupillary dilatation will be. When they progress to involve the entire circumference of the anterior lens capsule, a complete blockage of the aqueous humor passage from the posterior to the anterior chamber occurs. The consequence is an iris bombé with acute uveitic angle closure.

16.1.2 Peripheral Anterior Synechiae

Peripheral anterior synechiae (PAS) are a common complication of anterior uveitis, usually of the granulomatous type. Inflammatory debris accumulating at the inferior part of the iridocorneal angle can result in creation of adhesions between the iris periphery and the cornea. Another causative mechanism is a massive retinal detachment with forward movement of the iris–lens diaphragm.

These peripheral anterior synechiae can provoke a progressive closure of the angle. Even if they cover less than 360°, trabecular obstruction of pigmentary origin—liberated during the inflammatory process or through the use of mydriatics—can affect the open portion and exacerbate the situation. As more and more of the trabecular meshwork is sealed, the IOP begins to rise.

Among the risk factors for development of PAS are narrow angles, iris bombé secondary to posterior synechiae, anterior segment surgery, penetrating trauma of the anterior segment and neovascularization of the angle which can appear in the course of ocular inflammation, such as in Vogt-Koyanagi-Harada syndrome [2].

16.1.3 Forward Rotation of the Ciliary Body

This situation can be observed in severe cases of iridocyclitis, uveal effusion or posterior scleritis with swelling that leads to an anterior rotation of the ciliary body that can provoke acute angle-closure glaucoma without associated pupil block. In pronounced cases, the ciliary processes can be visualized through the pupil.

16.1.4 Ultrasound Biomicroscopy

Ultrasound biomicroscopy (UBM) is a useful method for differentiating various types of angle closure. In comparison to newer diagnostic methods such as the anterior segment OCT, this technique has the advantage of visualizing the ciliary body even in the presence of corneal opacification.

16.2 General Approach and Surgical Management

Treatment of uveitic glaucoma aims to control active inflammation, to prevent its damaging effects on aqueous outflow and to reduce elevated IOP. Reduction of the inflammation often allows for a spontaneous normalization of IOP. If this is not the case, and the level of IOP is considered harmful to the eye and unresponsive to medication, surgery becomes necessary. Indications for filtering surgery for glaucoma in uveitis patients are generally the same as those for any glaucoma. There are, however, differences in the choice of an appropriate surgical method. Furthermore, a well-coordinated combination of measures designed to lower the IOP, control the inflammatory activity and preserve the clarity of the cornea and lens is required in these patients.

16.2.1 Laser Peripheral Iridotomy

Laser peripheral iridotomy (LPI) is the procedure of choice in patients where a pupillary block is a contributing factor, such as an iris bombé. It is generally done after the failure of medical mydriatic therapy to break the posterior synechiae. LPI has proven to be an effective alternative to iridectomy. It can be performed easily on an out-patient basis and monitored for response to treatment.

This treatment has a low-risk profile. The most commonly encountered complication is a transient IOP elevation. To prevent this, topical alpha adrenoreceptor agonists (brimonidine or apraclonidine) should be administered 1 h before and immediately after the laser procedure. Before the patient can be discharged, IOP should be measured 45 minutes after the intervention. Tonometric pressure control and gonioscopy 1 week after treatment are required.

Other adverse events include microhemorrhage from the iridotomy site, lens damage and transient blurring of vision. Posterior segment complications, such as a macular hole, are extremely rare and generally related to direct laser-induced damage [3].

16.2.2 Iridectomy

Surgical peripheral iridectomy is only resorted to if LPI is not possible or is ineffective. It might be the better choice in Asian and African eyes with thick irides that resist iridotomy. This procedure has the potential to exacerbate an anterior uveitis with subsequent IOP rise.

Surgical iridectomy is a less aggressive procedure than filtering surgery, particularly in inflamed eyes. When iridectomy is unsuccessful, a subsequent filtering procedure can become necessary without altering the prognosis.

However, subsequent surgical intervention is often necessitated since in case of persistent inflammation, the opening made by laser photocoagulation may close itself. In addition, the angle can already be damaged to an extent where it requires first-line surgical management.

16.2.3 Filtering Surgery

Filtering surgery becomes necessary when the IOP cannot be controlled medically or with iridectomy. Minimal intraocular inflammatory activity at the time of surgery and during the postoperative period is a prerequisite for a successful operation.

Surgical success can be limited since the filtering area can close following the intervention. Development of autoimmunity is likely after severe or chronic inflammation and iris damage that leads to a breakdown of the blood–aqueous barrier. Intraocular operations, and particularly drainage operations, performed on inflamed eyes have the potential to initiate an autoimmune response that may not only increase the uveitic activity but, in theory, also induce sympathetic ophthalmia.

16.3 Trabeculectomy

Trabeculectomy may be performed to lower IOP in eyes with a chronic angle closure that is insufficiently responsive to laser or medical treatment. In these eyes, it is the surgical procedure of choice.

The success rate of trabeculectomy without antimetabolites has been reported to be 53% in a series of 32 eyes after 5 years [4]. Other reports that studied the outcome of trabeculectomy enhanced with antimetabolites in patients with uveitis reported success rates between 51 and 90% [5, 6]. Although there is substantial evidence for the benefit of adjunctive antimetabolites such as intraoperative 5-fluorouracil (5-FU) or mitomycin C (MMC), these agents are not universally used in uveitic glaucoma. There is controversy over the better antimetabolite regimen in uveitic glaucoma since MMC has not been clearly shown to have an advantage over 5-FU in terms of IOP control. Complication rates, however, are increased by the use of these agents, with hypotonous maculopathy and endophthalmitis from leaks through thin filtering blebs being the most serious ones.

Most of the cited studies looked either at uveitic patients with open angles or mixed groups of closed and open angles. Therefore, direct estimates of surgical success in uveitis-related glaucoma patients with closed angles are difficult to make.

Surgical intervention in uveitic glaucoma is sometimes delayed by surgeons due to concerns about precipitating an inflammatory relapse with its deleterious effects on IOP control and visual prognosis as reported in a series of 76 patients [7]. A number of studies have disproved this fear and shown an improvement in the pattern of uveitis after filtering surgery [8–11]. It is not clear, however, why remission of uveitis might occur after trabeculectomy, and the results of these studies suggest that it is not related to the use of antimetabolites. This warrants further research.

16.4 Nonpenetrating Glaucoma Surgery

There is little evidence on nonpenetrating surgical procedures in uveitis. Auer et al. have reported on deep sclerectomy with the collagen and T-flux implant in uveitic patients. In their series of 13 patients, they could achieve a qualified success rate of 90% after 1 year of follow-up. They argued that the low rate of surgical complications explained the better success rate of nonpenetrating glaucoma surgery (NPGS) compared to classical penetrating surgery [12]. In a recent study, deep sclerectomy without antimetabolites was performed on eight patients with medically uncontrolled IOP. After 42 months of follow-up, all eyes were controlled. One patient required a second operation. Use of medications was significantly reduced [13]. Milazzo and coworkers reported a case of scleral ectasia following deep sclerectomy in a 12-year-old patient with chronic arthritis and glaucoma secondary to a chronic uveitis [14]. However, all the published cases of nonpenetrating surgery in uveitic glaucoma have been performed on open angles. We do not have sufficient evidence at the moment to give specific recommendations on NPGS in closed-angle glaucoma secondary to uveitis.

16.5 Cataract Surgery

Cataract surgery may be considered as an option in eyes with a mild degree of angle closure (less than 180° of PAS).

16.6 Drainage Devices

The less than ideal success rates of filtering surgery in uveitis patients have led to alternative procedures. The use of valves and other setons, such as the Ahmed, Molteno, Baerveldt and Krupin implants, is increasingly gaining popularity. This trend has been supported by the fact that experienced surgeons achieve lower complication rates than previously believed.

The reported success rates are similar to those from filtering surgery without the use of antimetabolites [15]. In eyes with preserved vision, the use of valves is indicated when previous filtering surgery has failed. Intraoperative use of antimetabolites can improve the IOP reduction. Thresholds for the use of setons and reported success rates vary from center to center, but generally their IOP-lowering effect in uveitis patients is better than in other forms of refractory glaucoma. In uveitic glaucoma associated with juvenile idiopathic arthritis, the use of drainage devices is an appropriate primary surgical procedure [16]. They are also a good option in eyes with other risk factors, such as aphakia, failed previous filtering or vitreoretinal surgery.

16.6.1 Molteno Implant

The Molteno implant consists of a translimbal tube draining aqueous humor from the interior of the eye onto the outer surface of one or two circular episcleral plates. Molteno et al. have reported the long-term results in 40 eyes with uveitis after 5 and 10 years. At 5 years, 87% of 36 eyes were controlled with an average 0.44 medications; at 10 years, 93% of 14 eyes had a controlled IOP on 0.32 medications.

16.6.2 Ahmed Glaucoma Valve

The Ahmed valve was the first restrictive glaucoma implant with a genuine valve mechanism. In a retrospective study of 25 eyes, Da Mata et al. reported a 94% success rate after 1 year following Ahmed valve implantation with few postoperative complications [17]. In another study, Gil-Carrasco et al. achieved success in 8 out of 14 uveitic eyes after follow-ups of an average of 14 months [18].

16.6.3 Goniosynechiolysis

Nd:YAG goniosynechiolysis has been proposed as a therapeutic option in cases of angle synechiae in medically uncontrolled chronic angle-closure glaucoma without rubeosis. We identified two studies that reported on the use of this intervention in uveitic patients. They conclude that in selected cases, goniosynechiolysis may represent an effective management option [19, 20]. However, to date, there is not enough evidence to assess its efficacy of in the management of angle-closure glaucoma.

16.6.4 Cyclodestruction

These destructive techniques of an already-damaged ciliary epithelium were classically considered as a last resort when little visual potential remained. The procedures, per se, cause significant inflammation and have an unpredictable effect on IOP, with an significant risk of phthisis bulbi and a potential for sympathetic ophthalmia. One large retrospective study reported a 19% rate of hypotony in uveitis patients following diode laser cyclophotocoagulation ("cyclodiode") [21].

16.6.5 Cyclocryotherapy

There are different ways to conduct cyclocryotherapy [22]. Generally, the cryoprobe is used under local anesthesia. The inferior 180° of the eye are treated with two rows of "freezes" for 1 minute at −80°C in approximately three spots per quadrant. The first row begins about 2–3 mm back of the limbus, the "ice ball" extending away from the cornea. The second row is then placed immediately behind the first row. The eye is patched after instillation of a combined corticosteroid and antibiotic together with a cycloplegic. Analgesics should be given to reduce the substantial postoperative pain.

The technique is discussed in more detail in Chap. 17.

16.6.6 Goniotomy

Freedman et al. have reported on the success of goniotomy for juvenile idiopathic arthritis-associated uveitic glaucoma. Surgical success was achieved in 75% of the operated eyes and in 60% after a single goniotomy. Uveitis did not worsen during the early postoperative period [23].

16.7 Special Considerations

As a result of surgery, the inflamed eye may experience additional intraocular problems, such as hemorrhage and augmented inflammation. These factors highlight the importance of adequate postoperative follow-up to achieve long-term success.

> **Take Home Pearls**
>
> - Secondary glaucoma is a serious complication of intraocular inflammation.
> - Management is challenging, and medical therapy often fails to control IOP.
> - Mechanisms are often a combination of peripheral anterior synechiae, pupil block, and forward rotation of the ciliary body.
> - Iridotomy is the intervention of choice.
> - Trabeculectomy provides limited success. Little evidence is available on nonpenetrating surgery.
> - There is a promising role for drainage devices.

References

1. Kok H, Barton K. Uveitic glaucoma. Ophthalmol Clin North Am. 2002 Sep;15(3):375–87, viii
2. Gartner S, Henkind P. Neovascularization of the iris (rubeosis iridis). Surv Ophthalmol. 1978 Mar–Apr;22(5):291–312. Review
3. Anderson JE, Gentile RC, Sidoti PA, Rosen RB. Stage 1 macular hole as a complication of laser iridotomy. Arch Ophthalmol. 2006 Nov;124(11):1658–60
4. Stavrou P, Murray PI. Long-term follow-up of trabeculectomy without antimetabolites in patients with uveitis. Am J Ophthalmol. 1999 Oct;128(4):434–9
5. Jampel HD, Jabs DA, Quigley HA. Trabeculectomy with 5-fluorouracil for adult inflammatory glaucoma. Am J Ophthalmol. 1990 Feb 15;109(2):168–73
6. Towler HM, McCluskey P, Shaer B, Lightman S. Long-term follow-up of trabeculectomy with intraoperative 5-fluorouracil for uveitis-related glaucoma. Ophthalmology. 2000 Oct;107(10):1822–8
7. Okhravi N, Lightman SL, Towler HM. Assessment of visual outcome after cataract surgery in patients with uveitis. Ophthalmology. 1999 Apr;106(4):710–22
8. Weinreb RN. Adjusting the dose of 5-fluorouracil after filtration surgery to minimize side effects. Ophthalmology. 1987 May;94(5):564–70
9. Ophir A, Ticho U. Remission of anterior uveitis by subconjunctival fluorouracil. Arch Ophthalmol. 1991 Jan;109(1):12–3
10. Towler HM, McCluskey P, Shaer B, Lightman S. Long-term follow-up of trabeculectomy with intraoperative 5-fluorouracil for uveitis-related glaucoma. Ophthalmology. 2000 Oct;107(10):1822–8
11. Jampel HD, Jabs DA, Quigley HA. Trabeculectomy with 5-fluorouracil for adult inflammatory glaucoma. Am J Ophthalmol. 1990 Feb 15;109(2):168–73
12. Auer C, Mermoud A, Herbort CP. Deep sclerectomy for the management of uncontrolled uveitic glaucoma: preliminary data. Klin Monatsbl Augenheilkd. 2004 May;221(5):339–42
13. Souissi K, El Afrit MA, Trojet S, Kraiem A. [Deep sclerectomy for the management of uveitic glaucoma.] J Fr Ophtalmol. 2006 Mar;29(3):265–8
14. Milazzo S, Turut P, Malthieu D, Leviel MA. Scleral ectasia as a complication of deep sclerectomy. J Cataract Refract Surg. 2000 May;26(5):785–7
15. Hill RA, Nguyen QH, Baerveldt G, Forster DJ, Minckler DS, Rao N, Lee M, Heuer DK. Trabeculectomy and Molteno implantation for glaucomas associated with uveitis. Ophthalmology. 1993 Jun;100(6):903–8
16. Valimaki J, Airaksinen PJ, Tuulonen A. Molteno implantation for secondary glaucoma in juvenile rheumatoid arthritis. Arch Ophthalmol. 1997 Oct;115(10):1253–6
17. Da Mata A, Burk SE, Netland PA, Baltatzis S, Christen W, Foster CS. Management of uveitic glaucoma with Ahmed glaucoma valve implantation. Ophthalmology. 1999 Nov;106(11):2168–72
18. Gil-Carrasco F, Salinas-VanOrman E, Recillas-Gispert C, Paczka JA, Gilbert ME, Arellanes-Garcia L. Ahmed valve implant for uncontrolled uveitic glaucoma. Ocul Immunol Inflamm. 1998 Mar;6(1):27–37
19. Senn P, Kopp B. Nd:YAG laser synechiolysis in glaucoma due to iridocorneal angle synechiae. Klin Monatsbl Augenheilkd. 1990 Apr;196(4):210–3

20. Soheilian M, Aletaha M, Yazdani S, Dehghan MH, Peyman GA. Management of pediatric Vogt-Koyanagi-Harada (VKH)-associated panuveitis. Ocul Immunol Inflamm. 2006 Apr;14(2):91–8
21. Murphy CC, Burnett CA, Spry PG, Broadway DC, Diamond JP. A two centre study of the dose-response relation for transscleral diode laser cyclophotocoagulation in refractory glaucoma. Br J Ophthalmol. 2003 Oct;87(10):1252–7
22. Aaberg TM, Cesarz TJ, Flickinger RR. Treatment of peripheral uveoretinitis by cryotherapy. Am J Ophthalmol. 1973 Apr;75(4):685–8
23. Freedman SF, Rodriguez-Rosa RE, Rojas MC, Enyedi LB. Goniotomy for glaucoma secondary to chronic childhood uveitis. Am J Ophthalmol. 2002 May;133(5):617–21

Glaucoma / Chapter 17

Surgical Management of Open-Angle Glaucoma Associated with Uveitis

17

Herbert P. Fechter, Richard K. Parrish II

Core Messages

- Uveitic glaucoma poses special challenges for the internist, rheumatologist, uveitis specialist, glaucoma specialist and the patient.
- Exuberant inflammation, severe conjunctival scarring, iris neovascularization, corticosteroid-induced cataracts, medication side effects and the increased risk of hypotony make uveitic glaucoma especially difficult to manage.
- Careful preoperative evaluation insures that the correct diagnosis is made and an appropriate treatment plan is implemented. It is imperative that pre- and postoperative intraocular inflammation be controlled adequately with judicious medication use.
- When conservative measures fail, glaucoma drainage devices can provide an effective means of lowering intraocular pressure. Although several different, effective drainage implants are available, we prefer to use the modified 250 mm² BGDD for the majority of our uveitic patients with elevated IOP.
- Innovations in implantation technique and glaucoma drainage device modifications have improved our ability to achieve and maintain a low IOP in these challenging uveitic eyes.
- Careful preoperative planning and meticulous attention to operative technique can minimize complications and enhance surgical safety and efficacy.

Contents

17.1	Introduction	174	17.6.10	Patch Graft	185
17.2	Team Approach	174	17.6.11	Conjunctival Closure	185
17.3	Surgical Options	174	17.6.12	Conjunctival Closure with Extensive Scarring	185
17.4	Glaucoma Drainage Devices	175			
17.5	Preoperative Evaluation	177	17.6.13	Alternatives to Anterior Chamber Tube Placement—The Pars Plana Route	186
17.6	Principles	178			
17.6.1	Preoperative IOP Reduction	179	17.6.14	Drainage Implant Surgery in Combination with Other Procedures	186
17.6.2	Selection of Quadrant	181			
17.6.3	Conjunctival Incision	181	17.7	Postoperative Management	186
17.6.4	Preparation of the Scleral Site	181	17.7.1	Postoperative Day 1	186
17.6.5	The Implant	181	17.7.2	Postoperative IOP Management— Early	187
17.6.6	Reducing Immediate Postoperative Aqueous Outflow—Tube Ligation	182			
			17.7.3	Postoperative IOP Management— Weeks 2–6	187
17.6.7	Reducing Immediate Postoperative Aqueous Outflow—"Rip Cord" Technique	182			
			17.7.4	Postoperative IOP Management— Spontaneous Suture Absorption	188
17.6.8	Reducing Immediate Postoperative Aqueous Outflow—Prolene Suture Placement	183	17.8	Postoperative Complications	188
			17.8.1	Hypotony	188
			17.8.2	Tube Obstruction	191
17.6.9	Tube Position and Insertion	184	References		192

This chapter contains the following video clips on DVD: Video 12 shows Iris Bombe (Surgeons: Herbert Fechter, Greg Parkhurst), Video 13 shows Ahmed Implant (Surgeons: Herbert Fechter, Paul Palmberg), Video 14 shows Pulsating Fibrin Membrane (Surgeons: Herbert Fechter, Jennifer Cartwright), Video 15 shows Baerveldt Glaucoma Implant (Surgeons: Herbert Fechter, Brett Nelson), Video 16 shows Cataract Removal with Bearveldt Drainage Device (Surgeons: Herbert Fechter, Steven Donnelly), Video 17 shows Tube Fenestration (Surgeons: Herbert Fechter, Steven Gedde), Video 18 shows Relieving Pressure with a 30 Gauge Needle (Surgeons: Paul Palmberg, Herbert Fechter), Video 19 shows Burp Paracentesis (Surgeon: Herbert Fechter), Video 20 shows Cornea Patch Graft (Surgeons: Herbert Fechter, Donald Budenz), Video 21 shows Laser Suture Lysis of Ligated Baerveldt Tube (Surgeons: Paul Palmberg, Herbert Fechter), Video 22 shows Inferonasal Baerveldt Implant with Scarred Conjunctiva (Surgeons: Herbert Fechter, Steven Donnelly), Video 23 shows Baerveldt Implant with Retinal Detachment Repair (Surgeons: John Dick, Herbert Fechter, Greg Parkhurst, Mel Wagner), Video 24 shows Refenestrate Tube, Video 25 shows Cut Ligature with 30 Gauge Needle, Video 26 shows Healon V for Persistent Choroidals, Video 27 shows Permanent Ligature (Surgeon: Herbert Fechter), Video 28 shows Tying Off Baerveldt Tube and Draining Choroidals (Surgeons: Michael Mines, Herbert Fechter), Video 29 shows Fibrin Membranes (Surgeon: Herbert Fechter) and Video 30 shows Clearing Tube Tip (Surgeons: Eric Weichel, Benjamin Smith, Herbert Fechter).

17.1 Introduction

Chronic intraocular inflammation is often associated with wide fluctuations of intraocular pressure (IOP). Inflammation and associated treatment with topical and systemic corticosteroids can further compromise aqueous outflow and increase the risk of IOP-related optic neuropathy. When medical and laser therapy cannot achieve IOP control, surgical options should be considered. The operative options must be scrutinized carefully to insure that the management of elevated IOP minimizes early and late postoperative complications. Very low postoperative IOP can trigger the development of choroidal detachments and hypotony maculopathy, and persistently elevated IOP can cause progressive glaucomatous optic neuropathy. Medical treatment should be optimized to control intraocular inflammation prior to, during and after surgery. Special care must be taken to minimize postoperative hypotony that should be treated expeditiously if it occurs. Glaucoma drainage devices (GDD) have been more frequently used in patients with chronic intraocular inflammation, since trabeculectomy surgery is more likely to fail in these eyes [1].

17.2 Team Approach

Medical and surgical management of uveitic glaucoma requires a coordinated team approach. A rheumatologist, internist, uveitis specialist, pediatric ophthalmologist and glaucoma specialist may be required to provide optimal coordinated patient care. Other chapters discuss specific topical, local and systemic immunosuppressive treatment for control of intraocular inflammation. Ocular and systemic side effects of local and systemic medications must be closely monitored in the treatment of ocular inflammation prior to glaucoma surgery. Effective immunosuppressive therapy may obviate the need for glaucoma surgery by decreasing trabecular meshwork inflammation and normalizing aqueous humor outflow; however, if the ciliary body secretory function increases after permanent trabecular meshwork damage has occurred, then further medical and surgical management may be required. Intravitreal corticosteroids, used to treat posterior uveitis, such as the Retisert (fluocinolone acetonide intravitreal implant, Bausch and Lomb Inc., Rochester, NY) can also induce IOP elevation or a glucocorticoid response that may require surgical intervention [2].

17.3 Surgical Options

Surgical intervention to increase aqueous humor outflow, such as trabeculectomy or glaucoma drainage devices (GDD) should be delayed, when possible, until active intraocular inflammation is controlled and any pupillary block has been treated. Peripheral iridoplasty, laser peripheral iridotomy or surgical peripheral iridectomy are indicated when mydriatics fail to break posterior synechiae that cause acute pupillary block. Patients with uncontrolled open- and closed-angle glaucoma after resolution of pupillary block may require filtering surgery, cyclodestructive procedures, or GDD surgery.

Traditional filtering surgery, such as trabeculectomy, has a low success rate in uveitic eyes that is associated with robust postoperative fibroblast proliferation and subconjunctival fibrosis [3]. Trabeculectomy, even when performed with adjunctive anti-scarring drugs, such as mitomycin C or 5-fluorouracil, is prone to failure in uveitic eyes with extensive conjunctival scarring, intraocular inflammation or abnormal limbal anatomy. Conjunctival wound and bleb leaks increase the risk of

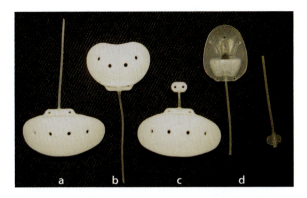

Fig. 17.1 Ahmed–Baerveldt comparison. (**a**) Baerveldt BG 101-350 (350 mm^2), (**b**) Baerveldt BG 103-250 (250 mm^2), (**c**) Baerveldt with Hoffman elbow BG 102-350 (350 mm^2) and (**d**) Ahmed FP7 (184 mm^2)

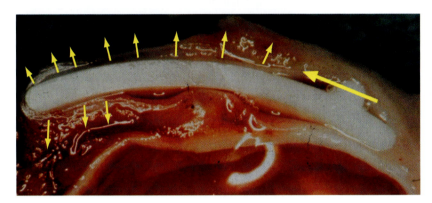

Fig. 17.2 Cross section of Baerveldt implant with arrows representing direction of aqueous flow through fibrous capsule (© Surgical Techniques in Ophthalmology – Glaucoma Surgery. Edited by Teresa Chen. Elsevier, 2007, ISBN 978-1-4160-3021-8)

hypotony, exacerbation of ocular inflammation, late-onset blebitis and endophthalmitis. In our opinion, in view of the poor prognosis for trabeculectomy in the long-term management of inflammatory glaucomas, these eyes are candidates for GDD surgery.

Cyclodestructive procedures that acutely increase intraocular inflammation are usually reserved for eyes that have failed both medical and surgical therapy and are poor candidates for further incisional glaucoma surgery. Thermal laser energy can be delivered either via the transscleral approach in the phakic eye or with an endophotocoagulator through the pupil or a pars plana incision in the pseudophakic or aphakic eye [4]. Large plate GDD, such as the 350 mm^2 Baerveldt glaucoma drainage implant (Advanced Medical Optics, Irvine, California), should not be used in eyes with a prior history of either cyclophotocoagulation or endocycloablation due to their decreased aqueous production and the risk of hypotony (Fig. 17.1).

17.4 Glaucoma Drainage Devices

We favor the use of GDD in uveitic eyes because the risk of failure or hypotony is less than that with either trabeculectomy or cyclophotocoagulation. Preoperative care and operative decisions must be executed to minimize postoperative hypotony. Glaucoma drainage implants are divided into two categories, *valved* and *nonvalved*. Valved devices employ some flow restriction mechanism, such as the Ahmed (New World Medical, Rancho Cucamonga, CA) and Krupin GDD (Hood Laboratories, Pembroke, MA). Nonvalved implants consist of an open tube connected to a plate reservoir. The Baerveldt glaucoma drainage device (BGDD) and the Molteno (IOP, Inc., Costa Mesa, CA,) are commercially available nonvalved implants. These devices lower IOP by draining aqueous humor from the anterior chamber into the potential subconjunctival or sub-Tenon space located superficial to the plate. This reservoir for aqueous humor is the potential space between the plate and the surrounding fibrovascular tissue. Aqueous humor diffuses through the acellular fibrous pseudocapsular wall, and periocular capillaries ultimately absorb the fluid (Fig. 17.2).

The Ahmed glaucoma valve is often selected for use in uveitic eyes due to its ease of insertion into one quadrant of the eye and the IOP control offered by the one-way valve [5]. In our experience, the Ahmed valve may be useful in the management of patients with juvenile idiopathic arthritis whose chronic intermittent uveitis is associated with periods of reduced aqueous secretion. When the Ahmed valve fails to restrict aqueous flow sufficiently, profound early hypotony may develop. Uveitic eyes are especially prone to postoperative fibrin formation, which can obstruct the Ahmed valve and lead to elevated IOP. We prefer the nonvalved 250 mm² Baerveldt glaucoma drainage device for the majority of our uveitic glaucoma patients. The Baerveldt GDD may provide effective long-term IOP control, requires fewer additional glaucoma medications, and may be less likely to develop late-onset failure than the Ahmed implant in nonuveitic eyes [6]. Individual surgeon preferences vary, and similar success rates have been reported with the Ahmed, Baerveldt, Krupin and Molteno GDDs [7].

Although many glaucoma implants have been used in managing uveitic glaucoma, we will concentrate primarily on BGDD implantation techniques and how to minimize intraoperative and postoperative complications. The BGDD principles apply to the other implants. As a detailed description of our BGDD insertion technique has been published elsewhere, we will focus on the pertinent aspects of uveitic glaucoma management with the BGDD [8].

The surgeon should consider several factors, such as the level of intraocular inflammation and extent of functional trabecular meshwork during the preoperative evaluation when deciding whether the 250-mm² or 350-mm² plate would provide the safest postoperative pressure control. The rate of aqueous humor production in uveitic eyes is often markedly reduced and can favor the use of the smaller 250-mm² plate (BG 103-250). The nonvalved tube, which offers very low resistance to aqueous humor outflow without occlusion, can lead to acute postoperative hypotony and subsequent flat anterior chamber. Surgeons must restrict aqueous humor passage through the device by ligating the tube with an absorbable suture, such as a 910 polyglactin (Vicryl, Ethicon, Somerville, NJ). Venting slits in the tube made with a spatulated needle can minimize undesirable IOP spikes in the early postoperative period. In addition to the plate's larger surface area, the BGDD's nonvalved tube may contribute to the long-term IOP lowering success by creating less resistance to flow.

> The following uveitic conditions are associated with glaucoma [9]:
> - Ocular conditions
>   - Episcleritis and scleritis
>   - Fuchs heterochromic cyclitis
>   - Glaucomatocyclitic crisis (Posner-Schlossman syndrome)
>   - Idiopathic anterior uveitis
>   - Intermediate uveitis
>   - Lens-induced uveitis
>   - Phacoanaphylactic glaucoma
>   - Phacolytic glaucoma
>   - Pseudophakic-inflammatory glaucoma
>   - Masquerade syndromes
>   - Intraocular neoplasm
>   - Retinal detachment
>   - Pars planitis (intermediate uveitis)
>   - Sympathetic ophthalmia
>   - Traumatic uveitis
> - Systemic diseases
>   - Arthritis
>   - Ankylosing spondylitis (Marie-Strumpell disease)
>   - Juvenile idiopathic arthritis (JIA)
>   - Acute systemic arthritis (Stills disease)
>   - Polyarticular JIA
>   - Pauciarticular JIA
>   - Reactive arthritis
>   - Behçet's disease
>   - Crohn's disease
>   - Dermatologic conditions
>   - Acne rosacea
>   - Erythema multiforme
>   - Poikilodermatomyositis
>   - Sweet's syndrome (acute febrile neutrophilic dermatosis)
>   - Sarcoidosis
>   - Vogt-Koyanagi-Harada syndrome
> - Infectious diseases
>   - Acute retinal necrosis
>   - AIDS
>   - Coccidiomycosis
>   - Gnathostomiasis
>   - Hansen disease (leprosy)
>   - Onchocerciasis
>   - Syphilis
>   - Acquired
>   - Congenital
>   - Toxoplasmosis
>   - Tuberculosis
>   - Viral
>   - Herpesvirus
>   - Herpes simplex
>   - Herpes zoster
>   - Human immunodeficiency virus (HIV)
>   - Influenza
>   - Mumps
>   - Rubella

17.5 Preoperative Evaluation

A thorough preoperative evaluation plays a critical role in surgical planning to reduce intraoperative risks and postoperative complications. The first decision is to determine the potential for useful vision. We operationally define *useful vision* as the ability to ascertain the outline of a door in the examination room and to ambulate without assistance. A filtering procedure on a blind painful eye with glaucomatous uveitis may provoke sympathetic ophthalmia in the fellow eye [10]. We, therefore, do not recommend GDD surgery if the patient does not have this visual potential. If the goal is simply to maintain a comfortable and cosmetically acceptable eye, then we do not recommend GDD surgery.

The surgeon should identify anterior segment characteristics that are associated with an increased risk of intraoperative and postoperative complications (Table 17.1). Each portion of the exam contributes to the development of an operative plan. The preoperative IOP level will guide the decision whether to alter the implantation technique to minimize an early postoperative IOP spike. Very high preoperative IOP, greater than 40 mmHg, in association with immediate postoperative hypotony increases the risk of delayed suprachoroidal hemorrhage in eyes without uveitis [11].

Table 17.1 Preoperative evaluation

Criteria	Notes
Prior ocular history	Type of uveitic glaucoma, operative intervention and location
Past medical history	Anticoagulants: risk for discontinuation?
Inflammation control	Medications and duration of quiescence
Assessment of visual potential	Useful vision?
Intraocular pressure	Level of IOP control on tolerated medical therapy
Motility	Phoria or tropia? Diplopia?
Posterior lid margin	Blepharitis
Lid position, lid closure and scleral exposure	Lid lag or lid retraction?
Conjunctival scarring and mobility	Prior incision for cataract extraction or pars plana vitrectomy, superior conjunctival mobility?
Corneal clarity and endothelial appearance	View sufficient for implantation?
Pachymetry	Possible endothelial dysfunction if greater than 600 μm
Gonioscopy	Extent and location of peripheral anterior synechiae: active neovascularization or vitreous in anterior chamber?
Anterior chamber depth (central and peripheral)	Sufficient for the drainage tube?
Lens: type and density of opacity	Affecting activities of daily living?
Optic nerve damage	Extent of glaucomatous optic neuropathy: ability to tolerate postoperative IOP spike?
Visual field status	Fixation splitting defect, risk of acute loss of central visual acuity "snuff-out"
Macular edema	Limiting visual acuity?
Retinal status	Requires treatment?

The preoperative upper lid position, extent of scleral exposure, and tear film stability determine if the implant will be adequately covered with moist, healthy conjunctiva. Uveitic patients with scleritis or high axial myopia may have ectatic sclera that is too thin to safely place anchoring sutures for the implant plate. In these eyes, the surgeon may elect to suture the plate to the muscle insertions. Scleral, corneal or pericardial patch graft erosion is often associated with poor lid closure, dry eyes, and conjunctival exposure. A careful eyelid examination for posterior marginal blepharitis is mandatory.

Assessment of preoperative peripheral corneal clarity is critical to planning the surgical strategy. A sufficiently clear peripheral cornea is necessary for visualization during anterior chamber tube placement. Corneal transparency limited by arcus senilis or stromal edema associated with endothelial dysfunction may prevent intraoperative confirmation of the exact tube location. Band keratopathy, commonly associated with uveitis, also may restrict the view. A shallow anterior chamber increases the likelihood of tube–endothelial cell touch and associated mechanical injury with resultant corneal edema. The surgeon may consider pars plana vitrectomy and pars plana tube insertion to reduce the risk of endothelial cell loss in pseudophakic eyes, in eyes with shallow anterior chambers, in eyes after penetrating keratoplasty or in eyes with marginal endothelial cell function associated with stromal thickening.

The anterior chamber should be examined before and after dilation for the presence of vitreous strands. We recommend vitrectomy, through either a limbal or pars plana route depending on the amount of vitreous anterior to the posterior capsule and pupillary border. Meticulous attention to the removal of residual vitreous is important particularly with pars plana tube insertion, as even small quantities can occlude the tube postoperatively. Nd:YAG laser vitreolysis seldom relieves the occlusion permanently. Pars plana tube insertion requires a complete vitrectomy, with special attention directed toward clearing the vitreous base in the quadrant of tube insertion. The effect of cataracts and associated visual disability should be assessed in phakic patients. Cataract removal and intraocular lens implantation may be performed concurrently with BGDD placement, if the lenticular opacity substantially limits visual-acuity-related activities of daily living. Oral, as well as topical, corticosteroids should be considered in the perioperative period to suppress the inflammation expected with a combined cataract and glaucoma surgery.

Gonioscopy should be performed to determine the location and extent of peripheral anterior synechiae and angle neovascularization. If possible, peripheral anterior synechiae should be avoided when choosing the site for tube insertion. Intraoperative goniosynechiolysis can be performed to open the trabecular meshwork or clear room for tube insertion. Alternatively, a cyclodialysis spatula inserted through a separate paracentesis can be used to elevate the tube above the iris plane. The underlying cause of neovascularization must be identified and treated preoperatively, usually with panretinal photocoagulation, to halt future new vessel growth. An off-label injection of one of the new humanized anti-VEGF antibody fragments (e.g., Lucentis (ranibizumab) and Avastin (bevacizumab), Genetech Inc., San Francisco, CA) that inhibit VEGF may be given prior to or during surgery to reduce the neovascularization [12]. Anticoagulants, such as warfarin (Coumadin), may be stopped preoperatively, if this does not pose a substantial medical risk to the general health of the patient. Miotics, like pilocarpine HCl and long-acting cholinesterase inhibitors, such as echothiophate (phospholine iodide) should be discontinued to reduce the risk of intraoperative bleeding and inflammation. Other preoperative glaucoma medications, with the exception of the prostaglandin analogs, should be continued preoperatively to reduce IOP.

17.6 Principles

Pre– and postoperative inflammation control is critical in management of uveitic eyes to normalize the rate of aqueous humor production before and after glaucoma surgery. Frequent use of topical, and often systemic, corticosteroids is required to manage intraocular inflammation. Control of preoperative intraocular inflammation may lessen postoperative fibrin formation, hypotony and subsequent choroidal effusions.

Several modifications of the originally described BGDD technique have been developed to minimize the profound postoperative hypotony reported with earlier nonvalved devices [13]. These techniques all restrict postoperative aqueous humor outflow temporarily, usually for 4–6 weeks, until a fibrous pseudocapsule forms around the plate. The thick-walled capsule is the primary site of long-term resistance to aqueous humor outflow. Two-stage implantation, reversible tube occlusion with simultaneous filtration surgery, intraluminal stents and tube fenestrations with an absorbable occluding suture have also been employed to minimize immediate postoperative hypotony [14]. We prefer to temporarily occlude the tube with a 7-0 coated 910 polyglactin suture tied around the tube. The suture completely blocks the passage of aqueous humor through the tube for the first 4–6 postoperative weeks or until it is absorbed. We perform multiple "through and through" tube fenestrations with a TG-140 or TG-160 spatula needle (Ethicon,

Somerville, NJ) between the suture and the tube tip to provide an egress site to achieve immediate postoperative IOP control (Fig. 17.3).

These fenestrations permit aqueous humor passage through the side wall of the tube until the 910 polyglactin suture dissolves and aqueous flow begins to the plate [15]. The surgical instruments usually required for BGDD implantation are listed in Table 17.2.

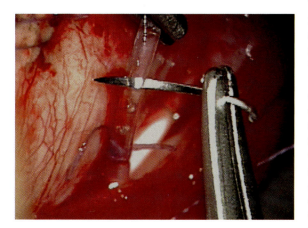

Fig. 17.3 Tube fenestration with the TG-140 needle. (© Surgical Techniques in Ophthalmology – Glaucoma Surgery. Edited by Teresa Chen. Elsevier, 2007, ISBN 978-1-4160-3021-8)

17.6.1 Preoperative IOP Reduction

The IOP should be measured in all patients with high preoperative IOP (greater than 30 mmHg) prior to giving retrobulbar or peribulbar anesthesia. A paracentesis, to reduce very high IOP, should be considered if the preoperative IOP is greater than 40 mmHg. The additional volume of the retrobulbar anesthetic may increase orbital pressure, impede blood flow through the central retinal artery, and can cause retinal ischemia. A gradual and step-wise decrease in IOP may reduce the risk of an intraoperative suprachoroidal hemorrhage associated with sudden decompression of the globe.

To safely lower IOP, we insert a 30-gauge needle on a tuberculin syringe without a plunger into the anterior chamber at the temporal limbus to permit the outflow of approximately 0.1 ml of aqueous humor. After approximately 10 s, the IOP usually falls to 10–15 mmHg and the needle can be removed through the self-sealing clear corneal tract. The paracentesis usually clears the corneal epithelial edema and minimizes a much larger IOP drop during tube insertion. A separate paracentesis site made with a sharp-angled blade can be used during the early postoperative period to lower IOP by depressing the posterior margin of the incision with a closed jeweler's forceps. If a sharp-angled blade is used for the paracentesis in the postoperative period instead of a 30-gauge

Table 17.2 Instruments and devices [8]

Instruments/devices	Notes
Topical medications	
Tetracaine HCl	Topical anesthesia
Lidocaine/bupivacaine mixture	Optional peribulbar anesthesia
Prednisolone acetate 1%	Postoperative medication
Atropine sulfate	Postoperative medication
Topical antibiotic	Postoperative medication
Subconjunctival medications	Optional injections at end of case
Antibiotic	Typically cefazolin or gentamicin
Steroids	Triamcinolone acetonide or dexamethasone sodium phosphate
Sutures and disposable supplies	
7-0 910 polyglactin on TG cutting needle	Tube ligature, corneal traction suture, tube occlusion, patch graft suture to sclera, conjunctival closure
8-0/9-0 nylon	Securing tube and plate to sclera

Table 17.2 *(continued)* Instruments and devices [8]

Instruments/devices	Notes
Cellulose sponges	Remove blood from surgical field
Super-sharp blade	Paracentesis, assist with peritomy
23-gauge needle	Enter anterior chamber for tube placement
22-gauge needle	Pars plana tube insertions
MVR blade	Hoffman elbow insertion into pars plana
30-gauge needle on tuberculin syringe with plunger removed	Preoperative anterior chamber paracentesis to reduce elevated pressure
30-gauge angled cannula on a tuberculin syringe	Check tube patency and occlusion
Pencil tip cautery	Hemostasis
Balanced salt solution	
Surgical instruments	
Smirmaul lid speculum with solid, broad blade	Exposure
Heavy-jaw needle holder (2)	Place traction suture, tie 7-0 910 polyglactin sutures
Needle holder	Titanium (fine), nonlocking preferred
Blunt-tipped Westcott scissors	Open conjunctiva and Tenon's fascia
Curved Stevens tenotomy scissors	Dissect Tenon's capsule
Glaucoma drainage implant	Baerveldt 250-mm² or 350-mm² plate
Small Stevens muscle hooks (2)	Isolate rectus muscles
Harms tying forceps (2)	Place plate beneath rectus muscles
Long Vannas scissors	Cut sutures, cut tube with bevel
Pierse-Hoskins forceps (or Max Fine)	
0.12 and 0.3 Castroviejo forceps	Manipulate sclera
Angled Kelman forceps or tube introducer (optional)	Place tube into anterior chamber
Tying forceps	
Calipers	Measure correct plate and tube placement
Patch graft	
Glycerin-preserved cornea, sclera or Tutoplast	
1 bottle of BSS with 40 mg of Gentamicin in sterile cup	Soak patch graft

needle, the larger wound can lead to unpredictable IOP lowering and hypotony.

17.6.2 Selection of Quadrant

Most surgeons prefer the superior temporal quadrant for primary BGDD placement. This approach facilitates tube placement by providing excellent exposure, permits complete scleral patch graft coverage by the upper lid, affords good cosmetic appearance, and reduces the incidence of postoperative motility problems compared with placement in the superior nasal quadrant [16]. When placed in the superior temporal quadrant, the nasal edge of the implant should be situated superficial to the superior oblique tendon insertion. When conjunctival scarring prevents dissection of a fornix-based flap without buttonhole formation in the superotemporal quadrant, the implant may be inserted in one of the other three quadrants. In order of preference, we select the inferior nasal, inferior temporal, and superior nasal locations. The low profile of the 350-mm^2 BGDD facilitates implantation in either of the inferior quadrants. The superonasal quadrant should be avoided for BGDD implantation, if possible, to prevent development of an acquired Brown syndrome [17]. If the superior nasal quadrant is selected as a last resort, then a smaller implant, the pediatric BGDD (BG 103-250, Advanced Medical Optics, Irvine, California) should be placed nasal to the superior oblique tendon to minimize postoperative motility problems.

17.6.3 Conjunctival Incision

A five clock-hour, fornix-based conjunctival peritomy gives the clearest view of limbal anatomy for tube placement. A fornix-based flap is easier to dissect than a limbus-based flap, especially when prior trauma or ocular surgery results in extensive anterior limbal scarring. If the conjunctiva adheres firmly to the underlying episclera, sterile balanced salt solution (BSS, Alcon, Ft. Worth, TX) injected through a 25-gauge needle into the subconjunctival space can be used to identify the location of mobile conjunctiva and define a dissection plane. The site of conjunctival perforation with the needle tip near the corneoscleral junction should be included in the fornix-based incision. To fashion an incision as anterior as possible, we often use a small, sharp, angled blade to incise the insertion of the conjunctiva into the peripheral corneal epithelium. With the blade held tangent to the scleral surface, we tease the anterior insertion from the underlying Tenon's capsule. This establishes an anterior site for conjunctival reattachment. We perform wide relaxing incisions angled inferiorly at the peritomy margins to allow visualization of the rectus muscles and to prevent inadvertent conjunctival tearing during the plate insertion. Conjunctival relaxing incisions should not be radially positioned at the 3 or 9 o'clock positions where they would overlie the implant plate and possibly predispose to plate exposure.

17.6.4 Preparation of the Scleral Site

We dissect Tenon's capsule from the underlying episclera with blunt Westcott scissors and Stevens tenotomy scissors. Cellulose sponges can be used to push Tenon's capsule from the lateral edges of the rectus muscles. Bleeding episcleral vessels should be cauterized with wet-field, bipolar cautery to maintain a clear operative field. Anterior limbal epithelial cells should be cauterized to stimulate limbal wound closure and to reduce the risk of fornix-based conjunctival flap wound dehiscence. When withdrawing the Stevens tenotomy scissors from the quadrant, we maintain the blades spread widely to mobilize and expose the Tenon's space posterior to the insertion of the recti. Care should be taken to avoid cutting Tenon's capsule during dissection that may predispose to orbital fat herniation and fibrosis with resultant restrictive scarring.

The sclera, at the site of planned plate fixation, should be carefully inspected for ectasia that could jeopardize safe suturing of the implant to the globe. If staphylomata or ectasia are present in the area of planned attachment, the plate should be sutured to the avascular superior or lateral rectus tendon near the point of insertion. The muscle insertions may also be selected to secure the plate in patients with quiescent scleritis to reduce the risk of inducing surgically related scleral melting. We use two small Stevens muscle hooks to isolate the rectus muscles and strip Tenon's capsule from its lateral borders to facilitate exposure and insertion. One muscle hook is used to secure the muscle insertion, while the other is placed under the muscle belly to lift and separate the lateral border from Tenon's capsule and the intramuscular septum.

17.6.5 The Implant

We handle the GDD with nontoothed forceps and inspect each implant for defects. We flush the tube with BSS on a 30-gauge cannula to insure tube patency. After the surgeon exposes first the superior and then the lateral rectus muscle with two small Stevens tenotomy muscle hooks, the assistant, usually seated temporal to the surgeon, inserts the tip of the plate beneath the muscle belly, approximately 5 mm posterior to the muscle insertion. Proper equatorial positioning of the implant reduces the chance of the eyelid rubbing the plate and minimizes the likelihood of conjunctival erosion. Calipers are used to verify that the anterior edge of the plate is situated approximately 10 mm posterior to the limbus. To obtain a clear view, we rotate the eye inferiorly with the corneal traction suture and retract the conjunctiva with a small muscle hook. We suture the plate to the sclera, 10 mm posterior to the corneoscleral junction, or to the muscle insertion with a 9-0-monofilament nylon suture on a spatula needle. The surgeon's knots are rotated into the two anterior fixation holes to minimize conjunctival erosion over the suture ends, and no suture end should be visible.

If the needle is passed too deeply when securing the plate to the globe and scleral perforation is suspected, the suture tract should be checked for vitreous with a cellulose sponge (Weck-cel Spear, Medtronic Xomed Ophthalmic Products, Jacksonville, FL) and any vitreous cut flush to the scleral surface. The surgeon should examine the peripheral retina with scleral depression. A peripheral retinal tear or hemorrhage may be treated with light cryotherapy. Postoperative monitoring is essential to determine if a retinal detachment develops.

17.6.6 Reducing Immediate Postoperative Aqueous Outflow—Tube Ligation

We tie off the tube with a surgeon's knot to minimize immediate postoperative hypotony and to allow a fibrous capsule to form around the silicone plate before aqueous humor flow begins. With two locking needle holders, we tie the 7-0 910 polyglactin suture in a watertight manner approximately 2 mm from the junction of the tube and the silicone plate. We use a double or triple throw on the first knot to prevent inadvertently cutting the tube (Fig. 17.4).

The knot should be rotated posteriorly to the scleral side of the tube so that only the suture indenting the tube is seen anteriorly. This will facilitate future laser suture lysis if required for IOP control. We verify complete tube occlusion by injecting BSS through a 30-gauge cannula into the tube tip after completing the first throw. No flow should be seen if the suture is watertight. Placement of a second suture may be necessary, if the initial ligature does not completely obstruct flow. The 7-0 910 polyglactin spontaneously absorbs after 4–6 weeks. In our experience for most patients, this occurs on postoperative day 35, +/− 3 days. We make venting slits or

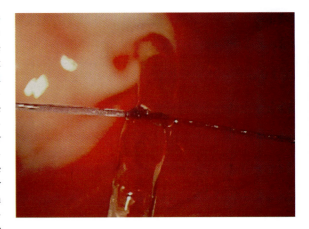

Fig. 17.4 Baerveldt tube occluded with a 7-0 910 polyglactin ligature. (© Surgical Techniques in Ophthalmology – Glaucoma Surgery. Edited by Teresa Chen. Elsevier, 2007, ISBN 978-1-4160-3021-8)

tube fenestrations whenever the preoperative pressure is judged to be dangerously elevated while on maximal medical therapy. We pass the TG-140 or TG-160 needle (Ethicon, Somerville, NJ) from the 7-0 910 polyglactin suture perpendicular to the long axis of the tube in a "through and though" manner, approximately 1 mm distal to the ligature. It is important to place the slits through the center of the tube to avoid cutting the tube in half (Fig. 17.3). We make three separate noncontiguous passes, if the preoperative pressure is greater than 30 mmHg, and two passes if the preoperative pressure is greater than 20 mmHg. If the slits are contiguous, profound immediate hypotony may occur. Ideally, the fenestrations maintain an IOP in the teens or low twenties for the first two postoperative weeks. The fibrous reaction and scarring around the tube usually prevents flow through the fenestrations by the time the occluding suture releases and aqueous humor flow begins.

17.6.7 Reducing Immediate Postoperative Aqueous Outflow—"Rip Cord" Technique

In our experience, patients with sarcoid uveitis, using frequent topical anti-inflammatory therapy on a chronic basis, have required more than 5 weeks to establish adequate scarring around the BGDD plate. In these patients, an optional "rip cord" technique can be employed to minimize immediate hypotony after spontaneous ligature absorption (Fig. 17.5).

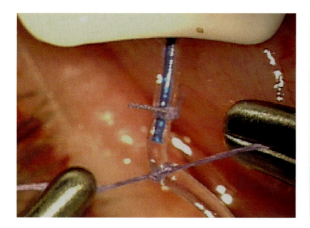

Fig. 17.5 Optional 3-0 Prolene rip cord inserted into the tube lumen and tube ligated with 7-0 polyglactin suture. (© Surgical Techniques in Ophthalmology – Glaucoma Surgery. Edited by Teresa Chen. Elsevier, 2007, ISBN 978-1-4160-3021-8)

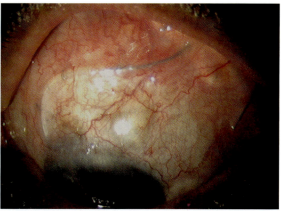

Fig. 17.6 Rip cord seen within tube lumen and extending to temporal subconjunctival space. (© Surgical Techniques in Ophthalmology – Glaucoma Surgery. Edited by Teresa Chen. Elsevier, 2007, ISBN 978-1-4160-3021-8)

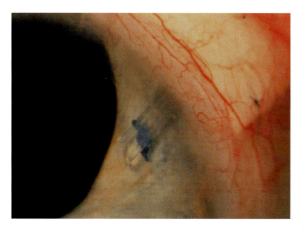

Fig. 17.7 Prolene suture ligating tube in anterior chamber. (© Surgical Techniques in Ophthalmology – Glaucoma Surgery. Edited by Teresa Chen. Elsevier, 2007, ISBN 978-1-4160-3021-8)

to 3-0 polypropylene or 3-0 mersiline (Mersed, Ethicon, Somerville, NJ). One end of the rip cord lies between the ligature aroun d the tube and the tube entry into the eye, such that it is included in the 910 polyglactin ligature around the tube and extends toward the limbus past the suture. The other end of the rip cord is then placed subconjunctivally near the limbus, so that it can be easily accessed after surgery (Fig. 17.6).

We cut the edge of the rip cord suture (bevel up) with Westcott scissors so that it is less likely to protrude or erode through the conjunctiva before suture removal. The suture is removed at the slit lamp by cutting the conjunctiva with Vannas scissors to expose the rip cord suture end and then removing it with tying or jeweler's forceps.

17.6.8 Reducing Immediate Postoperative Aqueous Outflow—Prolene Suture Placement

The rip cord can also be removed in the office as early as 2 weeks after surgery to lower the IOP prior to dissolution of the occluding 910 polyglactin suture [18]. The rip cord can be placed either adjacent to the external wall of the tube or within the lumen of the tube. Rip cord use may have a possibly higher endophthalmitis risk with intraluminal placement, since bacteria could migrate through the suture track into the anterior chamber if the suture is exposed at the conjunctival surface. Several sutures have been used for rip cords, such as 5-0 nylon

A 6-0 or 8-0 polypropylene (Prolene, Ethicon, Sommerville, NJ) suture can be tied around the tube for a more permanent occlusion, with the anticipation of future laser suture lysis. The Prolene suture knot can be positioned either beneath the conjunctiva, near the plate or inserted into the anterior chamber (Fig. 17.7). A scleral tunnel created with a 22-gauge needle may be required to insert the Prolene ligated tube into the anterior chamber. We use a slit lamp mounted argon laser (50-μm spot size, 0.5 W for 0.2 s) to "melt the belt" and release the

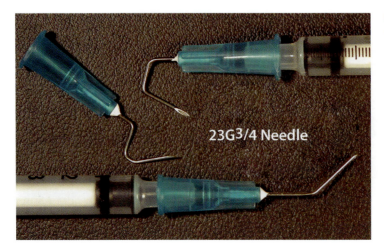

Fig. 17.8 Bent 23-gauge needles assist with tube insertion

ligature tension around the tube. This allows the flow of aqueous humor from the anterior chamber into the tube and around the drainage plate.

17.6.9 Tube Position and Insertion

The tube should be routed toward the 12 o'clock meridian, so the upper eyelid completely covers the tube and the patch graft. The uncut tube is draped over the cornea and cut so that its length and position are estimated to be at least 3 mm within the eye. The intraocular portion should be sufficiently long enough to prevent extrusion, but short enough to avoid cornea or iris touch. We use sharp suture scissors to cut the tube tip with the bevel facing anteriorly to minimize the chance of the iris occluding the orifice postoperatively. The bevel should face posteriorly whenever the tube is situated behind the iris or placed in the pars plana. The insertion site, just posterior to the mid limbus, should be treated lightly with application of thermal cautery and the residual strands of Tenon's capsule and episclera stripped away. A very anterior or clear cornea entry site should be avoided to reduce the risk of epithelial down-growth [14].

We use a 23-gauge needle on a tuberculin syringe to make a tract for tube insertion. To facilitate positioning, we bend the needle as shown in *c* of Fig. 17.8. The scleral entry site is located at the mid limbus in phakic eyes and at the posterior limbus in aphakic or pseudophakic eyes. For placement in the superior temporal quadrant, we bend the needle shaft toward the bevel so that the syringe may be held in the position of a pen (Fig. 17.8, *b*). If conjunctival scarring mandates inferior nasal insertion, the lateral nose and external nares often interfere with needle insertion. In this case, we bend the needle shaft in two places to form a U-shaped instrument with the needle tip directed toward the surgeon (Fig. 17.8, *a*).

The needle should enter the eye anterior to the iris insertion and parallel to the iris plane. The surgeon should exercise caution to avoid injuring the corneal endothelium with the needle tip. If the needle tract is placed too anteriorly, the tip should be withdrawn and a second tract made directly posterior to the first one. Pressure from the tube placed through the more posterior entry site will push anteriorly and close the first incision in a self-sealing manner [19]. The tube may also be placed posterior to the iris in aphakic or pseudophakic eyes, but anterior to the zonular apparatus and posterior capsule, if extensive peripheral anterior synechiae impede anterior chamber placement. The surgeon can position the tube orifice within a prior iridectomy to prevent tip occlusion with the iris (Fig. 17.9). Occasionally, we perforate the iris with the 23-gauge needle tip and place the tube through the iris. In eyes with anterior chamber lenses, the tube may be inserted over the haptic where the iris is pushed posteriorly from the entry site.

We enlarge slightly the external or scleral dimension of the tube tract with the needle tip as we withdraw it to facilitate tube insertion. This technique produces a watertight trapezoidal-shaped tract, which is widest at the scleral surface and narrowest at the endothelial entry site. In eyes with shallow anterior chambers or low IOP, we inject BSS through the paracentesis tract to facilitate tube placement and raise IOP. A normal or slightly elevated IOP makes the subsequent tube insertion easier.

Viscoelastic substances can be used; however, it is not possible to accurately judge the insertion site for watertight closure after implantation when they are employed. If the tube is completely occluded and the outflow resis-

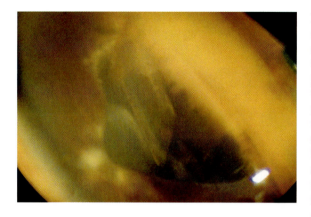

Fig. 17.9 Tube tip positioned within a prior iridectomy site

tance is high, then residual viscoelastic may cause a high IOP spike in the immediate postoperative period. We use nontoothed forceps or a Tube Inserter (New World Medical, Rancho Cucamonga, CA) or smooth-angled tying forceps to grasp the tube for insertion through the scleral tract. An excessively long tube that obscures the visual axis should be trimmed or redirected. Ideally, the tube tip should bisect the anterior chamber angle and not touch the cornea, iris or anterior lens capsule. Very short tubes that may extrude can be lengthened with a Tube Extender (New World Medical, Rancho Cucamonga, CA).

Eyes with epithelial down-growth or extensive neovascularization may require an extra long tube to preclude tip obstruction. Leakage around the tube at the insertion site indicates that the scleral incision is too wide. Placement of a single, interrupted 9-0 nylon suture at one end of the scleral tract, just adjacent to the tube, can be used to repair an oversized scleral incision. This effectively shortens the incision and pushes the tube snugly against the other end of the scleral tract. This watertight tube entry site greatly reduces the risk of early postoperative hypotony.

17.6.10 Patch Graft

After positioning the tube, we suture it to the sclera with a 9-0 nylon mattress suture and rotate the knot into the sclera. Postoperatively, a fibrous capsule will engulf the tube and prevent lateral displacement. We always place a patch graft over the tube to minimize eyelid friction and to diminish the chance of conjunctival erosion. We fashion a rectangular patch graft, approximately 5 mm × 6 mm, from either Tutoplast (Innovative Ophthalmic Products Inc., Costa Mesa, CA), glycerin-preserved sclera or donor cornea (Florida Lions Eye Bank). We suture the graft at each anterior corner with the tube in the middle, near the limbus with interrupted 7-0 910 polyglactin sutures. Split-thickness donor cornea, with the endothelial layer and posterior stroma removed, provides a cosmetically more appealing appearance than donor sclera or Tutoplast, especially in the inferior quadrant where exposure may be more obvious. The limbal margin of the patch graft should be trimmed as smoothly as possible to reduce the risk of corneal dellen formation. We do not use trabeculectomy-type scleral flaps for tube coverage because they are prone to erosion and do not stabilize the tube tip in the anterior chamber. Diode or argon laser suture lysis of the 7-0 910 polyglactin suture can be performed through the cornea patch graft or through the conjunctiva after postoperative hyperemia has subsided, if the IOP remains uncontrolled and the fenestrations have ceased to function.

17.6.11 Conjunctival Closure

We suture the conjunctiva to the anterior corneoscleral limbus and close the relaxing incisions at the lateral extent of the peritomy with two running 7-0 910 polyglactin sutures. After reforming the chamber with BSS, we inspect the tube for proper positioning. A visible bleb, located posterior to the patch graft, demonstrates that the fenestrations are functioning properly. We inject a broad spectrum antibiotic, such as cefazolin (50 mg) or gentamicin sulfate (20 mg) and a corticosteroid, such as dexamethasone sodium phosphate (2 mg) into the subconjunctival space directly opposite to the implant.

17.6.12 Conjunctival Closure with Extensive Scarring

Extensive subconjunctival scarring associated with pars plana vitrectomy incisions may limit tissue mobility and prevent the anterior advancement of the fornix-based flap to cover the patch graft. If fibrosis exists at the corneoscleral junction, then debridement and cauterization of the underlying episclera should be performed to minimize surface epithelial cell proliferation beneath the fornix flap and patch graft. We undermine and free healthy, unscarred conjunctiva posterior to the corneoscleral junction with blunt tip Westcott scissors to facilitate tissue mobility. Excessive dissection of Tenon's capsule posteriorly may injure the levator aponeurosis and cause ptosis or motility problems.

Autologous conjunctiva transplantation from the same or fellow eye is an infrequently employed alternative to cover the patch graft. If additional surgery is anticipated, then the options will be limited by the scarring at the donor site. Amniotic membrane graft (AmbioDry Amniotic Membrane Allograft, OKTO Ophtho Inc, Costa Mesa, CA, or Amniotic Graft, Bio-Tissue, Inc., Miami Fl) placed over the corneal or scleral patch graft can be used to provide scaffolding for epithelial cell proliferation. If extensive patch graft exposure cannot be resolved, a partial lateral tarsorrhaphy can be performed to promote surface epithelization. Pars plana tube insertion after pars plana vitrectomy may be necessary in extreme cases of perilimbal conjunctival scarring to assure graft coverage and to minimize tube exposure risk.

17.6.13 Alternatives to Anterior Chamber Tube Placement—The Pars Plana Route

Anterior chamber tube placement in eyes with narrow angles, marginal corneal endothelial cell function or after penetrating keratoplasty are at increased risk for corneal endothelial cell injury. Tube insertion through the pars plana into the vitreous cavity may minimize postoperative mechanical trauma to the endothelium. Pars plana vitrectomy, with special attention paid to clearing the vitreous base at the sclerotomy site must be performed to prevent postoperative occlusion. After the vitrectomy, a separate 23-gauge sclerotomy should be made 3.5 mm posterior to the corneoscleral limbus in pseudophakic or aphakic eyes for tube insertion. If the tube is inserted through the same pars plana site used for the vitrectomy instruments, the scleral wound usually cannot be closed in a watertight fashion around the tube.

A Hoffman elbow modification to the Baerveldt implant (model BG 102-350 Advanced Medical Optics, Irvine, California) can be used to maintain perpendicular entry of the tube into the vitreous cavity. The length of the tube peripheral to the Hoffman elbow is 4 mm. Surgeons who prefer avoiding blockage with any residual vitreous by using a longer tube that extends approximately 6 mm into the vitreous cavity should not use this implant. After a standard three-port pars plana vitrectomy, the infusion cannula should be left in place to maintain an elevated IOP during tube insertion through the separate sclerotomy. We confirm that the tube tip is free of vitreous and in the vitreous cavity with indirect binocular ophthalmoscopy and scleral depression. The surgeon should always tie off the tube in a watertight manner and make the decision for fenestration based on the same criteria used for the anterior chamber placement. The tube and pars plana entry site should be covered with a patch graft to prevent tube erosion.

17.6.14 Drainage Implant Surgery in Combination with Other Procedures

Long-term corticosteroid treatment of inflammatory eye disease often leads to posterior subcapsular cataract formation. Cataract surgery can be combined with the BGDD implantation. We usually remove the cataract through a temporal, clear cornea incision and insert the intraocular lens into the capsular bag. After lens implantation, we retain the viscoelastic in the anterior chamber and close the keratotomy with a 9-0-nylon suture. The BGDD implantation technique is described above. At the conclusion of the case, we remove the residual viscoelastic from the anterior chamber with the bimanual irrigation and aspiration hand pieces. Uveitic patients undergoing combined cataract removal and drainage implant surgery may receive intravenous corticosteroid injection at the time of surgery, in addition to postoperative topical, periocular and oral corticosteroids.

17.7 Postoperative Management

17.7.1 Postoperative Day 1

Patients with advanced glaucomatous optic neuropathy should be examined frequently to monitor IOP. If markedly elevated, the surgeon can lower the IOP by releasing aqueous humor or residual viscoelastic material, by depressing the posterior lip of the temporal paracentesis tract under direct visualization at the slit lamp. If a paracentesis was not made at the time of tube implantation, then oral carbonic anhydrase inhibitor therapy may be necessary to control IOP until the 7-0 polyglactin ligature spontaneously breaks. Alternatively, a paracentesis can be made with a 30-gauge needle as described earlier to lower IOP acutely. All patients are instructed to shield their eye when sleeping. Patients with very low postoperative IOP should avoid Valsalva maneuvers, such as lifting heavy lifting, straining on bowel movements or forceful coughing, which increases intraluminal blood pressure in the long posterior ciliary arteries and may cause delayed-onset suprachoroidal hemorrhage.

At each postoperative visit we assess visual acuity, IOP, lid position, bleb status, conjunctival closure (Seidel test), corneal clarity, tube position and anterior cham-

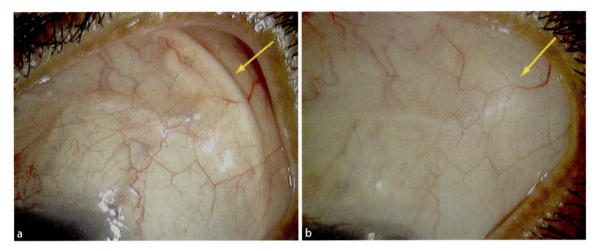

Fig. 17.10 a View of the Baerveldt ridge before tube ligature opens (3 weeks postoperation). **b** View of the Baerveldt ridge after the tube ligature opens (5 weeks postoperation)

ber depth and inflammation. Topical 1% prednisolone acetate drops are instilled hourly during the daytime and are tapered according to the level of inflammation. A broad spectrum antibiotic drop, such as polymyxin and trimethoprim or a third generation fluoroquinolone, is used until the conjunctival wound has healed, and usually discontinued after 1 week.

17.7.2 Postoperative IOP Management—Early

The tube fenestrations usually maintain an acceptable IOP during the early postoperative period. Aqueous humor flows through the fenestrations into the subconjunctival space anterior to the plate and adjacent to the tube until scarring blocks its egress. Topical glaucoma medications are usually required for IOP control until the tube ligature spontaneously opens, usually 5 weeks after surgery. Occasionally, the early postoperative IOP cannot be controlled, even with fenestrations and medications. The hallmark of an occluded tube is the visible ridge at the anterior margin of the plate (Fig. 17.10a). This ridge is not visible when aqueous humor flow elevates the conjunctiva over the implant (Fig. 17.10b).

If necessary, the surgeon can refenestrate the tube to lower the IOP. We instill a topical anesthetic; prep the lids, lashes and ocular surface with povidone iodine solution and place a lid speculum. While directly visualizing the tube at the slit lamp, we use a TG-160 needle (Ethicon, Somerville, NJ) held on a needle driver to perforate the tube in a through and through manner. The 9-0-nylon suture, previously placed to secure the tube to the sclera, minimizes movement and possible accidental withdrawal from the eye during refenestration. We insert the needle through the conjunctiva, about 5 mm lateral and distal to the tube and 910 polyglactin ligatures. The needle shank should be passed perpendicularly to the long axis of the tube lumen under direct visualization. A bleb overlying the tube should form spontaneously after removing the needle. A Seidel test, with a fluorescein strip, should be performed to determine if a conjunctival leak exists at the needle puncture site. If a leak is present, we apply direct pressure with a cotton tip applicator to compress the underlying Tenon's fascia and close the perforation. If the leak persists, light applications of a battery-powered cautery may be used to seal the perforation and stimulate wound healing.

17.7.3 Postoperative IOP Management—Weeks 2–6

Severely damaged optic nerves may not tolerate prolonged, elevated IOP. If the fenestrations and medication do not control the IOP, ligature release may be necessary prior to spontaneous absorption. When possible, the fibrous capsule around the implant plate should develop sufficient resistance to minimize acute postoperative hypotony prior to the unobstructed aqueous flow. We prefer waiting as long as possible, to permit conjunctival healing before performing suture lysis, but have cut the occluding suture as early as 2 weeks after implantation. Either a Hoskins or a Ritch nylon suture lens (Lantham and Phillips Ophthalmic Products, Grove City, OH) can be used to compress the conjunctival blood vessels and provide a clear view of the ligature. Argon green laser energy (50-μm spot size, 500-mW pulse, 0.02 s duration) is usually sufficient to thermally cut the 7-0 910 polyglactin suture. A bleb forms over the implant plate and obscures the ridge that traverses the long axis of the plate when the tube is patent. We perform a Seidel test to insure that the laser treatment did not perforate the conjunctiva. If the suture cannot be cut with laser energy, then a needle may be used to cut the suture or to refenestrate the tube.

17.7.4 Postoperative IOP Management—Spontaneous Suture Absorption

Patients usually experience mild ocular discomfort when the ligature opens. The tenderness is probably caused by the abrupt IOP reduction and the ensuing intraocular inflammatory response (Fig. 17.11).

The inflammation, often characterized by debris and fibrin strands, should be treated with frequent topical corticosteroids and occasionally oral corticosteroids. We begin cycloplegic drops, such as 1% atropine sulfate, to minimize the anterior chamber narrowing associated with acute hypotony. Topical glaucoma medications should be stopped immediately after the tube opens to reduce the risk of prolonged hypotony. After the tube opens and aqueous flow begins, the IOP must be monitored frequently, since most eyes go through an initial hypotonous period that is followed by a postoperative hypertensive phase that lasts between 2 and 4 months. During the hypertensive phase, associated with the inflammation and fibrosis of the capsule around the implant, topical glaucoma medications lower the IOP until the inflammation subsides and the capsule wall becomes more permeable to aqueous humor. The late postoperative IOP typically stabilizes in the mid-teens, although glaucoma medications are usually required in patients with a very high preoperative IOP.

Occasionally, the late postoperative IOP rises to a damaging level despite the addition of maximal medical therapy. The treatment options include revision of the existing implant, further glaucoma drainage implant surgery, cyclodestructive procedures or needling the capsule. Surgical excision of the thick bleb wall usually fails to permanently control IOP. Needling is most likely to succeed in eyes with encapsulated blebs that are neither thick nor vascularized after the postoperative inflammation has subsided [20]. We perform needling at the slit lamp with a bent 27-gauge needle on a 1-ml tuberculin syringe. After scrubbing the lids and lashes with povidone iodine solution and inserting a lid speculum, we pass the needle tip under direct visualization through the conjunctiva and advance it into the subconjunctival space to cut through the fibrous capsule or encysted bleb. The needling may be repeated, as needed, to achieve suitable IOP control. If multiple needlings do not reduce IOP adequately, we recommend implantation of a second BGDD, usually in the inferonasal quadrant, if the potential for useful vision still exists.

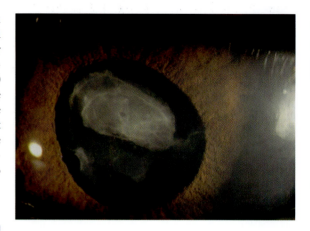

Fig. 17.11 Fibrin formation in anterior chamber after tube opens

17.8 Postoperative Complications

Chronically inflamed eyes often develop an exuberant fibrinous response in the anterior chamber associated with reduced aqueous humor production after glaucoma drainage device surgery. Postoperative complications usually result from inadequate preoperative evaluation or intraoperative technical problems. A comprehensive listing of complications based on the time of occurrence is provided in Table 17.3. We will focus primarily on the unique problems of glaucoma drainage implant surgery in eyes with inflammation: hypotony and tube obstruction.

17.8.1 Hypotony

Markedly reduced aqueous humor production associated with intraocular inflammation (often referred to as "ciliary body shutdown") or incomplete tube occlusion, or both, can result in early postoperative hypotony and a flat anterior chamber (Figs. 17.12 and 17.13).

Corneal–tube touch or cornea–lens touch, unless corrected, can damage the corneal endothelium and cause an acute cataract [22]. Early hypotony is associated with low resistance to aqueous humor outflow, such as larger than desired fenestrations, fenestrations that are placed contiguously, an oversized sclerotomy that permits aqueous to leak around the tube or incomplete occlusion of the tube. Eyes with very low IOP can be observed for spontaneous IOP elevation, if the tube tip is not in contact with the corneal endothelium or the crystalline lens. Topical or oral corticosteroids or both can be used with increased frequency if inadequately controlled inflammation is responsible for the hypotony. If tube–corneal touch develops, the chamber should be reformed immediately to prevent mechanical damage to the endothelium. We prefer injecting viscoelastic through the temporal paracentesis tract. If the ligature opens before the fibrous capsule has formed around the plate and resistance to aqueous humor flow has developed, hypotony may complicate the postoperative course. The extent of postoperative conjunctival healing, IOP level, anterior chamber depth and choroidal effusion will determine if the hypotony can be managed conservatively. An additional 7-0 910 polyglactin (temporary) or Prolene (permanent) ligature can be placed around the tube under topical anesthesia through a small conjunctiva incision to eliminate aqueous outflow through the tube. This cannot be performed

Table 17.3 Potential complications and causes

	Complications	Causes
Intraoperative	Hyphema	Iris root trauma during tube insertion
	Lens damage	Improper length or direction of tube
	Lens or corneal endothelial damage	23-gauge needle tip trauma
	Scleral perforation and retinal tear	Needle injury while suturing plate to globe
	Hypotony	23-gauge limbal sclerotomy site not watertight, incomplete tube occlusion, contiguous fenestrations and slit too large
Early Postoperative	Hypotony	Decrease in aqueous production, excessive aqueous run-off with flat anterior chamber and choroidal effusion
	Intraocular inflammation	Marked in eyes with chronic uveitis
	IOP spike before occluding suture absorbs	Risk for progressive optic neuropathy in discs with advanced damage
	Dellen	Elevated conjunctiva over patch graft with poor tear lubrication
	Suprachoroidal hemorrhage	Acute postoperative hypotony and high preoperative IOP
	Transient diplopia	Edema within the orbit and rectus muscles, injury to recti with peribulbar anesthesia
	Endophthalmitis	Direct intraoperative contamination
	Aqueous misdirection	Initial postoperative hypotony and annular choroidal swelling [21]

Table 17.3 (continued) Potential complications and causes

	Complications	Causes
Late Postoperative	Cataract progression	With or without direct mechanical injury, prolonged hypotony
	Chorioretinal folds	Prolonged hypotony
	Chronic iritis	History of uveitis or neovascularization
	Hypotony maculopathy	Excessive aqueous humor runoff, high axial myopia, young patients
	Tube occlusion	Blood, fibrin, iris or vitreous
	Corneal edema and graft failure	With or without tube–cornea touch
	Persistent elevated IOP after tube opens	Thick fibrous capsule with high resistance
	Inadequate IOP control with properly functioning BGDD	Hypertensive phase
	Motility disturbance, strabismus, diplopia	Bleb displacement of globe, muscle fibrosis
	Patch graft melting	Tube or plate erosion associated with poor lid closure, dry eye
	Retinal detachment	Scleral perforation, underlying disease, such as proliferative diabetic retinopathy
	Tube migration	Inadequate fixation of plate to sclera
	Endophthalmitis	Tube or plate exposure and positive Seidel test

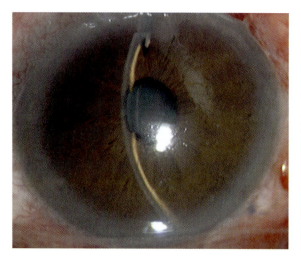

Fig. 17.12 Hypotonous eye with tube–corneal touch

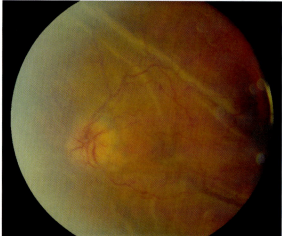

Fig. 17.13 Hypotonous eye with hypotony maculopathy

with slit lamp visualization and requires an operating microscope.

Acute postoperative hypotony is associated with an increased risk of developing choroidal effusion and suprachoroidal hemorrhage. Choroidal effusions tend to resolve rapidly and spontaneously, after the IOP is raised to a normal level. If an extensive choroidal effusion blocks the visual pathway (optical axis), drainage through an inferior scleral incision may be necessary. We use the Kelly punch to produce a circular scleral opening by cutting on each side of the scleral incision. This allows prolonged drainage of suprachoroidal fluid into the subconjunctival space during the immediate postoperative period.

Elderly, hypertensive patients with arteriosclerosis and prolonged hypotony are at increased risk for a suprachoroidal hemorrhage after glaucoma surgery [23]. Mechanical stress on the posterior ciliary arteries, produced by a choroidal effusion, can further contribute to a suprachoroidal hemorrhage [24]. Complete tube occlusion without aqueous flow into the plate is usually sufficient for a fibrous capsule to form around the plate. The encapsulated plate usually provides sufficient resistance to prevent hypotony after the tube opens, however, we have cared for three patients who developed suprachoroidal hemorrhages 6 weeks after implantation when the suture spontaneously released and the IOP fell precipitously to very low levels.

Patients with chronic or intermittent anterior uveitis are at particular risk for hypotony due to their markedly diminished aqueous production. As discussed earlier, we recommend the 250-mm² implant instead of the 350-mm² BGDD in these eyes. Similarly, a patient after a cyclodestructive procedure or initial implant surgery may require the smaller 250-mm² implant to avoid overfiltration. If a cyclodestructive procedure is planned in an eye with a drainage implant, less extensive ciliary body treatment may be necessary, since the outflow facility is already increased by the drainage implant.

17.8.2 Tube Obstruction

After the occluding ligature opens, a visible elevation forms over the plate (Fig. 17.10b). If this is not seen, then echography can be performed to determine if fluid is present overlying the implant. If the IOP remains elevated after 6 weeks without a visible bleb, then tube occlusion should be suspected. The tube tip should be inspected for possible obstruction with blood, fibrin, vitreous or iris. Digital pressure over the plate can occasionally dislodge inflammatory or fibrin debris occluding the tube orifice. If the tube is clogged with blood products or fibrin, a 0.1-µg solution (10 µg/0.1 ml) of tis-

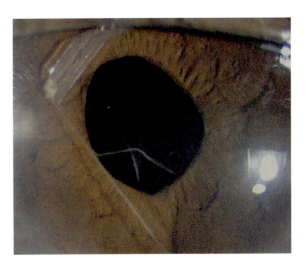

Fig. 17.14 Fibrin in anterior chamber obstructing tube. (© Surgical Techniques in Ophthalmology – Glaucoma Surgery. Edited by Teresa Chen. Elsevier, 2007, ISBN 978-1-4160-3021-8)

sue plasminogen activator (TPA) (Activase, Genentech, San Francisco, CA) can be injected into the tube to dissolve the fibrin. The use of TPA may further complicate matters by dissolving fresh clots before the postoperative vascular endothelial cell repair has been completed and lead to an intraocular hemorrhage. If the tube tip is blocked by iris, inflammatory debris, or vitreous, argon laser or Nd:YAG laser energy delivered through a gonioprism can be used to cut the tissue (Fig. 17.14).

If a large amount of tissue occludes the tube tip, surgical revision is usually necessary. It is also possible to clear inflammatory debris by flushing the tube with BSS that is delivered through a 30-gauge cannula placed through the paracentesis, across the anterior chamber, and into the tube tip under direct visualization. Tubes obstructed with vitreous almost always require a vitrectomy to clear the blockage, lower IOP, and reduce the risk of a retinal detachment from vitreous traction.

Uveitic glaucoma poses special challenges for the internist, the rheumatologist, the uveitis specialist, the glaucoma specialist, and the patient. Exuberant inflammation, severe conjunctival scarring, iris neovascularization, corticosteroid induced cataracts, medication side-effects, and the increased risk of hypotony make uveitic glaucoma especially difficult to manage. Careful preoperative evaluation insures that the correct diagnosis is made and an appropriate treatment plan is implemented. It is imperative that pre and postoperative intraocular inflammation be controlled adequately with judicious medication use. When conservative measures fail, glaucoma drainage devices can provide an effective means of lowering intraocular pressure. Although several different, effective drainage implants are available, we prefer to use the modified 250 mm² BGDD for the majority of our uveitic patients with elevated IOP. Innovative revisions in implantation technique and glaucoma drainage device modifications have improved our ability to achieve and maintain a low IOP in these challenging uveitic eyes. Careful preoperative planning and meticulous attention to operative technique can minimize complications and enhance surgical safety and efficacy.

References

1. Hill RA, Nguyen QH, Baerveldt G, Forster DJ, Minckler DS, Rao N, Lee M, Heuer DK: Trabeculectomy and Molteno implantation for glaucomas associated with uveitis. Ophthalmology. 1993;100:903–8
2. Jaffe GJ, Martin D, Callanan D: Fluocinolone acetonide implant (Retisert) for noninfectious posterior uveitis. Ophthalmology. 2006;113:1020–7
3. Skuta GL, Parrish RK: Wound healing in glaucoma filtering surgery. Surv Ophthalmol. 1987;32:149–70
4. Chen J, Cohn RA, Lin SC: Endoscopic photocoagulation of the ciliary body for treatment of refractory glaucomas. Am J Ophthalmol. 1997;124:787–96
5. Ozdal PC, Vianna RNG, Deschenes J: Ahmed valve implantation in glaucoma secondary to chronic uveitis. Eye. 2006;20:178–83
6. Tsai JC, Johnson CC, Kammer JA, Dietrich MS: The Ahmed shunt versus the Baerveldt shunt for refractory glaucoma II: longer-term outcomes from a single surgeon. Ophthalmology. 2006;113:913–7
7. Schwartz KS, Lee RK, Gedde SJ: Glaucoma drainage implants: a critical comparison of types. Curr Opin Ophthalmol. 2006,17.181–9
8. Fechter HP, Parrish RK II: Preventing and treating complications of Baerveldt glaucoma drainage device surgery. Int Ophthalmol Clin. 2004;44:107–36
9. Krupin T, Feitl M, Karalekas D: Glaucoma associated with uveitis. In: Ritch R, Shields MB, Krupin T: The Glaucomas. 1996; St Louis: Mosby, p 1232
10. Shammas HF, Zubyk NA, Stanfiedl TF: Sympathetic uveitis following glaucoma surgery. Arch Ophthalmol. 1977;95:638–41
11. The Fluorouracil Filtering Surgery Study Group: Risk factors for suprachoroidal hemorrhage after filtering surgery. Am J Ophthalmol. 1992;113:501–7
12. Rosenfeld PJ. Intravitreal Avastin: the low cost alternative to Lucentis? Am J Ophthalmol. 2006;142:141–3
13. Lloyd ME, Baerveldt G, Heuer DK, et al.: Initial clinical experience with the Baerveldt implant in complicated glaucomas. Ophthalmology. 1994;101:640–50
14. Wax M, Kass M: Glaucoma surgery. In: Krupin T, Kolker A, Rosenberg L, editors: Complications in ophthalmic surgery. 1999; St Louis: Mosby, pp 162–70
15. Emerick GT, Gedde SJ, Budenz BL: Tube fenestrations in Baerveldt glaucoma implant surgery: 1 year results compared with standard implant surgery. J Glaucoma. 2002;11:340–6
16. Eid T, Spaeth GL, Heuer D: The glaucomas: concepts and fundamentals. 1999; Philadelphia: Lippincott Williams and Wilkins, pp 294–9
17. Hodkin MJ, Goldblatt WS, Burgoyne CF, et al.: Early clinical experience with the Baerveldt implant in complicated glaucomas. Am J Ophthalmol. 1995;120:32–40
18. Breckenridge RR, Bartholomew LR, Crosson CE, Kent AR: Outflow resistance of the Baerveldt glaucoma drainage implant and modifications for early postoperative IOP control. J Glaucoma. 2004;13:396–9
19. Baerveldt G. Implantation of glaucoma drainage devices. Audio Dig Ophthalmol. 2002;40(17)
20. Chen PP, Palmberg PF: Needling revision of glaucoma drainage device filtering blebs. Ophthalmology. 1997;104:1004–10
21. Dugel PU, Heuer DK, Thach AB: Annular peripheral choroidal detachment simulating aqueous misdirection after glaucoma surgery. Ophthalmology. 1997;104:439–44
22. Tanji T, Heuer D: Aqueous shunts. In: Spaeth G: Ophthalmic surgery: principles and practice. 2003; Philadelphia: Elsevier, pp 297–308
23. Law SK, Kalenak JW, Connor TB Jr, et al.: Retinal complications after aqueous shunt surgical procedures for glaucoma. Arch Ophthalmol. 1996;114:1473–80
24. Nguyen QH, Budenz DL, Parrish RK: Complications of Baerveldt glaucoma drainage implants. Arch Ophthalmol. 1998;116:571–5

Glaucoma / Chapter 18

Cyclodestructive Procedures

Torsten Schlote

Core Messages

- The main advantages of transscleral cyclodestructive procedures compared to other glaucoma surgical procedures are (a) ease of performance and (b) possibility of retreatments.
- Both transscleral cyclocryocoagulation and cyclophotocoagulation using either Nd:YAG or diode laser are characterized by (a) a comparable success rate and (b) no linear dosage–efficacy relationship.
- Because transscleral cyclophotocoagulation acts more selectively (by melanin absorption) than cyclocryocoagulation, (a) postoperative inflammatory reaction is less intense and (b) the risk of further scleral damage, such as scleral atrophy from scleritis, is lower.
- There is a strong age-dependent probability of success for all cyclodestructive procedures, which is independent of the underlying type of glaucoma.
- Transscleral cyclophotocoagulation has not only a lower risk profile, but also a lower success rate than other surgical procedures in pediatric glaucoma, including secondary glaucoma in pediatric uveitis. It remains a surgical procedure of last choice in children.
- Transscleral cyclophotocoagulation offers a good therapeutic opportunity in older patients with uveitic glaucoma after other glaucoma surgery has failed. Probably it has the best benefit–risk ratio in scleritis-associated glaucoma if parameters of application are reduced.
- Endoscopic cyclophotocoagulation is an intraocular procedure, which allows more precise diode laser application under direct visualization of the ciliary processes. Whereas the results in refractory glaucoma are encouraging, success rate is much lower in pediatric glaucoma. More experience is needed with this treatment modality concerning inflammatory glaucoma.

Contents

18.1	Introduction	194
18.2	Effectivity and Safety of Transscleral Cyclocryocoagulation in Advanced Glaucoma	194
18.3	Effectivity and Safety of Transscleral Cyclophotocoagulation in Advanced Glaucoma	194
18.4	Transscleral Cyclophotocoagulation in Inflammatory Eye Disease	195
18.5	Endoscopic Cyclophotocoagulation	196
18.6	Risk Factors for Failure of Treatment	196
18.6.1	Age	196
18.6.2	Aphakia and Other Previous Ocular Surgery	196
18.6.3	Secondary Angle-Closure Glaucoma	197
18.7	Practical Approach	197
18.7.1	Anesthesia	197
18.7.2	Transscleral Cyclocryocoagulation	197
18.7.3	Transscleral Cyclophotocoagulation	197
18.8	Complications and Management	198
References		199

This chapter contains the following video clip on DVD: Video 31 shows Transscleral Diode Laser Cyclophotocoagulation (Surgeon: Torsten Schlote).

18.1 Introduction

Secondary glaucoma is a common, frequently serious complication of inflammatory ocular disease. Glaucoma in inflammatory eye disease is characterized by its heterogeneity in etiology, pathogenesis, and a wide range of different clinical pictures and circumstances, such as scleritis, episcleritis, uveitis, keratouveitis, previous surgical intervention, response to steroids, and others. Surgical procedures such as trabeculectomy are associated with the risk of failure or activation of the inflammatory process.

Cyclodestructive procedures are typically indicated in patients with advanced and refractory glaucoma as a treatment option of second or last choice and are one way of treating severe glaucoma as a result of an underlying, usually persistent, inflammatory eye disease. Different transscleral procedures have been developed, including cyclocryocoagulation and contact and noncontact laser procedures using the diode laser, Nd:YAG, or ruby laser. Today, clinically relevant transscleral cyclodestructive procedures are:

- Contact diode laser cyclophotocoagulation
- Contact Nd:YAG laser cyclophotocoagulation
- Cyclocryocoagulation

Transscleral cyclocryocoagulation still remains a widely used cyclodestructive procedure since its introduction in clinical practice by Bietti in 1950 [19]. The principal mechanism is destruction of epithelial as well as vascular and stromal components with hemorrhagic microcirculatory infarction of the ciliary body resulting in ciliary body atrophy [15].

Nd:YAG and diode laser are the energy sources of choice for transscleral cyclophotocoagulation. Cyclodestruction is achieved by transscleral application of infrared light (wavelength diode laser 805–810 nm, Nd:YAG 1,064 nm), which is mainly absorbed by the pigmented epithelium of the ciliary body, resulting in destruction of the ciliary epithelium and coagulative necrosis of the ciliary body stroma [27]. Hemorrhagic infarction by photothrombosis and rarefication of the ciliary body microvasculature is probably a strong synergistic mechanism in the decrease of intraocular pressure (IOP) [24].

A relatively new way of cyclodestruction is endoscopic cyclophotocoagulation under direct visualization of the ciliary processes by fiber-optic systems. The diode laser is the energy source of choice for fiber-optic systems.

18.2 Effectivity and Safety of Transscleral Cyclocryocoagulation in Advanced Glaucoma

Transscleral cyclocryocoagulation has been an established clinical method for lowering the IOP in advanced, mostly secondary glaucoma for more than 50 years. In heterogeneous glaucoma populations, a success rate between 30% and 100% (depending on different success criteria, study criteria, glaucoma subtypes, follow-up periods, and so on) has been reported in the literature [4, 6]. The retreatment rate is between 17% and 43%. In different types of *pediatric glaucoma*, a success rate of 66% was reported. However, an average number of 4 treatment sessions per eye was needed to obtain this result [30]. Most of the serious complications (hypotonia, phthisis bulbi, anterior segment ischemia) were found after 360° cyclocryotherapy. After 180° cyclocryotherapy, bulbus hypotonia has been reported in up to 10%, phthisis bulbi between 3% and 12%.

18.3 Effectivity and Safety of Transscleral Cyclophotocoagulation in Advanced Glaucoma

In heterogeneous glaucoma populations, overall success rates of transscleral cyclophotocoagulation between 35% and 85% were reported on midterm follow-up periods [1, 5, 12, 25]. Both transscleral contact laser procedures (Nd:YAG or diode laser) seem comparable in efficacy and risk profile. Today, the risk of severe complications such as hypotonia and phthisis bulbi is probably less than 1% after initial transscleral cyclophotocoagulation using established parameters for application. Therefore the use of transscleral cyclophotocoagulation has been extended to various types of glaucoma, including eyes with good visual acuity or eyes with primary and secondary open-angle glaucoma even as a primary or secondary treatment [1, 12]. On the other hand, no linear dosage–efficacy relationship exists, although higher dosages are more effective, including a higher risk of overdosage/complications, than lower dosages [7].

In cases of refractory pediatric glaucoma, a useful reduction in IOP was reported in 72% of treated eyes after a mean of 2.3 treatment sessions in one study [16]. Taking all experiences together, transscleral cyclophotocoagulation shows a clear age-dependent component, resulting in a much lower success rate in children compared to adults (see Sects. 18.4 and 18.6).

Cyclocryocoagulation and cyclophotocoagulation probably are equally effective in decreasing the intraocular pressure in patients with refractory, uncontrolled glaucoma [11]. The risk of side effects is significantly lower with transscleral laser cyclophotocoagulation than with cyclocryocoagulation (see Sect. 18.8).

> Complications of transscleral cyclocryocoagulation and cyclophotocoagulation in advanced (mostly secondary) glaucoma include:
> – Mild anterior uveitis (50–100%)
> – Severe iridocyclitis (seldom)
> – Conjunctival hyperemia/chemosis (cyclocryocoagulation)
> – Conjunctival burns (cyclophotocoagulation)
> – Scleral atrophy/thinning
> – Scleral perforation (seldom)
> – Intraocular pressure rise
> – Hypotonia
> – Phthisis bulbi
> – Decrease in visual acuity
> – Intraocular hemorrhage
> – Cystoid macular edema
> – Corneal transplant decompensation/reaction
> – Pupil distortion (cyclophotocoagulation)
> – Choroidal detachment (with flat anterior chamber—malignant glaucoma)
> – Exudative retinal detachment
> – Anterior segment ischemia
> – Neuroparalytic keratitis/corneal ulceration
> – Sympathetic ophthalmia

18.4 Transscleral Cyclophotocoagulation in Inflammatory Eye Disease

No large or long-term studies have investigated the efficacy and safety of transscleral cyclophotocoagulation in inflammatory glaucoma.

So far, only one prospective study has been published [23]. In this study, 22 eyes of 20 consecutive patients (9–77 years, mean age 50.3 ± 20.6 years) with inflammatory, medically uncontrollable glaucoma, secondary to chronic uveitis, chemical injury, episcleritis, and necrotizing scleritis with inflammation (see case report) were treated by diode laser cyclophotocoagulation and followed over one year after the initial treatment. Nearly 40% of the eyes had previous failed glaucoma surgery. Within 12 months after the first treatment, intraocular pressure was controlled in 77% of all eyes (72% in uveitic glaucoma). No serious side effects were observed. More than one treatment was necessary in 64% of the patients (mean of 2.0 treatments per eye). The procedure failed in five eyes with uveitic glaucoma (mean of 3.0 treatments in these 5 eyes). Two of the five eyes were aphakic; three eyes had previous failed cyclocryocoagulation (including the child with JCA-associated uveitis) and two had a previous failed trabeculectomy.

In eyes with thin/atrophic sclera (e.g., after scleritis) parameters for application should be reduced to avoid further scleral damage and tissue disruption (see case report). Scleral perforation has been observed in only a few patients after cyclophotocoagulation [2, 10].

> **Case Report**
> A 60-year-old female patient developed a severe secondary glaucoma due to recurrent anterior necrotizing scleritis with inflammation in her right eye (Fig. 18.1) [22].
> Scleral thinning with focal staphyloma was present circumferentially. At first, control of the inflammatory activity was achieved by immunosuppression using methotrexate. Persistently high IOP values up to 40 mmHg were observed despite maximal medical treatment. Diode laser cyclophotocoagulation (Oculight SLx 810 nm, Iris Med Instruments, CA, USA) was performed under general anesthesia using reduced laser parameters (12 applications, 1 s, 1.25 W per application). Postoperatively, IOP decreased to normal values between 14 and 18 mmHg within a few days and remained stable. No retreatment was needed. Mild anterior uveitis was seen for a few days. No serious complications, especially scleral perforation, occurred. No reactivation of scleritis was seen.

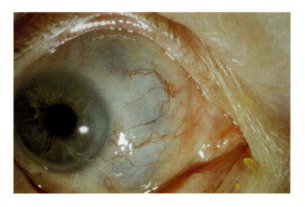

Fig. 18.1 Diode laser cyclophotocoagulation using reduced parameters of application in an eye with anterior, necrotizing scleritis with inflammation after control of inflammatory activity by immunosuppression

Recently, Heinz and coworkers first reported about the results of diode laser cyclophotocoagulation as a primary treatment in *children* with chronic anterior uveitis (pediatric glaucoma associated with chronic juvenile arthritis) and secondary open-angle glaucoma [14]. In this retrospective study, 19 eyes of 12 patients received diode laser cyclophotocoagulation (retreatment rate nearly 80%) and were followed for a mean time of 10 months. Qualified success was achieved in only 32% despite this high retreatment rate. However, no serious complications were observed. In conclusion, cyclophotocoagulation has a much lower success rate in children with uveitic glaucoma than in adults and has a much lower success rate as a primary surgical treatment compared to other surgical techniques (e.g.; goniotomy, trabeculectomy). On the other hand, a very low complication rate is seen.

In conclusion, cyclophotocoagulation seems to be a safe procedure for the treatment of refractory inflammatory glaucoma, but seems to be associated with a lower success rate—especially in children—than other surgical procedures. Therefore cyclophotocoagulation should be regarded as a surgical procedure of second choice in the management of uveitic glaucoma in younger patients with uveitis. It might be helpful to gain time before surgical treatment is performed. Diode laser cyclophotocoagulation may become the surgical procedure of choice in treating secondary glaucoma due to chemical injury and also in scleritis-associated glaucoma, using reduced parameters for application.

18.5 Endoscopic Cyclophotocoagulation

The predictability of transscleral cyclophotocoagulation is limited by the surgeon's inability to visualize the target tissue and to assess completeness of treatment. Endoscopic cyclophotocoagulation using a diode laser is an intraocular procedure to treat the ciliary processes under direct endoscopic visualization. Endoscopic cyclophotocoagulation can be performed through a limbal incision via the anterior chamber (in pseudophakic patients) or a pars plana incision.

Early results showed a successful outcome in more than 80% of the treated eyes within 2 years of follow-up in patients with refractory glaucoma of different origin [8].

Direct prospective comparison between endoscopic cyclophotocoagulation and the Ahmed glaucoma valve showed a comparable success rate of 74% and 71% respectively in patients with refractory glaucoma at 2 years of follow-up [18]. Endoscopic cyclophotocoagulation is a moderately effective procedure in the treatment of pediatric glaucoma. Neely and Plager (2001) reported a success rate of only 43% in pediatric glaucoma of different origin [20]. All significant postoperative complications, including retinal detachment, occurred in aphakic patients.

No study has been performed concerning the efficacy/safety of the procedure in secondary glaucoma due to inflammatory eye disease.

18.6 Risk Factors for Failure of Treatment

18.6.1 Age

It has been reported by several authors that patients with repeated cyclophotocoagulation or cyclocryoagulation are significantly younger than those with only one successful treatment [6, 28]. Furthermore, a clear relationship between success of treatment using diode laser cyclophotocoagulation and age of patients has been demonstrated [25]. Success rate was significantly better in patients above the age of 50 years than in patients below the age of 50 years. This age-dependent success rate of cyclophotocoagulation is not confined to very young patients (children or adolescents) only. A recently published work by Heinz and coworkers demonstrated also poor results of diode laser cyclophotocoagulation in children with uveitis, which may be predominantly associated with age of these patients more than the type of secondary glaucoma [14].

The reason for the relationship between age and success of cyclodestruction is not clear. Age-dependent changes in structure and function of the ciliary body epithelium and stroma may explain why the ciliary epithelium seems to be more susceptible to cyclodestruction in the elderly. Additionally, longstanding increase of IOP in chronic glaucoma results in pronounced atrophy of ciliary body structures, which may predispose to further damage.

18.6.2 Aphakia and Other Previous Ocular Surgery

Previous ocular surgery may be a risk factor for failure of cyclophotocoagulation in primary as well as secondary glaucoma [12, 25]. Aphakia, especially, is a significant risk factor for failure of cyclodestruction.

18.6.3 Secondary Angle-Closure Glaucoma

Subtotal or total secondary angle-closure glaucoma as a result of peripheral anterior synechiae is a special risk factor for failure, because of the overwhelming amount of subtotal destruction of the ciliary body epithelium that must be achieved to lower IOP efficiently. A higher failure rate that leads to retreatment may be ultimately associated with a higher risk of hypotonia and phthisis. Nevertheless, good clinical results using diode laser cyclophotocoagulation have been reported in chronic angle-closure glaucoma [17].

18.7 Practical Approach

18.7.1 Anesthesia

In cyclocryocoagulation, parabulbar or retrobulbar anesthesia is used, but subconjunctival anesthesia using cocaine, lidocaine 2%, or mepivacaine 2% is also effective.

In transscleral cyclophotocoagulation, *subconjunctival anesthesia* is a simple but effective and very safe method of anesthesia [26]. Oxybuprocaine (or another topical anesthetic eye drop), approximately 4–6 drops, is instilled in the eye. Then, 1–1.5 ml of 2% mepivacaine/2% lidocaine is placed beneath the conjunctiva (Fig. 18.2). The needle is carefully placed 6–8 mm from the limbus to avoid bleeding at the injection site. The eye is patched for 10 minutes with a low-pressure bandage. In general, no oral or intravenous sedation is needed.

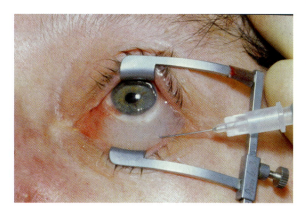

Fig. 18.2 Subconjunctival anesthesia using scandicaine 2% before diode laser cyclophotocoagulation. Bleeding of conjunctiva should be avoided by careful application and a limbal distance of 6 mm or more (see Fig. 18.3)

General anesthesia may be needed in children or noncompliant adults, or eyes with high risk of perforation by parabulbar or subconjunctival anesthesia (e.g., scleral staphyloma).

18.7.2 Transscleral Cyclocryocoagulation

Usually, six applications lasting 60 s each at –80°C on the inferior or superior 180° of the globe are performed [21]. The anterior edge of a 2.5 mm probe tip should be placed at a distance of about 1 mm from the anterior border of the limbus inferiorly, temporally, and nasally and about 1.5 mm superiorly. At the end of the operation subconjunctival steroid injection should be given in all eyes with uveitis, and steroid ointment should be instilled. Acetazolamide and osmotic agents can be used to control early postoperative IOP peaks in sighted eyes. If no adequate IOP response is obtained 4 weeks after the first treatment, the procedure can be repeated.

18.7.3 Transscleral Cyclophotocoagulation

Transscleral contact *Nd:YAG laser cyclophotocoagulation* using the Microruptur 3 (Meridian, Bern, Switzerland) is performed with a laser power of 10 W, exposure duration of 0.2–0.4 s (corresponding to 2–4 J/pulse) and 10–20 applications per treatment session [9].

For transscleral cyclophotocoagulation using a diode laser, the laser energy is delivered through a contact fiber-optic G-probe (IRIS Endoprobe®) attached to the *Oculight SLx semiconductor diode laser* (IRIS Medical Instruments, Inc., CA, USA) (Fig. 18.3).

Typical treatment consists of approximately 20 applications of 2.0 W energy applied for 2.0 s, for not more than 270° (not more than 180° in glaucoma secondary to chemical injury). Energy and duration (1.5 s, 1.5 W) should be reduced in cases of thinned sclera (e.g., necrotizing scleritis) and if audible pops are heard, indicating disruption of the ciliary body epithelium. After surgery, 0.5 ml of dexamethasone is applied subconjunctivally, and topical corticosteroids, rimexolone or prednisolone acetate 1%, are administered for at least 2 weeks. Antiglaucoma medication is continued and gradually withdrawn during the follow-up period, starting with oral carboanhydrase inhibitors. If inadequate IOP response is obtained 4 weeks after the first treatment, the procedure can be repeated.

In normal eyes the use of *transillumination* does not seem to be necessary for exact placement of the laser or cryo probe over the pars plicata. However, transillumi-

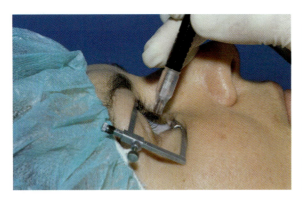

Fig. 18.3 The "G-probe" is placed parallel to the optical axis with the anterior edge of the probe at the anatomical limbus

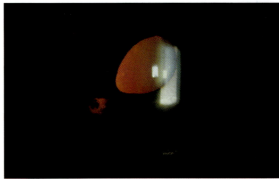

Fig. 18.5 Anterior displacement of laser energy to the iris root may result in irreversible pupil distortion and severe iritis

nation may be used for better localization of the ciliary band in eyes with abnormal dimensions or pathological changes of the anterior segment of the eye [29]. In retreatments, transillumination helps identify atrophic areas from previous cyclodestruction and permits more focused application.

18.8 Complications and Management

Severe complications after cyclodestructive procedures are relatively rare, especially after transscleral cyclophotocoagulation. However, early complications such as severe iridocyclitis and decompensated IOP may occur and cause pain (Figs. 18.4 and 18.5). Therefore, frequent follow-up of all patients is mandatory in the early postoperative phase.

Early postoperative *increase of IOP* can be treated by short-term use of acetazolamide and, rarely, by administration of osmotic substances. A steroid-responsive effect does not occur within the first days of treatment, so reduction of topical corticosteroids is probably not helpful in managing an early increase in intraocular pressure.

Early iritis is seen in nearly 50–100% of all patients after cyclodestructive treatment within the first few days after treatment. It is most often a bland, transient inflammatory reaction and should be manageable with topical prednisolone acetate 1% three to five times daily for 1–2 weeks postoperatively. A *severe iridocyclitis* associated with fibrinous reaction and pain may occur, most often some days after the cyclodestructive treatment has been performed. A more intensive treatment using prednisolone acetate 1% every hour for some days and occasionally high-dose systemic steroid treatment may be necessary to control the inflammation.

Scleral perforation is a very rare complication after transscleral cyclodestruction and can be avoided by reduction of application parameters in patients with preoperative scleral thinning. If scleral perforation occurs, a scleral patch is indicated to avoid hypotonia and endophthalmitis.

Hypotonia and phthisis bulbi are late and rare complications after cyclophotocoagulation and cyclocryocoagulation. In severe cases of prolonged hypotonia, the therapeutic options are limited. An inapparent cyclodialysis cleft should be considered. Intensive topical steroid therapy, discontinuation of all IOP-reducing medication, and occasionally injection of viscoelastic substances into the anterior chamber may be helpful to induce recovery of IOP.

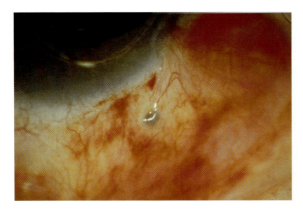

Fig. 18.4 Application of diode laser energy using the G-probe in an area of subconjunctival bleeding. Conjunctival burning occurred due to stronger absorption of laser energy by the conjunctiva

Sympathetic ophthalmia, malignant glaucoma, and *retinal detachment* have been reported in some patients after cyclophotocoagulation as well as after cyclocryocoagulation [3, 13]. A causal relationship between cyclodestructive procedures and sympathetic ophthalmia is doubtful.

Take Home Pearls

- Cyclodestructive procedures remain important treatment options in advanced glaucoma of different origins after medical antiglaucoma therapy or surgical procedures have failed.
- In comparison to cyclocryotherapy, transscleral cyclophotocoagulation (Nd:YAG or diode laser) shows comparable efficacy but a significantly lower risk profile.
- Transscleral cyclophotocoagulation is a relatively safe procedure in eyes without active inflammatory process. Cyclodestruction should only be performed in eyes with chronic intraocular inflammation if an adequate anti-inflammatory regimen is in place.
- Transscleral cyclophotocoagulation may be the surgical procedure of choice in treating secondary glaucoma caused by chemical injury and in scleritis-associated glaucoma.
- Factors which limit success of cyclophotocoagulation are: age < 50 years, aphakia, previous ocular surgery, and total or subtotal secondary angle-closure glaucoma.
- Since many patients with chronic intraocular inflammation and secondary glaucoma are younger, the effect of cyclodestruction is often transient with a high rate of retreatment. The hypotensive response to cyclodestruction is especially poor in children with persistent anterior uveitis. Cyclodestruction remains a procedure of second choice in younger patients with glaucoma.
- Moderate improvement of the surgical success rate can probably be achieved by endoscopic cyclophotocoagulation in adult refractory glaucoma because of the direct visual control of the location and intensity of the cyclodestructive effect. More experience is needed with this procedure to refine the risk–benefit ratio. The procedure is probably only moderately effective in pediatric glaucoma.

References

1. Ansari E, Gandhewar J (2007) Long-term efficacy and visual acuity following transscleral diode laser photocoagulation in cases of refractory and non-refractory glaucoma. Eye 21: 936–940
2. Beadles KA, Smith MF (1994) Inadvertent sclerotomy during transscleral Nd:YAG cyclophotocoagulation. Am J Ophthalmol 118: 669–670
3. Bechrakis NE, Müller-Stolzenburg NW, Helbig H, Foerster MH (1994) Sympathetic ophthalmia following laser cyclocoagulation. Arch Ophthalmol 112: 80–84
4. Benson MT, Nelson ME (1990) Cyclocryotherapy: a review over a 10-year period. Br J Ophthalmol 74: 103–105
5. Bloom PA, Tsai JC, Sharma K, Miller MH, Rice NSC, Hitchings RA, Khaw PT (1997) "Cyclodiode" transscleral diode laser cyclophotocoagulation in the treatment of advanced refractory glaucoma. Ophthalmology 104: 1508–1520
6. Brindley G, Shields MB (1986) Value and limitations of cyclocryotherapy. Graefes Arch Clin Exp Ophthalmol 224: 545–548
7. Chang SH, Chen YC, Li CY, Wu SC (2004) Contact diode laser cyclophotocoagulation for refractory glaucoma: comparison of two treatment protocols. Can J Ophthalmol 39: 511–516
8. Chen J, Cohn RA, Lin SC, Cortes AE, Alvarado JA (1997) Endoscopic photocoagulation of the ciliary body for treatment of refractory glaucomas. Am J Ophthalmol 124: 787–796
9. Fankhauser F, Kwasniewska S, van der Zypen E (2004) Cyclodestructve procedure. I. Clinical and morphological aspects: a review. Ophthalmologica 218:77–95
10. Gaasterland DE, Pollack IP (1992) Initial experience with a new method of laser transscleral cyclophotocoagulation for ciliary ablation in severe glaucoma. Trans Am Ophthalmol Soc 90: 225–246
11. Goldenberg-Cohen N, Bahar I, Ostakinski M, Lusky M, Weinberger D, Gaten DD (2005) Cyclocryotherapy versus transscleral diode laser cyclophotocoagulation for uncontrolled intraocular pressure. Ophthalmic Surg Lasers Imaging 36: 272–279
12. Grüb M, Rohrbach JM, Bartz-Schmidt KU, Schlote T (2006) Transscleral diode laser cyclophotocoagulation as primary and secondary surgical treatment in primary open-angle and pseudoexfoliative glaucoma. Graefes Arch Clin Exp Ophthalmol 244: 1293–1299
13. Hardten DR, Brown JD (1991) Malignant glaucoma after Nd:YAG cyclophotocoagulation. Am J Ophthalmol 111: 245–247
14. Heinz C, Koch JM, Heiligenhaus A (2006) Transscleral diode laser cyclophotocoagulation as primary surgical treatment for secondary glaucoma in juvenile idiopathic

15. Howard GM, de Roetth AJ (1967) Histopathologic changes following cryotherapy of the rabbit ciliary body. Am J Ophthalmol 64: 700–701
16. Kirwan JF, Shah P, Khaw PT (2002) Diode laser cyclophotocoagulation: role in the management of refractory pediatric glaucomas. Ophthalmology 109: 316–323
17. Lai JS, Tham CC, Chan JC, Lam DS (2005) Diode laser transscleral cyclophotocoagulation as primary surgical treatment for medically uncontrolled chronic angle closure glaucoma: long-term clinical outcomes. J Glaucoma 14: 114–119
18. Lima FE, Magacho C, Carvalho DM, Susanna R Jr, Avila MP (2004) A prospective, comparative study between endoscopic cyclophotocoagulation and the Ahmed drainage implant in refractory glaucoma. J Glaucoma 13: 233–237
19. Matrobattista JM, Luntz M (1996) Ciliary body ablation: where are we and how did we get here? Surv Ophthalmol 41: 193–213
20. Neely DE, Plaqer DA (2001) Endocyclophotocoagulation for management of difficult pediatric glaucomas. J AAPOS 5: 221–229
21. Prost M (1983) Cyclocryotherapy for glaucoma. Evaluation of techniques. Surv Ophthalmol 28: 93–100
22. Schlote T, Mielke J, Zierhut M, Jean B, Thiel H-J (1998) Zyklophotokoagulation als effektive und sichere Methode zur Therapie des Sekundärglaukoms bei anteriorer, nekrotisierender Skleritis. Klin Monatsbl Augenheilkd 213: 306–308
23. Schlote T, Derse M, Zierhut M (2000) Transscleral diode laser cyclophotocoagulation for the treatment of refractory glaucoma secondary to inflammatory eye diseases. Br J Ophthalmol 84: 999–1003
24. Schlote T, Beck J, Rohrbach JM, Funk RHW (2001a) Alteration of the vascular supply in the rabbit ciliary body by transscleral diode laser cyclophotocoagulation. Graefes Arch Clin Exp Ophthalmol 239: 53–58
25. Schlote T, Derse M, Rassmann K, Nicaeus T, Dietz K, Thiel H-J (2001b) Efficacy and safety of contact transscleral diode laser cyclophotocoagulation for advanced glaucoma. J Glaucoma 10: 294–301
26. Schlote T, Derse M (2001c) Subconjunctival anesthesia in contact diode laser cyclophotocoagulation. Ophthalmic Surg Lasers 32: 289–293
27. Simmons RB, Prum BE, Shields SR, Echelmann DA, Shields MB (1994) Videographic and histologic comparison of Nd:YAG and diode laser contact transscleral cyclophotocoagulation. Am J Ophthalmol 117:337–341
28. Threlkeld AB, Johnson MH (1999) Contact transscleral diode laser cyclophotocoagulation for refractory glaucoma. J Glaucoma 8: 3–7
29. Vesti E, Rong-Guang W, Raitta C (1992) Transillumination guided cyclocryotherapy in the treatment of secondary glaucoma. Eur J Ophthalmol 2: 190–195
30. Wagle NS, Freedman SF, Buckley EG, Davis JS, Biglan AW (1998) Long-term outcome of cyclocryotherapy for refractory pediatric glaucoma. Ophthalmology 105: 1921–1927

II Posterior Segment

Chapter 19

Macular Surgery for Posterior Segment Complications of Uveitis

Janet L. Davis

Core Messages

- Surgical management of uveitic macular complications utilizes standard vitreoretinal surgical techniques.
- Medical management of uveitic macular complications utilizes intraocular corticosteroids and anti-angiogenic factors in common use for other diseases.
- Either medical or surgical management of posterior segment complications requires control of uveitis. Systemic corticosteroids or immunosuppression without surgery can be effective treatment for macular complications.
- Imaging with OCT provides more useful information than fluorescein angiography in assessing uveitic macular disease.
- Factors predictive of surgical success in macular edema are unknown, but probably relate to anatomic features such as status of posterior hyaloid, configuration of epiretinal membranes, and vitreomacular traction.

Contents

19.1	Posterior Segment Complications of Uveitis	203
19.2	Surgery for Posterior Segment Disease	203
19.2.1	Nonuveitic Macular Disease	203
19.2.2	Uveitic Macular Disease	204
19.3	Adjunctive Medical Therapy for Macular Disease	204
19.4	Imaging in the Assessment of Macular Disease	204
19.4.1	Patterns of Uveitic Macular Edema	204
19.4.2	Measuring Uveitic Macular Edema	205
19.4.3	OCT Parameters	205
19.4.4	Future Research	205
References		206

This chapter contains the following video clips on DVD: Video 32 shows Removal of subretinal membrane and Video 33 shows ILM-Peeling (Surgeon: Marc de Smet).

19.1 Posterior Segment Complications of Uveitis

Macular complications are common in uveitis. Inflammation due to immune recovery in eyes with cytomegalovirus retinitis markedly increases macular edema and epiretinal membranes [1]. In multifocal choroiditis, choroidal neovascularization, cystoid macular edema, or epiretinal membrane occur at a rate of 0.13 per eye year [2]. Macular edema or atrophy accounts for most of the visual loss in birdshot and occurs [3] in one third to one half of patients with birdshot chorioretinopathy; an additional 10% have epiretinal membrane [4]. In pediatric uveitis, macular complications occur in up to 70% of patients [5] despite the common belief that children are more resistant to macular disease.

19.2 Surgery for Posterior Segment Disease

19.2.1 Nonuveitic Macular Disease

Pars plana vitrectomy (PPV) is well established in the management of macular disease. Classic examples are the removal of adherent vitreous strands in postcataract cystoid macular edema, removal of epiretinal membrane (ERM) with or without macular edema (ME), and release of vitreomacular traction (VMT) [6]. More recently, PPV has been proposed as a treatment for diabetic macular edema (DME) [7–9]. Concomitant peeling of the internal limiting membrane (ILM) in DME may be beneficial [10–15] but is controversial [16–18]. Patients with diabetic macular edema with intraoperative detachment of the posterior hyaloid may benefit more from PPV than patients with preexisting posterior vitreous detachment (PVD) [19]. Simple PPV with detachment of the posterior hyaloid can lead to improvement on multiple measures in patients with DME [20, 21]. The need for more complicated procedures, such as internal limiting membrane peeling, to achieve a therapeutic result is therefore uncertain and has not been explored in uveitis.

19.2.2 Uveitic Macular Disease

Vitreoretinal surgical techniques developed for other conditions should be applicable to uveitis. This is especially true for macular edema, the most prevalent macular complication in uveitis patients and long a focus of surgical therapy of uveitis. There is fair evidence from older observational case series for a possible benefit in the reduction of macular edema from PPV [22]. The most common surgical technique is simple PPV with peeling of surface membranes and complete separation of the posterior hyaloid, or core vitrectomy in eyes with PVD. Two recent case series of PPV with ILM peeling for ME included patients with uveitic macular edema (UME) as well as DME and reported improvement in some patients [23, 24].

Macular edema was the indication for PPV in 5 of 20 eyes (15 patients) with Behçet's disease; macular edema resolved in 3 of the 5 eyes [25]. Retrospective case series limited to patients with macular complications have focused primarily on ERM peeling in sarcoid-related uveitis [26]. Vitreous surgery in uveitis patients may not be as inflaming as anterior segment surgery and need not be avoided for this reason. In a small case series of eight patients, PPV for vitreous opacities in sarcoidosis did not lead to worsened inflammation or macular edema [27] whereas 5% of a much larger series undergoing phacoemulsification in pars planitis had progression of macular edema [28]. Anterior chamber inflammation did not worsen in patients undergoing therapeutic vitrectomy in one series [29]; however, suppression of all anterior chamber inflammation with topical corticosteroids is advised before PPV.

Tranos and associates [29] studied surgical vs. medical treatment of uveitic macular edema in a small, underpowered, randomized clinical trial. Twenty-three patients were accrued over a 5-year period. Patients entered the trial only if they had already been determined to have cystoid macular edema resistant to medical therapy. The vast majority of patients were pseudophakic, limiting the applicability of study results to phakic patients. This may also indicate selection bias to avoid cataract progression, which occurs in 30–50% of phakic patients by 6 months after PPV and ERM peeling [30]. Although the authors felt that surgical therapy was better than medical treatment, their methodology limits the generalizability of this conclusion.

19.3 Adjunctive Medical Therapy for Macular Disease

Medical treatment with corticosteroids or other agents should be emphasized prior to surgical management when macular edema is present in uveitis patients. Treatment with immunosuppressive medication alone reduces macular edema and development of choroidal neovascularization in patients with multifocal choroiditis [2] and birdshot chorioretinopathy [31]. Even if medical treatment is not successful, it is presumed that ongoing inflammation is detrimental to recovery and may also lead to reaccumulation of edema fluid. Alternative treatments with intravitreal triamcinolone injections may be very useful in controlling uveitic macular edema [32, 33]. Intravitreal triamcinolone has also resolved macular edema that failed to respond to PPV [34]. Intravitreal injection of anti-angiogenic factors has almost certainly replaced the use of submacular surgery to extract choroidal neovascular membranes from uveitic eyes [35] and shows promise as a treatment for some patients with uveitic macular edema [36].

19.4 Imaging in the Assessment of Macular Disease

19.4.1 Patterns of Uveitic Macular Edema

Markomichelakis and coworkers analyzed patterns of macular edema in 70 patients with uveitis [37] and subdivided them into diffuse edema, cystoid edema, and subretinal fluid based on OCT findings. Diffuse edema was the most common pattern, present in greater than 50% of patients. One quarter had cystoid edema. Subretinal fluid was present in another 20%, split 2:1 between cystoid and diffuse edema. Epiretinal membrane was present in 40% of eyes and vitreomacular traction in almost 10%. Thus, nearly half of patients had anatomic findings suggesting a mechanical factor that might contribute to macular edema and be treatable with surgery. Correlation between pattern and surgical outcomes is a logical extension of this classification scheme.

19.4.2 Measuring Uveitic Macular Edema

The optimal method for grading macular edema in clinical trials or clinical care is not clear. Angiographic assessment of macular edema is almost surely not adequate as it is semiquantitative and cannot reveal important structural characteristics [37], although confirmation of active leakage can be important. Most descriptive studies use OCT-derived central retinal thickness measures [37]. An alternative of confocal scanning laser has been proposed [38] to measure macular volume. B-scan ultrasonography detection of macular edema also has good correlations with vision, fluorescein angiographic findings, and OCT thickness measures [39].

19.4.3 OCT Parameters

For OCT documentation of macular edema, use of the central subfield thickness is more reproducible than the central point thickness, and central point thickness measures with greater than 10% variability indicate poor fixation and are unreliable [40]. Both central retinal thickness and total macular volume have been used in recent studies of therapeutic interventions for macular edema [41]. Intraobserver variability of total macular volume measurements by OCT is less than for foveal zone thickness measurements, which are operator-dependent [42]. Machine-generated values for both parameters are reliable when compared to manual grading and suitable for clinical trials [43].

19.4.4 Future Research

Factors predictive of surgical success may ultimately be identified so that medical therapy can be tried for a defined period of time before proceeding to surgery. Potential indicators favoring surgical intervention are vitreomacular traction, taut membranes with rippling of the underlying retina, thick membranes that may blur vision, and persistence of edema despite medical control of inflammation. Cystic retina with minimal leakage on fluorescein angiography may indicate severe structural damage. Three-dimensional ultra-high-resolution OCT, currently investigational, provides information that may be extremely useful in determining whether epiretinal membrane peeling is likely to be of benefit in that it can display traction lines extending from surface membranes into the retina [44].

> **Take Home Pearls**
>
> Although surgical techniques are standard, there are some observations pertinent to vitrectomy surgery in uveitic eyes with macular complications.
>
> **When you can't see the macula preoperatively, you don't know yet what the visual potential might be.** Preoperative assessment of macular potential may be difficult in eyes with vitreous opacification or cataract. Irregular reflections from the retinal surface are very common yet may not indicate significant macular disease. Epiretinal membrane peeling or ILM peeling in patients with unknown central acuity may be unnecessary; thick or distorting membranes that are encountered should be removed. OCT can help visualize gross macular status in (nearly) opaque eyes.
>
> **Visualize the vitreous with triamcinolone acetonide during surgery.** A 3:1 dilution is extremely helpful in removal of the posterior hyaloid. Vitreoretinal attachments are often patchy in uveitic eyes and schisis of the posterior cortical hyaloid may be common. There is risk of retention of the posterior leaflet of the hyaloid to the macula, which may increase later epiretinal membrane, macular edema, or create tangential traction with macular hole formation. Separation of residual vitreous attachments postoperatively can produce troublesome floaters.
>
> **Be aware that epiretinal membranes can adhere tightly to focal chorioretinal lesions.** Care should be taken in peeling them. The membrane often ramifies well beyond the vascular arcades and adheres to focal scars. Similarly, disc adhesions may be so tight as to risk injury to the nerve fiber layer if the attachment is forcibly broken. Conversely, Weiss rings adherent to, but slightly separated from, the optic nerve can often be gently elevated with an angled pick.

Remember that uveitis can alter the structural integrity of the macula. Eyes with long-standing edema may both have limited visual potential and a more fragile retinal structure with less elasticity. Tangential stretching during epiretinal membrane peeling should be minimized. Membranes with good retinal separation at least in some areas are probably the best candidates for peeling. Some cases may need to be abandoned if excessive traction from the surgical instruments is noted. Unroofing of central macular cysts can occur and should be treated as a macular hole.

Don't confuse clarity of the ocular media with control of the uveitis. Clearing the ocular media by PPV is an important confounder in observational series that report good results from surgical therapy because vitreous haze is one of the signs used to grade intraocular inflammation. Removal of vitreous opacities may or may not help control uveitis, but it certainly does not eliminate the need for control. Progressive anterior segment disease and uveitic complications after PPV must be monitored and treated.

References

1. Kempen JH, Min YI, Freeman WR, et al. Risk of immune recovery uveitis in patients with AIDS and cytomegalovirus retinitis. Ophthalmology 2006;113:684–94
2. Thorne JE, Wittenberg S, Jabs DA, et al. Multifocal choroiditis with panuveitis incidence of ocular complications and of loss of visual acuity. Ophthalmology 2006;113:2310–6
3. Rothova A, Berendschot TT, Probst K, et al. Birdshot chorioretinopathy: long-term manifestations and visual prognosis. Ophthalmology 2004;111:954–9
4. Kiss S, Ahmed M, Letko E, Foster CS. Long-term follow-up of patients with birdshot retinochoroidopathy treated with corticosteroid-sparing systemic immunomodulatory therapy. Ophthalmology 2005;112:1066–71
5. Rosenberg KD, Feuer WJ, Davis JL. Ocular complications of pediatric uveitis. Ophthalmology 2004;111:2299–306
6. Aylward GW. The place of vitreoretinal surgery in the treatment of macular oedema. Doc Ophthalmol 1999;97:433–8
7. Grigorian R, Bhagat N, Lanzetta P, et al. Pars plana vitrectomy for refractory diabetic macular edema. Semin Ophthalmol 2003;18:116–20
8. Ma J, Yao K, Jiang J, et al. Assessment of macular function by multifocal electroretinogram in diabetic macular edema before and after vitrectomy. Doc Ophthalmol 2004;109:131–7
9. Thomas D, Bunce C, Moorman C, Laidlaw DA. A randomised controlled feasibility trial of vitrectomy versus laser for diabetic macular oedema. Br J Ophthalmol 2005;89:81–6
10. Kuhn F, Kiss G, Mester V, et al. Vitrectomy with internal limiting membrane removal for clinically significant macular oedema. Graefes Arch Clin Exp Ophthalmol 2004;242:402–8
11. Stefaniotou M, Aspiotis M, Kalogeropoulos C, et al. Vitrectomy results for diffuse diabetic macular edema with and without inner limiting membrane removal. Eur J Ophthalmol 2004;14:137–43
12. Kimura T, Kiryu J, Nishiwaki H, et al. Efficacy of surgical removal of the internal limiting membrane in diabetic cystoid macular edema. Retina 2005;25:454–61
13. Kolacny D, Parys-Vanginderdeuren R, Van Lommel A, Stalmans P. Vitrectomy with peeling of the inner limiting membrane for treating diabetic macular edema. Bull Soc Belge Ophtalmol 2005;15–23
14. Rosenblatt BJ, Shah GK, Sharma S, Bakal J. Pars plana vitrectomy with internal limiting membranectomy for refractory diabetic macular edema without a taut posterior hyaloid. Graefes Arch Clin Exp Ophthalmol 2005;243:20–5
15. Yanyali A, Horozoglu F, Celik E, et al. Pars plana vitrectomy and removal of the internal limiting membrane in diabetic macular edema unresponsive to grid laser photocoagulation. Eur J Ophthalmol 2006;16:573–81
16. Bahadir M, Ertan A, Mertoglu O. Visual acuity comparison of vitrectomy with and without internal limiting membrane removal in the treatment of diabetic macular edema. Int Ophthalmol 2005;26:3–8
17. Kamura Y, Sato Y, Isomae T, Shimada H. Effects of internal limiting membrane peeling in vitrectomy on diabetic cystoid macular edema patients. Jpn J Ophthalmol 2005;49:297–300
18. Patel JI, Hykin PG, Schadt M, et al. Pars plana vitrectomy with and without peeling of the inner limiting membrane for diabetic macular edema. Retina 2006;26:5–13
19. Terasaki H, Kojima T, Niwa H, et al. Changes in focal macular electroretinograms and foveal thickness after vitrectomy for diabetic macular edema. Invest Ophthalmol Vis Sci 2003;44:4465–72
20. Yamamoto S, Yamamoto T, Ogata K, et al. Morphological and functional changes of the macula after vitrectomy and creation of posterior vitreous detachment in eyes with diabetic macular edema. Doc Ophthalmol 2004;109:249–53
21. Yamamoto T, Hitani K, Sato Y, et al. Vitrectomy for diabetic macular edema with and without internal limiting membrane removal. Ophthalmologica 2005;219:206–13

22. Becker M, Davis J. Vitrectomy in the treatment of uveitis. Am J Ophthalmol 2005;140:1096–105
23. Avci R, Kaderli B, Avci B, et al. Pars plana vitrectomy and removal of the internal limiting membrane in the treatment of chronic macular oedema. Graefes Arch Clin Exp Ophthalmol 2004;242:845–52
24. Radetzky S, Walter P, Fauser S, et al. Visual outcome of patients with macular edema after pars plana vitrectomy and indocyanine green-assisted peeling of the internal limiting membrane. Graefes Arch Clin Exp Ophthalmol 2004;242:273–8
25. Sullu Y, Alotaiby H, Beden U, Erkan D. Pars plana vitrectomy for ocular complications of Behcet's disease. Ophthalmic Surg Lasers Imaging 2005;36:292–7
26. Kiryu J, Kita M, Tanabe T, et al. Pars plana vitrectomy for epiretinal membrane associated with sarcoidosis. Jpn J Ophthalmol 2003;47:479–83
27. Ieki Y, Kiryu J, Kita M, et al. Pars plana vitrectomy for vitreous opacity associated with ocular sarcoidosis resistant to medical treatment. Ocul Immunol Inflamm 2004;12:35–43
28. Ganesh SK, Babu K, Biswas J. Phacoemulsification with intraocular lens implantation in cases of pars planitis. J Cataract Refract Surg 2004;30:2072–6
29. Tranos P, Scott R, Zambarajki H, et al. The effect of pars plana vitrectomy on cystoid macular oedema associated with chronic uveitis: a randomised, controlled pilot study. Br J Ophthalmol 2006;90:1107–10
30. Rizzo S, Genovesi-Ebert F, Murri S, et al. 25-gauge, sutureless vitrectomy and standard 20-gauge pars plana vitrectomy in idiopathic epiretinal membrane surgery: a comparative pilot study. Graefes Arch Clin Exp Ophthalmol 2006;244:472–9
31. Thorne JE, Jabs DA, Peters GB, et al. Birdshot retinochoroidopathy: ocular complications and visual impairment. Am J Ophthalmol 2005;140:45–51
32. Angunawela RI, Heatley CJ, Williamson TH, et al. Intravitreal triamcinalone acetonide for refractory uveitic cystoid macular oedema: longterm management and outcome. Acta Ophthalmol Scand 2005;83:595–9
33. Kok H, Lau C, Maycock N, et al. Outcome of intravitreal triamcinolone in uveitis. Ophthalmology 2005;112:1916
34. Gutfleisch M, Spital G, Mingels A, et al. Pars plana vitrectomy with intravitreal triamcinolone: effect on uveitic cystoid macular oedema and treatment limitations. Br J Ophthalmol 2007;91:345–8
35. Holekamp NM, Thomas MA, Dickinson JD, Valluri S. Surgical removal of subfoveal choroidal neovascularization in presumed ocular histoplasmosis: stability of early visual results. Ophthalmology 1997;104:22–6
36. Cordero CM, Sobrin L, Onal S, et al. Intravitreal bevacizumab for treatment of uveitic macular edema. Ophthalmology 2007;114:1574–9
37. Markomichelakis NN, Halkiadakis I, Pantelia E, et al. Patterns of macular edema in patients with uveitis: qualitative and quantitative assessment using optical coherence tomography. Ophthalmology 2004;111:946–53
38. Bartsch DU, Aurora A, Rodanant N, et al. Volumetric analysis of macular edema by scanning laser tomography in immune recovery uveitis. Arch Ophthalmol 2003;121:1246–51
39. Lai JC, Stinnett SS, Jaffe GJ. B-scan ultrasonography for the detection of macular thickening. Am J Ophthalmol 2003;136:55–61
40. Reproducibility of Macular Thickness and Volume Using Zeiss Optical Coherence Tomography in Patients with Diabetic Macular Edema. Ophthalmology 2007;
41. Costa RA, Jorge R, Calucci D, et al. Intravitreal bevacizumab (Avastin) for central and hemicentral retinal vein occlusions: IBeVO study. Retina 2007;27:141–9
42. Browning DJ. Interobserver variability in optical coherence tomography for macular edema. Am J Ophthalmol 2004;137:1116–7
43. Sadda SR, Joeres S, Wu Z, et al. Error correction and quantitative subanalysis of optical coherence tomography data using computer-assisted grading. Invest Ophthalmol Vis Sci 2007;48:839–48
44. Schmidt-Erfurth U, Leitgeb RA, Michels S, et al. Three-dimensional ultrahigh-resolution optical coherence tomography of macular diseases. Invest Ophthalmol Vis Sci 2005;46:3393–402

Chapter 20

Surgical Treatment of Retinal Vasculitis with Occlusion, Neovascularization or Traction

Jose M. Ruiz-Moreno, Javier A. Montero

Core Messages

- Fluorescein angiography should be performed in any case of retinal vasculitis as soon as the media are transparent enough to allow it.
- The affected area revealed by fluorescein angiography is usually greater than what is suspected by ophthalmoscopy.
- We must pay special attention to the retina distal to the area affected by vasculitis: this will frequently be affected by ischemia.
- Treatment should be started as soon as possible in ischemic cases in order to prevent neovascularization.
- Concomitant steroidal therapy and adequate dosage are of utmost importance in order to control vasculitis.

- The ischemic area should be treated by laser ablation under topical anesthesia in order to prevent neovascularization or to reduce it.
- Posterior three-port vitrectomy should be performed in case of recurrent or persistent vitreous hemorrhage, vitreoretinal traction with macular distortion, or tractional retinal detachment.
- Posterior three-port vitrectomy is useful to remove hemorrhages, perform resection of new vessels and associated traction and perform endophotocoagulation.
- New technology such as 25-gauge vitrectomy should be considered in order to reduce surgical trauma.
- The development of new antiangiogenic drugs (anti-VEGF) may offer a new therapeutic alternative to these cases.

Contents

20.1	Introduction	209
20.2	Types of Retinal Vasculitis	210
20.3	Signs and Symptoms	210
20.4	Diagnosis	210
20.5	Occlusive Retinal Vasculitis	210
20.6	Pathogenesis of Neovascularization	211
20.7	Inflammation and VEGF	211
20.8	Treatment	211
20.8.1	Background Therapy	212
20.8.2	Management of Complications	212
20.8.2.1	Argon Laser Photocoagulation	212
20.8.2.2	Indications for Conventional Vitrectomy	212
20.8.2.3	25-Gauge Vitrectomy	213
20.9	Case Report	213
References		217

This chapter contains the following video clips on DVD: Video 34 shows Insertion of 23G trocar, Video 35 shows Pars plana vitrectomy and Video 36 shows Endolaser (Surgeon: Jose Ruiz-Moreno).

20.1 Introduction

Retinal vasculitis (RV) is an ocular inflammatory disease affecting the vessels of the retina, the uveal tract and the vitreous gel. It is a potentially blinding condition usually affecting young patients and may appear either as an isolated form (idiopathic vasculitis) or associated with infections, neoplasm, or systemic inflammatory diseases [2, 37].

The inflammation of the retinal vessels may induce retinal ischemia leading to occlusive RV [10]. New vessels may appear surrounding these ischemic areas and be followed by vitreous hemorrhages and, occasionally, vitreoretinal traction and retinal detachment [10].

20.2 Types of Retinal Vasculitis

RV may be classified into ischemic and nonischemic forms, according to fluorescein angiographic (FA) findings. From an etiological point of view, it may be classified as idiopathic or secondary, and these may be associated with infections, neoplasm, neurological diseases and systemic inflammatory diseases [2, 37].

20.3 Signs and Symptoms

RV affecting only retinal periphery and leaving the vitreous undamaged may be asymptomatic. Posterior retinal vessels vasculitis and/or vitreous affection with cellular infiltrates and opacities will cause a reduction in visual acuity and/or the perception of floaters [2].

Retinal ischemia may cause perception of scotomata in the visual field. The apparition of new vessels secondary to ischemia may lead to vitreous hemorrhages with a potentially severe decrease in visual acuity. Macular ischemia and edema are additional causes of vision loss [2, 9, 37].

Ophthalmoscopy shows retinal vessels sheathing and vitreous cellularity during the acute phase of the disease. Involvement of macular vessels is usually associated with macular edema. Vascular occlusion secondary to vasculitis shows cotton wool spots as manifestation of retinal microinfarctions, intraretinal hemorrhages and edema.

> Changes in retinal vascularization such as telangiectasia and microaneurysms appear in later stages of the disease [2]. As the condition progresses, retinal ischemia gives way to new retinal vessels and vitreous hemorrhages. Occasionally the new vessels may be associated with a marked fibrous component that induces retinal distortion and/or tractional retinal detachment [10].

Venous retinal vasculitis is usually associated with Behçet's disease, tuberculosis, sarcoidosis, multiple sclerosis, pars planitis, Eales disease (retinal vasculitis associated with tuberculoprotein hypersensitivity) or AIDS. Retinal vasculitis predominantly affecting arteries is commonly found in association with systemic erythematous lupus, polyarteritis nodosa and viral retinopathies. Intraretinal infiltrates may be found in relationship with infectious agents [2].

20.4 Diagnosis

The etiological study of retinal vasculitis should be considered from a multidisciplinary point of view [23, 40]. Even though ophthalmoscopy may be diagnostic, FA should be performed if the clarity of the media allows it. In this way we may find fluorescein leakage caused by inner blood–retinal barrier breakdown and vessel wall staining.

> The area affected by RV is usually found to be greater by FA than it was suspected by ophthalmoscopy, and FA may also provide information on the presence of vessel occlusions. The diagnosis of an occlusive or nonocclusive vasculitis will condition our therapeutic decision.

Optical coherence tomography (OCT) is of great utility in the evaluation and quantification of macular edema.

> Macular edema is second only to vitreous hemorrhage to cause vision loss among these patients [10]. OCT will also allow us to determine the efficacy of the therapy.

20.5 Occlusive Retinal Vasculitis

Occlusive retinal vasculitis (ORV) can be found in association with recurrent vitreous hemorrhages in cases of tuberculosis or in vasculitis with tuberculoprotein hypersensitivity (Eales disease) [4, 16], Lyme disease [47] and cat-scratch disease (usually affecting arterioles and venules) [36]. ORV may appear less frequently in toxoplasmosis [48] and in Mediterranean spotted fever (with venous and arterial occlusion), in which choroidal neovascularization has been described as a complication of vasculitis [5, 27, 42]; as retinal periphlebitis in multiple sclerosis, which may progress into occlusive periphlebitis with neovascularization and retinal traction and detachment [52]; and in Behçet's disease, in which repeated vascular occlusive episodes may cause important vision loss [35, 43, 51]. Vasculitis is seldom occlusive in sarcoidosis [33, 41]. Other frequent associations of ORV are erythematous systemic lupus (SLE) with arteriolar occlusion [3, 2 6], Wegener's granulomatosis, polyarteritis nodosa with arterial and choroidal occlusion [13, 24, 25, 32] and Crohn's disease with occlusive arteritis and phlebitis [44, 45].

ORV has been described less frequently in frosted branch angiitis [1, 12, 28], idiopathic retinal vasculitis aneurysms and neuroretinitis (IRVAN) [14], acute retinal hemorrhagic retinal vasculitis [11] and idiopathic recurrent branch retinal arterial occlusion [20].

20.6 Pathogenesis of Neovascularization

Tissue ischemia and/or inflammation induce the production of proangiogenic molecules in pathological neovascularization. This proangiogenic signal activates a proteolytic cascade in the vascular endothelial cells [38]. This enzymatic sequence causes local digestion of the vascular endothelium, allowing the migration and proliferation of endothelial cells towards the angiogenic stimulus [38]. At a later stage, a new membrane appears surrounding these endothelial cells, forming a new vessel [38, 39]. Enzymatic extracellular proteolysis following the activation of the extracellular matrix proteinases is key in this process [38, 39].

The predominant role of the vascular endothelial growth factor (VEGF-A) in the development of pathological angiogenesis has been demonstrated in the last few years for different conditions such as cancer, ischemia and inflammation. VEGF-A has been found in the synovial fluid in rheumatoid arthritis and in psoriasis. Hypoxia plays another important role in the regulation of angiogenesis [53].

Inflammation and hypoxia trigger the formation and growth of new vessels in ORV in which inflammation is a primary factor, and retinal hypoxia secondary to vascular occlusion aids in the production and release of VEGF.

VEGF (or VEGF-A), is a cytokine, a secreted protein which induces neovascularization in different conditions. It is a powerful cellular mitogen and inhibitor of apoptosis, increasing survival of endothelial cells, attracting endothelial cell precursors and promoting their mobilization and differentiation from the bone marrow. It also increases vascular permeability and up-regulates the expression of metalloproteinases and down-regulates the expression of metalloproteinases inhibitors in the endothelial cells. VEGF also activates the endothelial cell nitric oxide synthetase, which is a powerful mediator of VEGF-induced endothelial cell proliferation [8].

> Four biologically active human isoforms of VEGF are known, containing 121, 165, 189 and 208 amino acids respectively. VEGF 165 is the isoform involved in pathological neovascularization [18, 19].

Three tyrosine-kinase mediated receptors for VEGF are known: VEGFR-1, VEGFR-2 and VEGFR-3. VEGFR-1 plays a key role in embryogenesis. VEGFR-2 has less affinity for VEGF than VEGFR-1, and is considered to be the main mediator of the mitogenic, angiogenic and permeability enhancing effects of VEGF [18, 19]. The blockade of VEGFR-2 phosphorylation inhibits the formation of new vessels in an animal model of neovascularization in the mouse [31]. VEGFR-3 is located in the endothelium of veins in early stages of embryogenesis. In later stages it is located only in lymphatic vessels. In the adult human is can only be detected in lymphatic endothelium and in some venous endothelium [30].

> The association of retinal vasculitis with posterior vitreous detachment is a positive prognostic factor because of the elimination of the scaffold upon which the new vessels appear.

20.7 Inflammation and VEGF

The role of VEGF has been demonstrated in different inflammatory conditions [15, 29]. Van Bruggen et al. reported the beneficial effect of VEGF antagonists in an animal model of cortical ischemia, reducing the edema of the tissue immediately after the start of ischemia and the infarcted area measured several weeks later [49].

Inflammation is also mediated by the H-factor protein, which is involved in the activation of the complement cascade. Inflammation induces pathological angiogenesis, releasing proangiogenic molecules which induce new vessels formation in tissues with inflammatory processes [17, 22].

20.8 Treatment

> Management of ORV should be in two different steps: background anti-inflammatory therapy and treatment of the complications of vascular occlusion (neovascularization, vitreoretinal traction and retinal detachment).

Vascular occlusion induces ischemia, which in association with inflammation originates a proliferative retinopathy with new vessels formation, recurrent vitreous hemorrhage, tractional retinal detachment, and rubeosis iridis with neovascular glaucoma, which may occasionally lead to loss of visual function [46].

20.8.1 Background Therapy

Medical therapy to treat retinal vasculitis is useful to prevent vessel occlusion and subsequent ischemia. Additionally, new vessels may regress with medical treatment.

Patients with limited forms of retinal vasculitis or affected with macular edema and/or ischemia secondary to vascular occlusion should be managed by systemic steroid therapy such as 1.0–1.5 mg/kg/day methyl prednisolone or an equivalent dosage of any other steroid, which should be slowly tapered after 5–7 days [46].

Intravenous pulses and higher doses of methyl prednisolone should be used in cases more severely affected, followed by oral steroids. Steroid dosage and duration of treatment should be managed in accordance to the risk of visual loss and the response to therapy [46].

Immunomodulation and immunosuppression with Azathioprine or Cyclosporine A can be used either isolatedly or associated with steroids to reduce their side effects [46].

20.8.2 Management of Complications

20.8.2.1 Argon Laser Photocoagulation

> The main indications of laser photocoagulation in retinal vasculitis are persistent neovascularization, vitreous hemorrhage and, less frequently, neovascular glaucoma. Some authors suggest it should be used once immunosuppressive treatment has been started, especially since there is a high risk of increasing the inflammation (21), while other recommend its early use, even in absence of neovascularization [34].

Retinal neovascularization in uveitis is associated both with ischemia and inflammation, and its behavior shares some characteristics of other proliferative conditions. It is unlikely that neovascularization induced by retinal ischemia should not respond to photocoagulation as is the case with diabetic retinopathy or occlusive venous disease.

Argon laser photocoagulation is the first-line therapy for eyes with retinal ischemia secondary to vessel occlusion in the course of retinal vasculitis. Fluorescein angiography is useful to perform photocoagulation to the ischemic areas.

Argon laser photocoagulation can be performed under topical anesthesia in the office, as an outpatient procedure. We prefer to use a wide field lens, which easily allows treating all the ischemic areas following FA.

Photocoagulation can be performed with any of the usual thermal lasers. Most frequently it is a green or blue-green argon laser, but we can also use green Nd:YAG, dye yellow, red or diode. We usually start photocoagulation with a 100-μm-diameter spot to treat the area posterior to the temporal arcades, and with a greater spot to treat areas farther from the posterior pole (200–500 μm). The duration of the laser pulse can be set at 0.1–0.2 s with intensity enough to achieve moderately intense retinal burns in the form of scattered photocoagulation.

Photocoagulation is performed not only in non-perfused areas, but also in areas of flat neovascularization, microaneurysms and arteriovenous shunt vessels. Elevated neovascularization is preferably not directly treated, though some authors advocate treatment to the feeder vessels. Panretinal photocoagulation is reserved for cases with optic disk neovascularization [7].

Panretinal photocoagulation and early vitrectomy have demonstrated an ability to improve the anatomic and visual outcome in patients with Eales disease. However, they are useful in controlling neovascularization, but not as much in controlling the inflammation [4, 6].

Another fact to be considered regarding ischemia is the possible procoagulant effect of immunosuppressors, which might aggravate the poor perfusion of the retina [50]. Anticoagulant therapy should be considered in patients with ischemic forms of retinal vasculitis receiving a potentially procoagulant therapy with immunosuppressors [37].

Laser therapy is frequently followed by the apparition of macular edema, occasionally associated to the formation of epiretinal membranes (ERM). These cases may later need epiretinal membrane removal by vitrectomy (ERM peeling).

20.8.2.2 Indications for Conventional Vitrectomy

Posterior pars plana vitrectomy should be performed in cases of persistent or recurrent vitreous hemorrhages secondary to new vessel formation after retinal ischemia. Even though initial vitreous hemorrhages tend to settle inferiorly and be absorbed, their recurrence and the appearance of traction bands and membranes in the vitreous are indications for vitrectomy. Final outcome is better among patients who have suffered less vitreous hemorrhages and of less duration, and those who have undergone photocoagulation prior to vitrectomy than patients with longstanding vitreous hemorrhages [6]. Difficulties in performing office photocoagulation are not uncommon due to the presence of residual vitreous hemorrhage or opacities, and due to retinal edema. The purpose of vitrectomy is to improve the quality of vision of the patient by removing vitreous opacities and blood, and to allow an adequate photocoagulation of ischemic areas.

Vitrectomy is also the therapy of choice to treat new vessels not responding to photocoagulation (inflammation is frequently involved in the development of neovascularization associated with ischemia) or the presence of vitreoretinal tractions caused by the fibrotic component of the neovascularization. Vitreoretinal traction may cause macular distortion and tractional retinal detachment. Vitrectomy and removal of the fibrous component should be performed, as well as removal of the neovascular tuft.

It is not uncommon that additional procedures may be required at the time of vitrectomy (these patients usually have posterior capsule opacities induced by steroidal therapy) such as phacoemulsification (preferred to lensectomy) to improve visualization and to allow a more complete vitrectomy; scleral buckling procedures in order to reduce vitreoretinal traction; and occasionally cryotherapy, in spite of the concern of increasing intraocular inflammation.

We usually perform a pars plana vitrectomy under peribulbar anesthesia in an outpatient regime. The first step of the surgery should be to remove all the remnants of vitreous hemorrhage as well as the vitreous opacities and as much vitreous as is possible. Afterward, the posterior hyaloid should be removed if still adhered to the posterior pole. Posterior hyaloid removal will prevent its eventual retraction and the distortion of the retinal surface. Furthermore, the presence of the hyaloid may facilitate the growth of new vessels with a fibrovascular component. Any tractional component should also be removed. The surgery finishes with endophotocoagulation of the affected area as previously described.

20.8.2.3 25-Gauge Vitrectomy

> Twenty-five-gauge vitrectomy is a useful new therapeutic option for patients with retinal vasculitis. This procedure is less aggressive to the eye than conventional vitrectomy, what may be of importance: the lesser trauma we induce in the eye, the lesser the postoperatory inflammation will be. Adequate 25-gauge instruments such as forceps and orientable laser probes allow a less aggressive surgery, reducing the risk of crystalline lens damage.

Twenty-five-gauge surgery starts with the insertion of the scleral trocars. The infusion is inserted first, in the inferior temporal quadrant 3.5–4.5 mm from the sclerocorneal limbus. A complete vitrectomy is then performed, removing as much opacified vitreous as possible. Any traction should be removed with the forceps. Finally, endophotocoagulation is performed to the whole extent of the ischemic retina or to the areas affected by neovascularization, and the trocars are removed. This new technology reduces the surgical trauma and subsequent inflammation.

20.9 Case Report

A 34-year-old male patient was attended at our clinic (Instituto Oftalmologico de Alicante VISSUM). He had been diagnosed with bilateral retinal vasculitis. Familiar, systemic and ophthalmic antecedents were not relevant. Laboratory work-up was negative.

Best corrected visual acuity (BCVA) was 0.8 for the right eye and 0.7 for the left eye. Slit lamp examination was normal for both eyes without any sign of ocular inflammation, and intraocular pressure was normal. The examination of the posterior segment after pharmacological dilation of the pupil was compatible with bilateral retinal vasculitis, which was demonstrated by FA (Fig. 20.1).

Indirect ophthalmoscopy showed remnants of vitreous hemorrhage in the left eye. FA showed retinal periphlebitis next to nonperfused areas in the temporal sector of the equatorial retina in both eyes

Systemic steroid therapy was started with 1 mg/kg prednisone, which was slowly tapered after the resolution of the inflammation.

Argon laser photocoagulation was performed to the ischemic areas in the peripheral retina. However, a vitreous hemorrhage appeared in the left eye 5 months later. Ophthalmoscopy revealed a moderately severe vitreous hemorrhage, which allowed retinal visualization, with retinal traction in the superior temporal vascular arcade and a neovascular tuft growing from the optic disc and the superior temporal vessels. FA showed previous laser

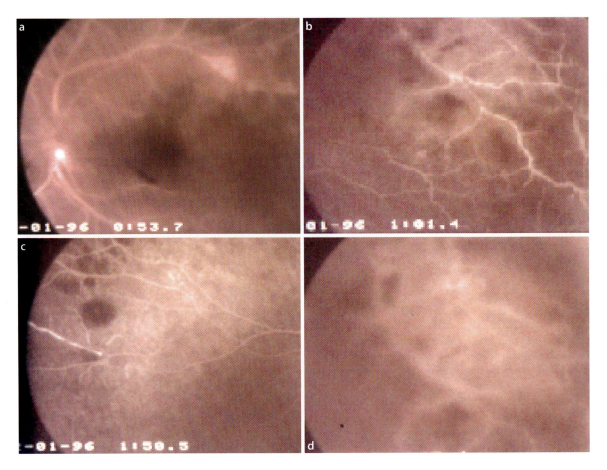

Fig. 20.1 **a** Left eye fluorescein angiography (FA). Remnants of vitreous hemorrhage can be appreciated with marked infiltration of the superior temporal vein. **b** FA of the left eye peripheral retina demonstrates the presence of hypoperfused areas. **c** FA of the right eye peripheral retina shows venous damage and hypoperfused areas. **d** Late phase FA of the right eye peripheral retina shows fluorescein leakage, with remnants of vitreous hemorrhage and ischemic areas

photocoagulation, nonperfused areas and inflammatory signs of retinal vasculitis (Fig. 20.2).

A surgical treatment with pars plana vitrectomy, traction and new vessels delamination, and endophotocoagulation of the ischemic area was performed. Two months later the patient progressed adequately with BCVA 0.8 in the left eye and stabilization of funduscopic findings (Fig. 20.2).

The patient returned 2 months later with visual decrease in his right eye. At the moment, BCVA was 0.3 in his right eye, with signs of an active retinal vasculitis with intraretinal hemorrhages and retinal edema next to the inferior temporal vein with a marked periphlebitis (Fig. 20.3).

Systemic steroid therapy was started as previously described, and BCVA improved to 0.5 2 months after the last episode (Fig. 20.3) and 0.7 at 4 months. However, 8 months after this episode, neovascularization and vitreous hemorrhages appeared in the right eye. Vitrectomy with removal of tractional components and of the new vessels and endophotocoagulation were performed to the right eye (Fig. 20.3).

Final BCVA was 1 in both eyes 8 years after the last vitrectomy. Presently, retinal vasculitis is stable without new inflammatory episodes (Fig. 20.4).

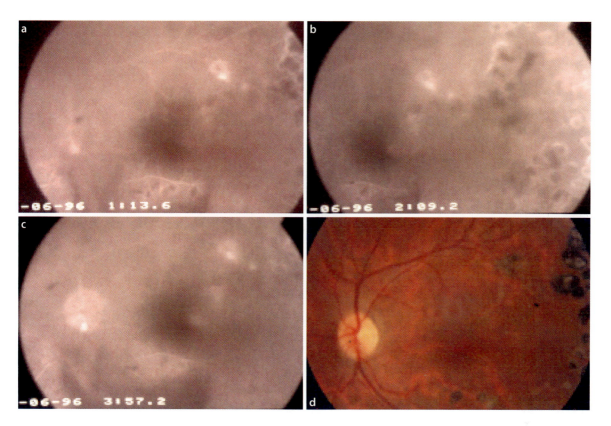

Fig. 20.2 a Left eye middle phase FA showing laser scars from previous photocoagulation procedures, remnants of vitreous hemorrhage and vascularization to the superior temporal arcade. **b** Middle phase FA of the left eye peripheral retina showing similar findings: laser scars, vitreous hemorrhage and neovascularization to the superior temporal retina. **c** Late phase FA of the same eye. **d** Color retinography shows outcome after vitrectomy

Take Home Pearls

- Indications for vitrectomy:
  — Persistent or recurrent vitreous hemorrhage
  — Neovascularization nonresponsive to photocoagulation
  — Vitreoretinal traction and tractional retinal detachment
  — Epiretinal membranes
  — Consider the need to associate phacoemulsification, cryotherapy, buckling surgery
- Indications for laser photocoagulation:
  — Persistent neovascularization
  — Vitreous hemorrhage
  — Neovascular glaucoma

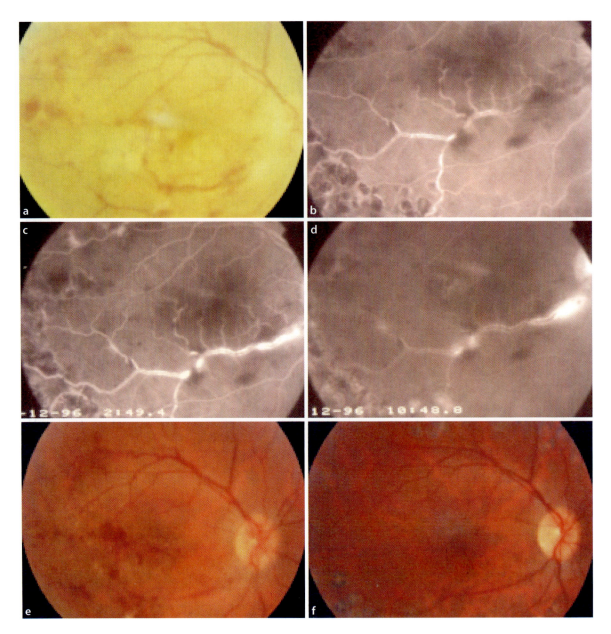

Fig. 20.3 **a** Retinography of the right eye shows active vasculitis with intraretinal hemorrhages and a marked inflammation of the inferior temporal vein. **b, c** Middle phases FA of the right eye showing marked infiltration of inferior temporal vein with vessel wall staining, and venous dilation and tortuosity. **d** Late phase FA of the right eye showing venous wall staining and occluded vessels. **e** The retinography shows the outcome after systemic steroid therapy, with residual retinal hemorrhages and signs of ischemia (cotton wool spots). **f** Retinography shows final outcome after vitrectomy

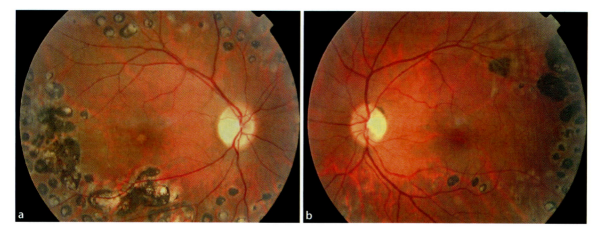

Fig. 20.4 **a** Final results eight years later of the right eye. **b** Left eye eight years later. Good results in both eyes after vitrectomy and endophotocoagulation

References

1. Abu El-Asrar AM, Al-Obeidan SA, Abdel G, et al. (2003). Retinal periphlebitis resembling frosted branch angiitis with nonperfused central retinal vein occlusion. Eur J Ophthalmol 13: 807–812
2. Abu El-Asrar AM, Herbort P, Tabbara KF (2005). Retinal vasculitis. Ocul Immunol Inflamm 13:415–433
3. Abu El-Asrar AM, Naddaf HO, Al-Momen AK, et al. (1995). Systemic lupus erythematosus flare-up manifesting as a cilioretinal artery occlusion. Lupus 4:158–160
4. Abu El-Asrar AM, AL-Kharashi SA (2002). Full panretinal photocoagulation and early vitrectomy improve prognosis of retinal vasculitis associated with tuberculoprotein hypersensitivity (Eales' disease). Br J Ophthalmol 86:1248–1251
5. Alio J, Ruiz-Beltran R, Herrero-Herrero JI, et al. (1987). Spotted fever. Ophthalmologica 195:31–37
6. Atmaca L, Nagpal P (1998). Eales´ disease: medical, laser and surgical treatments. Ophthalmol Clin North Am 11:619–626
7. Ayliffe W (2002). Retinal vasculitis. In: Foster CS, Vitale AT. Dianosis and treatment of uveitis. Philadelphia, Saunders
8. Barouch FC, Miller JW (2004). Anti-vascular endothelial growth factor strategies for the treatment of choroidal neovascularisation from age-related macular degeneration. Int Ophthalmol Clin 44:23–30
9. Bentley CR, Stanford MR, Shilling JS, et al. (1993). Macular ischaemia in posterior uveitis. Eye 7:411–414
10. Brockhurst RJ, Schepens CL (1968). Uveitis IV. Peripheral uveitis, the complication of retinal detachment. Arch Ophthalmol 80:747–753
11. Blumenkranz MS, Kaplan HJ, Clarkson JG, et al. (1988). Acute multifocal hemorrhagic retinal vasculitis. Ophthalmology 95:1663–1672
12. Borkowski LM, Jampol LM (1999). Frosted branch angiitis complicated by retinal neovascularization. Retina 19:454–455
13. Bullen CL, Liesegang TJ, McDonald TJ, et al. (1983). Ocular complications of Wegener's granulomatosis. Ophthalmology 90:279–290
14. Chang TS, Aylward W, Davis JL, et al. (1995). The Retinal Vasculitis Study Group. Idiopathic retinal vasculitis, aneurysms, and neuro-retinitis. Ophthalmology 102:1089–1097
15. Dvorak HF, Brown LF, Detmar M, et al. (1995). Vascular permeability factor/vascular endothelial growth factor, microvascular hyperpermeability and angiogenesis. Am J Pathol 146:1029–1039
16. Eales H (1880). Cases of retinal hemorrhage associated with epistaxis and constipation. Birmingham Med Rev 9:262
17. Edwards AO, Ritter R, Abel KJ, et al. (2005). Complement factor H polymorphism and age-related macular degeneration. Science 308:421–424
18. Ferrara N (2004). Vascular endothelial growth factor: basic science and clinical progress. Endocr Rev 25:581–611
19. Ferrara N, Gerber HP, LeCouter J (2003). The biology of VEGF and its receptors. Nat Med 9:669–676
20. Gass JDM, Tiedeman J, Thomas MA (1986). Idiopathic recurrent branch retinal arterial occlusion. Ophthalmology 93:1148–1157
21. Graham E, Stanford MR, Shillings JS, et al. (1987). Neovascularization associated with posterior uveitis. Br J Ophthalmol 71:826–833

22. Hageman GS, Anderson DH, Johnson LV, et al. (2005). A common haplotype in the complement regulatory gene factor H (HF1/CFH) predisposes individuals to age-related macular degeneration. Proceedings of the National Academy of Sciences, USA 102:7227–7232
23. Herbort CP, Cimino L, Abu El-Asrar AM (2005). Ocular vasculitis: a multidisciplinary approach. Curr Opin Rheumatol 17:25–33
24. Hsu CT, Kerrison JB, Miller NR, et al. (2001). Choroidal infarction, ischemic optic neuropathy, and central retinal artery occlusion from polyarteritis nodosa. Retina 21:348–351
25. Iida T, Spaide RF, Kantor J (2002). Retinal and choroidal arterial occlusion in Wegener's granulomatosis. Am J Ophthalmol 133:151–152
26. Jabs DA, Fine SL, Hochberg MC, et al. (1986). Severe retinal vaso-occlusive disease in systemic lupus erythematosus. Arch Ophthalmol 104:558–563
27. Khairallah M, Ladjimi A, Chakroun M, et al. (2004). Posterior segment manifestations of Rickettsia conorii infection. Ophthalmology 111:529–534
28. Kleiner RC, Kaplan HJ, Shakin JL, et al. (1988). Acute frosted retinal periphlebitis. Am J Ophthalmol 106:27–34
29. Koch AE, Polverini PJ, Kumkel SL, et al. (1992). Interleukin-8 as a macrophage-derived mediator of angiogenesis. Science 258:1798–1801
30. Kukk E, Lymboussaki A, Taira S, et al. (1996). VEGF-C receptor binding and pattern of expression with VEGRR-3 suggest a role in lymphatic vascular development. Development 122:3829–3837
31. Kwak N, Okamoto N, Wood JM, Campochiaro PA (2000). VEGF is major stimulator in model of choroidal neovascularization. Invest Ophthalmol Vis Sci 41:3158–3164
32. Morgan CM, Foster CS, Gragoudas ES (1986). Retinal vasculitis in polyarteritis nodosa. Retina 6:205–209
33. Nicholas J (2002). Sarcoidosis. Curr Opin Ophthalmol 13:393–396
34. Nussenblatt R, Whitcup S, Palestine A (1996). Retina vasculitis. In: Uveitis: Fundamentals and Clinical Practice. St Louis, Mosby
35. Okada AA (2000). Drug therapy in Behçet's disease. Ocul Immunol Inflamm 8:85–91
36. Ormerod LD, Dailey JP (1999). Ocular manifestations of cat-scratch disease. Curr Opin Ophthalmol 10:209–216
37. Palmer HE, Stanford MR, Sanders MD, et al. (1996). Visual outcome of patients with idiopathic ischaemic and non-ischaemic retinal vasculitis. Eye 10:343–348
38. Parfyonova YV, Plekhanova OS, Tkachuk VA (2002). Plasminogen activators in vascular remodelling and angiogenesis. Biochem (Moscow) 67:139–156
39. Pepper MS (2001). Role of the matrix metalloproteinase and plasminogen activator-plasmin systems in angiogenesis. Arterioscler Thromb Vasc Biol 21:1104–1117
40. Perez VL, Chavala SH, Ahmed M, et al. (2004). Ocular manifestations and concepts of systemic vasculitides. Surv Ophthalmol 49:399–418
41. Rothova A (2000). Ocular involvement in sarcoidosis. Br J Ophthalmol 84:110–116
42. Ruiz-Moreno JM (1997). Choroidal neovascularization in the course of Q fever. Retina 17:553–555
43. Sakane T, Takeno M (2000). Novel approaches to Behçet's disease. Expert Opin Investig Drugs 9:1993–2005
44. Saatci OA, Koçak N, Durak I, et al. (2002). Unilateral retinal vasculitis, branch retinal artery occlusion and subsequent retinal neovascularization in Crohn's disease. Int Ophthalmol 24:89–92
45. Salmon JF, Ursell PG, Frith P (2000). Neovascular glaucoma as a complication of retinal vasculitis in Crohn's disease. Am J Ophthalmol 130:528–530
46. Secchi AG, Tognon MS, Piermarocchi S, et al. (1999). Idiopathic retinal vasculitis. In: BenEzra D, Ocular inflammation. London, Martin Dunitz, pp 267–274
47. Smith JL, Winward KE, Nicholson DF, et al. (1991). Retinal vasculitis in Lyme borreliosis. J Clin Neuroophthalmol 11:7–15
48. Theodossiodis P, Kokolakis S, Ladas I, et al. (1995). Retinal vascular involvement in acute toxoplasmic retinochoroiditis. Int Ophthalmol 19:19–24
49. Van Bruggen N (1999). VEGF antagonism reduces edema formation and tissue damage after ischemia/reperfusion injury in the mouse brain. J Clin Invest 104:1613–1620
50. Vanrenterghem Y, Roels L, Lerut T, et al. (1985). Thromboembolic complications and haemostatic changes in cyclosporin-treated cadaveric kidney allograft recipients. Lancet 8436:999–1002
51. Verity DH, Wallace GR, Vaughan RW, et al. (2003). Behçet's disease: from Hippocrates to the third millennium. Br J Ophthalmol 87:1175–1183
52. Vine AK (1992). Severe periphlebitis, peripheral retinal ischemia, and preretinal neovascularization in patients with multiple sclerosis. Am J Ophthalmol 113:28–32
53. Yancopoulos GD, Davis S, Gale NW, et al. (2000). Vascular-specific growth factor and blood vessel formation. Nature 407:242–248

Chapter 21

Surgical Treatment of Uveitic Complications: Retinal Detachment

Heinrich Heimann

Core Messages

- Patients with uveitis have a higher rate of retinal breaks and retinal detachment than the normal population. The risk is often underrated; in patients with uveitis and symptomatic floaters, a thorough examination of the fundus periphery should be performed.
- Retinal detachment in patients with uveitis is often accompanied by pre- and postoperative proliferative vitreoretinopathy (PVR). In addition, there are significantly higher failure and complication rates than in nonuveitic patients. Because of the increased complication rate and concomitant anterior and posterior segment problems, the functional outcome of retinal detachment surgery is on average significantly worse in patients with uveitis.
- Treatment of retinal breaks or localized detachments with laser retinopexy, pneumatic retinopexy or scleral buckling surgery might be feasible. However, in cases complicated by epiretinal tractions, PVR or extensive retinal necrosis, pars plana vitrectomy is the surgical method of choice. Additional advantages of vitrectomy are retrieval of specimen for diagnostic purposes, removal of vitreous opacities, installation of intraocular drugs and long-term internal tamponades.
- The addition of 5-fluorouracil and low molecular weight heparin to the infusion fluid decreases the risk for postoperative PVR in cases with uveitis and retinal detachment.
- Treatment of retinal detachment has to be adjusted to the underlying disease and the patient's age, general status and treatment, overall prognosis and concomitant eye disease.
- Viral retinitis is associated with an extremely high rate of retinal detachment that is often difficult to treat. Acute retinal necrosis syndrome usually requires vitrectomy with silicone oil tamponade. Since the introduction of HAART, the number of patients with cytomegalovirus retinitis and retinal detachment has fallen significantly. However, this problem still exists in patients with longstanding AIDS or those nonresponsive to HAART.

Contents

21.1	Introduction	220
21.2	Diagnostic Workup	220
21.3	Pathophysiology	221
21.3.1	Rhegmatogenous Retinal Detachment	221
21.3.2	Tractional Retinal Detachment	221
21.4	Treatment	221
21.4.1	Laser Retinopexy and Cryotherapy	222
21.4.2	Pneumatic Retinopexy and Scleral Buckling Surgery	222
21.4.3	Pars Plana Vitrectomy	223
21.4.4	Concomitant Therapy and Combined Surgery	224
21.5	Entities Associated with a Higher Incidence of Retinal Detachment	224
21.5.1	Intermediate Uveitis	225
21.5.2	Acute Retinal Necrosis	225
21.5.2.1	Surgical Technique	226
21.5.2.2	Results	226
21.5.3	Cytomegalovirus Retinitis	226
21.5.4	Endophthalmitis	227
21.5.5	Eales Disease	227
References		227

21.1 Introduction

The occurrence of a retinal detachment in a patient with uveitis signifies a considerable challenge to the vitreoretinal surgeon. Compared to nonuveitic retinal detachment, the following differences can be seen [9, 11, 28, 38, 40, 50]:

- Patients are on average younger.
- They more frequently have other significant pathologies in the affected and/or the fellow eye.
- The detachments are more difficult to treat. They often resemble a combination of exudative, rhegmatogenous and tractional retinal detachment with proliferative vitreoretinopathy (PVR) already present preoperatively in about one third of all cases.
- Uveitis is the single most important risk factor for the development of postoperative PVR.
- There is a higher rate of pre- and postoperative hypotony.
- There is a higher rate of primary and final failures.
- There are more secondary complications (e.g., glaucoma, hypotony, synechiae, pupillary membranes and cataract).
- The combination of these factors on average leads to a worse functional outcome with a higher rate of functional blindness or no light perception compared to nonuveitic retinal detachment.

Due to the relative scarcity of the combination of retinal detachment and uveitis, the considerable differences between the individual cases, the small number and low power of studies on this subject, no clear guidelines on the use of different surgical techniques and tools have been established to date. Treatment, therefore, is still applied in a very individual way according to the patient's age and general condition, the severity of the patient's situation and the surgeon's experience. In this chapter, the characteristics of retinal detachment associated with uveitis and the different treatment strategies are reviewed.

21.2 Diagnostic Workup

Firstly, retinal detachment associated with uveitis has to be differentiated from secondary intraocular inflammation due to longstanding retinal detachment that can mimic uveitis [33, 36]. Secondly, the etiology of the uveitis has to be established or confirmed; treatment of the underlying condition might have to be initiated before or together with the surgical treatment of retinal detachment. If necessary, retrieval of diagnostic specimen or intraocular drug application can be combined with the surgical intervention of retinal detachment. Further, the necessity, urgency and extent of the planned surgical procedure have to be adjusted to the patient's status, e.g., age, general health, long-term prognosis and associated systemic treatments. Thirdly, the subtype of retinal detachment has to be specified, which is not always straightforward, and combinations of the various types of retinal detachment can be present. Occasionally, treatment of the underlying condition might lead to an improvement in the situation of the retinal detachment, and surgery can be avoided or less invasive surgical methods might be used.

Although slit-lamp examination of the posterior segment with noncontact lenses is gaining popularity, the "gold standard" for the identification and characterization of retinal breaks and retinal detachments is indirect ophthalmoscopy with scleral depression [37]. The shape of the retinal detachment, the shifting of subretinal fluid, the stiffness of the retina on eye movements, the presence and configuration of retinal breaks and/or vitreous infiltrations and vitreoretinal tractions can be seen in greater detail when this dynamic examination method is used. Exudative retinal detachments are characterized by bullous accumulations of subretinal fluid that does not extend to the ora serrata, a smooth appearance of the retinal surface, shifting of subretinal fluid according to the patient's positioning and gravity, and the absence of epiretinal proliferations despite sometimes marked intraocular and longstanding inflammation. The failure to detect a retinal break does not exclude the diagnosis of a rhegmatogenous retinal detachment.

One has to bear in mind that in even with careful ophthalmoscopy, a break cannot be identified correctly in 9% of all rhegmatogenous retinal detachments and in 30% of pseudophakic retinal detachments [17]. Due to the often impaired view of the fundus periphery, this rate is likely to be higher in patients with uveitis. In cases of dense vitreous opacities, ultrasound echography can be of value to detect a peripheral retinal detachment, vitreous tractions or large breaks [41]. In some cases, fluorescein angiography might aid in the detection of retinal or subretinal leakage associated with retinal detachment, e.g., in Vogt-Koyanagi-Harada syndrome or peripheral vasoproliferative changes, and help in the differential diagnosis of retinal detachment.

21.3 Pathophysiology

All three types of retinal detachment (exudative, rhegmatogenous and tractional) occur more often in patients with uveitis compared to the normal population. Exudative retinal detachment seems to be the most common; it is usually treated according to the underlying inflammatory process and does not need surgical intervention. However, it is of clinical importance to differentiate exudative from rhegmatogenous or tractional retinal detachment. On the one hand, surgical treatment of exudative detachment is usually not successful but may aggravate the disease process; on the other hand, if rhegmatogenous or tractional retinal detachment are mistaken for exudative retinal detachment, medical treatment of these subtypes of retinal detachment will lead to a delay in the necessary surgical treatment and might result in a worse anatomical and functional outcome.

Although rhegmatogenous and tractional retinal detachment associated with uveitis are rare, the combination of these disease processes seems to be more common than one would expect by pure coincidence alone. In one series of 1,387 patients with uveitis, retinal detachment could be diagnosed in 3.1% (43/1,387) compared to an incidence of around 0.01% in the general population [28]. This higher incidence is in part due to ocular changes in uveitic eyes that can lead to the development of rhegmatogenous or tractional retinal detachment [2, 28, 38].

21.3.1 Rhegmatogenous Retinal Detachment

Possible factors that increase the risk for retinal detachment in patients with uveitis are:

- A higher incidence of posterior vitreous detachment (one of the main changes preceding development of a retinal detachment) [25].
- Morphological changes within the vitreous base, e.g., following intermediate uveitis and pars planitis [22], that can increase the strength of vitreoretinal adhesions and, in consequence, increase the adherences and tractional forces between the vitreous and the retina.
- Inflammatory processes involving the retina that can destroy retinal cells and weaken the intercellular adhesions of the retinal cells and pigment epithelium. This, in consequence, may lead to lesser resistance to counter vitreoretinal traction, resulting in a higher rate of retinal breaks, or can cause retinal breaks directly through necrotic destructions, mostly within previously inflamed retina or at the border of unaffected retina to scarred tissue.
- Normal retinal attachment is in part dependant on the intraocular pressure. Ocular hypotony occurs more often in patients with uveitis, is associated with a higher rate of retinal detachment and is a significant risk factor for anatomical and functional failure in eyes with retinal detachment [21].

21.3.2 Tractional Retinal Detachment

Two different pathways can lead to the development of tractional retinal detachment in patients with uveitis:

- Preretinal traction can develop in a way comparable to other retinal diseases associated with retinal ischemia, e.g., proliferative diabetic retinopathy and retinal venous occlusions. Subsequent to retinal ischemia, intraretinal vascular anomalies and or teleangiectasia develop at the border of ischemic to nonischemic retina, followed by preretinal proliferations and by the development of retinal tractions. An example for this pathway is tractional retinal detachment associated with Eales disease [4].
- Tractional retinal detachment that resembles proliferative vitreoretinopathy (PVR) can develop in patients with uveitis, with or without the presence of retinal breaks. The partial breakdown of the blood–retina barrier and the organization of inflammatory debris can lead to formation of cyclitic membranes and fibrous vitreous bands [22]. This is not only true for primary cases but resembles a particular problem postoperatively following initial retinal detachment surgery in patients with uveitis [38].

21.4 Treatment

With the exception of pars plana vitrectomy for retinal detachment associated with viral retinitis, no large patient series examining the value of different surgical methods for retinal detachment associated with uveitis have been published to date. The rationale for the choice of operating method can therefore only be based on small retrospective series or can be extrapolated from the different approaches to nonuveitic retinal detachment. In addition, particular advantages and disadvantages of the individual techniques have to be considered in patients with uveitis.

Overall, significantly worse outcomes compared to nonuveitic retinal detachment independent of the choice of the surgical method can be expected. In one series, primary success rates were only around 60% compared to 80% in retinal detachment not associated with uveitis [28]. Final anatomical success was achieved in 88% compared to ≥95% in nonuveitic retinal detachment. A final visual acuity of ≤20/200 was seen in 67% of patients with no light perception in 11% of all patients.

21.4.1 Laser Retinopexy and Cryotherapy

Laser retinopexy and cryotherapy have been used in a number of different ways in the treatment of retinal detachment associated with uveitis. In analogy to nonuveitic retinal detachment, it can be applied for the treatment of retinal breaks or in areas of retinal changes predisposing to the development of retinal breaks and subsequent retinal detachment. Clinical experience and comparative trials tell us that the use of cryotherapy is associated with increased intraocular inflammation compared to laser retinopexy [48]. In addition, laser retinopexy usually is less painful than cryotherapy, which is of particular advantage in children and younger patients. On the other hand, visualization of the retinal periphery is often impaired in patients with uveitis due to media opacifications. Cryotherapy is easier to apply in these cases and has the additional advantage of treating larger areas of affected retina more efficiently. This cannot only be used to treat retinal breaks but can also destroy areas of diseased retina in order to diminish the production of growth factors. However, because of the differences in postoperative inflammation, laser retinopexy should be preferred over cryotherapy wherever possible.

Prophylactic laser retinopexy to prevent retinal detachment has been advocated in patients with viral retinitis [34, 44]. In patients with uveitis other than viral retinitis, no large trials regarding prophylactic treatment of retinal lesions predisposing to retinal detachment (lattice degeneration, cystic degenerations, round holes) have been published to date. In these cases, it therefore seems advisable to apply the recommendations for the prophylactic treatment of nonuveitic patients [51].

21.4.2 Pneumatic Retinopexy and Scleral Buckling Surgery

Pneumatic retinopexy and scleral buckling surgery are the two most popular operating methods for the treatment of localized retinal detachments. There is no data available comparing both methods in patients with retinal detachment and uveitis. A meta-analysis comparing studies of both methods in nonuveitic retinal detachment revealed higher primary anatomical success rates for scleral buckling with comparable functional and final anatomical results [39].

The choice of operating method shows a strong regional variation. In the USA, pneumatic retinopexy is the preferred first-line treatment [6]. In Europe, this method has not gained widespread popularity, and scleral buckling is the most popular method to treat localized retinal detachment [31]. Only case reports or small case series have been published on the use of pneumatic retinopexy or scleral buckling in retinal detachment associated with uveitis [7, 18, 34, 43, 51]. Due to the intravitreal injection of gas, pneumatic retinopexy is associated with more pronounced postoperative changes in the vitreous cavity with more postoperative vitreous traction and a higher incidence of new retinal breaks [29, 39]. In contrast, scleral buckling, particularly if it is not combined with drainage of the subretinal fluid, is an extraocular procedure and results in less intraocular inflammation. On the downside, scleral buckling can be associated with postoperative exposure, infection and inflammation around the buckling material in a significant number of patients; this can be of particular disadvantage in cases associated with uveitis. In addition, cataract progression is more commonly seen after scleral buckling surgery compared to pneumatic retinopexy.

There is no evidence-based recommendation regarding the preference of pneumatic retinopexy or scleral buckling in patients with uveitis and localized retinal detachment. Pneumatic retinopexy seems to be an alternative in cases with single breaks in the superior periphery. The higher anatomical success rate of scleral buckling and the lower grade of postoperative inflammation, particularly when combined with laser retinopexy, speak in favor of scleral buckling for localized retinal detachment in patients with uveitis. Both surgical methods, however, should be chosen only in detachments limited to a small area, especially in cases with viral retinitis [30]; there seem to be lower success rates with these methods in patients with uveitis, and vitrectomy might achieve better results [7]. Therefore, pneumatic retinopexy and scleral buckling should be chosen with caution if preoperative PVR-type reactions or dense vitreous infiltrates are present in patients with uveitis.

21.4.3 Pars Plana Vitrectomy

Pars plana vitrectomy seems to be the logical choice in the treatment of retinal detachment associated with uveitis. The rationale is to combine the treatment of retinal detachment with the additional advantages of vitrectomy for uveitis (removal of floaters, diagnostic workup of the vitrectomy specimen, application of drugs intravitreally). Other advantages of vitrectomy in these cases are the removal of traction bands in the vitreous, cyclitic membranes over the ciliary body, the ability to manipulate opacifications of the lens capsule, pupillary membranes or synechiae, the application of long-term tamponades in cases with extensive retinal damage and the theoretical advantage of removing the vitreous as a depot for vasoproliferative substances; this may have a positive influence on disease activity, the incidence of postoperative cystoid macular edema and PVR. In some retrospective series, better anatomical and functional results could be achieved with vitrectomy compared to scleral buckling [7, 28, 34].

However, several drawbacks of vitrectomy have to be considered as well:

- Cataract formation will occur in almost all eyes with a clear lens preoperatively. On average, patients with uveitic retinal detachment are younger, and the loss of accommodation poses a noteworthy clinical problem. Cataract formation significantly influences postoperative refraction and visual acuity with a higher incidence of macular edema and associated retinal problems. Patients with uveitis already have, on average, a lower visual acuity and will be affected more significantly by any cataract development and change in refraction. Lens opacities can also make ophthalmoscopy for the postoperative monitoring of posterior uveitis and chorioretinal disease more difficult. Finally, the surgical treatment of cataract in uveitis is also associated with more problems compared to nonuveitis patients.
- Ocular hypertension and secondary glaucoma are two of the complications of any vitrectomy that over a long period of time have not received the necessary attention and occur in about 10% of uncomplicated cases [12]. The use of intraocular tamponades can lead to short-term and long-term rises in intraocular pressure; while this will not result in significant clinical problems in the majority of patients with nonuveitic retinal detachment, it might amplify preexisting IOP problems in patients with uveitis as they already have a higher rate of acute and chronic IOP rises leading to acute glaucoma and long-term glaucomatous damage.
- The induction or completion of a posterior vitreous detachment together with the shaving of the vitreous base or the opposite, incomplete shaving of the vitreous base, can lead to the development of iatrogenic or new postoperative breaks.
- Vitrectomy in itself is a risk factor for the occurrence of a retinal detachment. In fact, previous vitrectomy in patients with uveitis was one of the major risk factors for retinal detachment in one retrospective series [28].
- Particularly in young female and myopic patients with round holes, a posterior vitreous detachment is not always present, despite typical signs of a rhegmatogenous retinal detachment [47]. Induction of a PVD can be extremely difficult or even impossible in these cases. Attempts to force separation of the vitreous from the retina might worsen the situation and increase the retinal detachment. If not removed completely, remnant vitreous can be a good starting point and scaffold for postoperative PVR development.

One of the hypothetical advantages of vitrectomy in retinal detachment surgery has been that with the removal of the vitreous and the included vasoproliferative substances and cells, the rate of postoperative PVR can be reduced. On the other hand, vitrectomy is associated with a higher rate of postoperative intraocular inflammation compared to scleral buckling, and it might be that surgical manipulation close to the retina and the vitreous base might accelerate inflammatory processes within these structures. As documented in the "Scleral buckling versus primary vitrectomy in rhegmatogenous retinal detachment study" (SPR study) that examined more complicated types of retinal detachment without associated uveitis, vitrectomy is not associated with a lower PVR rate compared to scleral buckling [19]. The study has shown that in phakic cases, scleral buckling still has an advantage over vitrectomy with better functional outcomes and fewer secondary surgeries, in particular cataract surgery. In pseudophakic patients, however, vitrectomy yielded better functional results and a slightly lower postoperative PVR rate. The use of an additional encircling element increased the success rates in pseudophakic patients but failed to yield better results in phakic cases [20].

Again, no evidence-based recommendations can be drawn from the current literature regarding the choice of operating method in the treatment of more complicated retinal detachment associated with uveitis. In complicated cases of retinal detachment associated with acute retinal necrosis, vitrectomy seems to achieve better results than scleral buckling. If tractional components are a significant feature of the retinal detachment present in patients with uveitis or other factors have to be considered (e.g. diagnostic workup of vitreous biopsy, floaters), PV seems to be the preferable operating method. Based on the results of the SPR study, this recommendation can also be extended to pseudophakic patients with retinal detachment. However, if these factors do not play a significant role, scleral buckling still seems to be a feasible method of treating retinal detachment in localized or even more complex cases of uveitic retinal detachment without major PVR.

21.4.4 Concomitant Therapy and Combined Surgery

With uveitis being a strong risk factor for the development of postoperative PVR, several studies have looked at the combination of vitrectomy with adjunctive therapy. In a prospective series of retinal detachment with established risk factors for postoperative PVR, Asaria et al. found a significant reduction of postoperative PVR when adding 5-fluorouracil (5-FU, 200 µg/ml) and low molecular weight heparin (LMWH, 5 IU/ml) to the infusion fluid [3]. Interestingly, further studies by the same group revealed that application of 5-FU and LMWH does not lower postoperative PVR when applied to all primary cases with retinal detachment or those with already established PVR [13]. However, with more than 70% of uveitis patients in the group that benefited from this treatment, the recommendation is to combine vitrectomy with 5-FU and LMWH in cases of primary vitrectomy for retinal detachment.

There are a large number of studies investigating other pre-, peri- and postoperative adjuvant therapy when performing vitrectomy in patients with uveitis. Patients with retinal detachment differ in that the surgical intervention usually cannot be delayed significantly to allow preoperative control of the intraocular inflammation. In the majority of patients, an increased dosage of topical and/or systemic steroids is incorporated into the postoperative treatment. In cases of infectious retinal detachment, it is of importance to include the adequate antimicrobiological therapy into the pre-, peri- and postoperative management.

In phakic retinal detachment, the combination of cataract surgery with vitrectomy facilitates the clearing of the vitreous base from preexisting membranes or vitreous remnants. However, combined surgery may lead to increased anterior chamber inflammation, posterior synechiae, development of pupillary membranes and a higher incidence of postoperative macular edema. Especially in the treatment of viral retinitis, recommendations differ between combined clear lens extraction in all cases [34] to preservation of the lens whenever possible [29]. It seems to be reasonable to perform combined surgery in cases with decreased visualization of the retinal periphery or the necessity of extensive surgical manipulation in the area of the vitreous base. In cases with a clear lens preoperatively, a two-step approach with secondary cataract surgery following retinal reattachment appears to be a sensible approach due to the lower rate of anterior segment inflammation with associated secondary problems.

As in nonuveitic retinal detachment, the issue of additional scleral buckling in combination with vitrectomy has its advocates [30] as well as its opponents [1]. The presumed advantages of additional buckling are the relief of traction at the vitreous base, enhanced trimming of the vitreous base and the support of old, iatrogenic or developing retinal breaks at the vitreous base. The disadvantages are anterior segment ischemia, myopic shift, choroidal effusion and intrusion/extrusion of the exoplant. No evidence-based data is available for patients with retinal detachment and uveitis. In nonuveitic retinal detachment, the SPR study has shown that additional buckling is of no benefit in phakic patients. However, in pseudophakic patients with more complicated types of retinal detachment, higher anatomical success rates could be achieved when combining vitrectomy with additional buckling [19, 20].

21.5 Entities Associated with a Higher Incidence of Retinal Detachment

Some patients with uveitis carry a higher risk for rhegmatogenous and tractional retinal detachments (Table 21.1). In general, all types of infectious uveitis involving the retina carry an increased risk for retinal detachment. The highest rates can be found after viral retinitis. However, bacterial, fungal and parasitic infectious diseases are also at risk for the development of retinal detachment that sometimes can occur years after the initial infection. This is particularly true for patients with fungal infections, toxoplasmosis, toxocariasis and syphilis.

Table 21.1 Entities with uveitis and an increased risk for the development of retinal breaks and retinal detachment [9, 11, 28, 38, 40, 50]

High risk for retinal detachment:	
Infectious uveitis	Viral retinitis (acute retinal necrosis, cytomegalovirus retinitis)
Increased risk for rhegmatogenous retinal detachment:	
Infectious uveitis	Toxoplasmosis
	Toxocariasis
	Syphilis
	Borreliosis
	Endophthalmitis (bacterial/fungal)
Noninfectious uveitis	Intermediate uveitis
	Behçet's disease
	Vogt-Koyanagi-Harada
	Multiple sclerosis
	Intraocular lymphoma
	Sarcoidosis
	Juvenile chronic arthritis
	Eales disease

21.5.1 Intermediate Uveitis

In the group of noninfectious uveitis, patients with intermediate uveitis, multiple sclerosis, sarcoidosis and intraocular lymphoma seem to have an increased risk for the development of retinal breaks and retinal detachment [28]. Although a rare disease, there also seems to be an increased risk for patients with sympathetic ophthalmia [28]. Intermediate uveitis associated with Behçet's disease [2] also has a higher incidence of retinal breaks and retinal detachment. It can be speculated that changes in the ultrastructure of the vitreous base in these patients might predispose to retinal detachment [22]. The message to be transferred to clinical practice is that, in patients with intermediate uveitis or pars planitis and symptomatic floaters, there might be reasons other than vitreous opacities causing symptomatic floaters, that is, retinal breaks. A careful fundus examination of the vitreous base regarding the possibility of retinal breaks or a peripheral detachment should therefore always be performed in these patients.

21.5.2 Acute Retinal Necrosis

Acute retinal necrosis (ARN) usually arises in otherwise healthy and immunocompetent patients and is characterized by uveitis, retinal vasculitis and retinal necrosis [8]. The mean age of the patients in most series is in the fourth decade. Diagnosis is based on clinical criteria [23]; a viral etiology can be found in the majority of patients with the most commonly isolated viruses of herpes simplex and varizella-zoster in about two thirds of patients and cytomegalovirus and Epstein-Barr in the remaining third [46]. Nonviral infections or noninfectious uveitis can also display clinical signs of necrotizing retinitis, e.g., toxoplasmosis, syphilis, fungal infections, Behçet's disease and intraocular lymphoma [5]. The fellow eye will be affected in about one to two thirds of patients, usually within 6 weeks after the initial diagnosis. Retinal detachment is a major complication of ARN in up to 75% of patients and occurs typically within 6–8 weeks following the onset of the disease. One of the major problems of retinal detachment in ARN is the fact that, in contrast to retinal detachment secondary to CMV retinitis, it usually is associated with advanced and anterior PVR and marked anterior and posterior segment inflammation [30].

21.5.2.1 Surgical Technique

In eyes with ARN and attached retina, prophylactic laser retinopexy to prevent development of retinal detachment has been advocated [44]. In addition, a barrier-type coagulation to wall off already detached peripheral retina has also been encouraged [49]. However, progression of retinal detachment despite photocoagulation in a significant number of patients and the development of considerable complications despite laser photocoagulation have been reported [24, 34]. In addition, laser photocoagulation is often difficult in patients with marked vitreous infiltrations and reduced visibility of the periphery. Retinal detachment in ARN is commonly associated with vitreous tractions and membrane formation that cannot be influenced by photocoagulation. Therefore, the exact role of prophylactic laser treatment in ARN remains to be defined.

Some authors have reported successful treatment of localized retinal detachment associated with ARN with scleral buckling or pneumatic retinopexy [7, 34]. In the more advanced stages, however, results of scleral buckling are disappointing, and vitrectomy is the preferred treatment option [30, 34]. The surgical technique should be tailored to the extent of the disease. Because many cases are associated with widespread disease, multiple breaks, vitreous infiltrations and anterior PVR, a more aggressive approach is often needed. This might include combined lensectomy or cataract surgery to enable a thorough cleaning of the vitreous base and an encircling band to support the vitreous base circumferentially [30].

Gas tamponades have been employed after vitrectomy for ARN, but in the majority of cases reported in the literature, silicone oil tamponade has been advocated due to widespread retinal disease. If possible, silicone oil should be removed after 3–6 months to prevent secondary problems associated with this tamponade.

21.5.2.2 Results

With the advances of surgical techniques, the anatomical results of surgical interventions for retinal detachment associated with ARN have improved over the past years. A retinal reattachment can nowadays be achieved in the majority of cases (e.g., Ahmadieh et al. achieved anatomical reattachment in 18 of 18 cases)[1]; however, the treatment is still complicated by an extremely high rate of postoperative PVR that develops in one form or another in almost all cases [1]. In addition, the disease is often complicated by optic neuropathy, macular pucker and macular edema that all significantly lower visual acuity. In a series by Blumenkranz et al., five out of six patients had a visual acuity of 20/200 or better with three patients reaching 20/40 or better [7]. Comparable results were achieved by McDonald et al. [34]. Sadly, a significant proportion of patients still lose ambulatory vision despite successful retinal reattachment. In the series by Ahmadieh et al., 7 of 18 eyes had a final visual acuity ≤ 5/200 [1].

21.5.3 Cytomegalovirus Retinitis

Since the introduction of highly active antiretroviral therapy (HAART) in patients with the acquired immunodeficiency syndrome (AIDS), the number of patients suffering from cytomegalovirus (CMV) retinitis has decreased significantly. Not only has HAART resulted in a reduction of new cases with CMV retinitis of about 75%, but it also has reduced the number of secondary retinal detachment in those affected by CMV retinitis by 60–80% [27]. This is due to the improved immune response that apparently results in a better scar formation in and around affected retinal areas and a stronger retinal attachment. However, CMV retinitis has not been eliminated completely, particularly in patients with longstanding AIDS and in those that do not respond to or tolerate HAART. Thus, there continues to be a number of patients with AIDS and HAART that suffer from advanced visual loss, predominantly secondary to CMV retinitis and its associated problems, including retinal detachment [45].

In patients with CMV retinitis, second eye involvement is seen in about 26% of patients; in about 20% of eyes, retinal detachment can develop [27]. In contrast to retinal detachment associated with ARN, the detachment develops later during the course of the disease and is rarely associated with a significant PVR reaction. However, this might change in the era of HAART; an up-regulated immune reaction might lead to more PVR reactions compared to CMV retinitis before the introduction of HAART [26]. In cases with CMV retinitis and attached retina, the value of prophylactic laser photocoagulation has been discussed [14, 49]; its value has also been questioned [29] and has not been proven in a prospective randomized trial. In rare cases of isolated breaks or localized detachments, pneumatic retinopexy or scleral buckling might be successful [30].

Because of the widespread destruction of retinal tissue and the decreased immune response in patients with AIDS, retinal detachment associated with CMV has traditionally been treated with vitrectomy and silicone oil tamponade. In cases of vitrectomy with silicone oil, preimplanted Ganciclovir implants can be left in situ, and new implants can be set in at the time of vitrectomy [30]. With the much-improved immune response and prognosis of patients under HAART, the mandatory use of vitrectomy plus silicone oil is likely to change within the next years, and treatment strategies will have to be adapted to the extent of the disease, the patient's immune status and general prognosis. Vitrectomy with gas tamponade or early removal of silicone oil has been considered [10, 35]; however, retinal redetachments could still be noted in about half of the patients after silicone oil removal [35].

21.5.4 Endophthalmitis

The incidence of endophthalmitis can be expected to rise over the next years with the worldwide increase in the number of cataract surgeries and, in particular, with the introduction of intravitreal injections for the treatment of age-related macular degeneration. Retinal detachment associated with endophthalmitis is a complication that is commonly underestimated. In the "Endophthalmitis Vitrectomy Study" it occurred in 8% of patients postoperatively and was associated with an extremely poor visual outcome [15]. Other groups of patients at risk of developing retinal detachment at the time of endophthalmitis or secondary to endophthalmitis are patients with ocular trauma and patients with endogenous endophthalmitis. In one series of posttraumatic endophthalmitis, retinal detachment occurred in 19% of patients and was a significant risk factor for a bad visual outcome [32]. Endogenous endophthalmitis is most commonly caused by fungal organisms; these can be associated with the development of intravitreal fibrotic strands and tractional retinal detachment some time after the start of the infection.

If retinal detachment is associated with endophthalmitis at the initial diagnosis, vitrectomy with intravitreal installation of antibiotics and silicone oil tamponade is usually indicated. In secondary retinal detachments, the choice of operating method should be adapted to the configuration of causative breaks, the extent of the retinal detachment, the presence of additional vitreous pathology, and the state of the intraocular infection and inflammation.

21.5.5 Eales Disease

Eales disease (periphlebitis retinae) is a vasoproliferative disease that typically occurs in otherwise healthy young males; both eyes are affected in about 80% of patients. The disease is characterized by an obliterative peripheral periphlebitis with secondary complications of vascular proliferations and vitreous hemorrhage. A tractional retinal detachment and/or rhegmatogenous retinal detachment can be seen in about 8% of patients [16]. Treatment of Eales disease consists of laser photocoagulation and systemic immunosuppressive therapy. A peripheral tractional retinal detachment does not need to be treated surgically in every case; comparable to a peripheral localized detachment in proliferative diabetic retinopathy, the localized detachments might settle following regression of vascular proliferations and the exudative component of the retinal detachment after photocoagulation or medical treatment. In the advanced stages, especially when combined with vitreous hemorrhage, early vitrectomy with delamination of vasoproliferative adhesions and combined with laser photocoagulation might achieve better results [16, 42].

References

1. Ahmadieh H, Soheilian M, Azarmina M, et al. (2003) Surgical management of retinal detachment secondary to acute retinal necrosis: clinical features, surgical techniques, and long-term results. Jpn J Ophthalmol 2003;47(5):484–91
2. Akova YA, Yilmaz G, Aydin P (1999) Retinal tears associated with panuveitis and Behcet's disease. Ophthalmic Surg Lasers 1999;30(9):762–5
3. Asaria RH, Kon CH, Bunce C, et al. (2001) Adjuvant 5-fluorouracil and heparin prevents proliferative vitreoretinopathy: results from a randomized, double-blind, controlled clinical trial. Ophthalmology 2001;108(7):1179–83
4. Atmaca LS, Batioglu F, Atmaca Sonmez P (2002) A long-term follow-up of Eales' disease. Ocul Immunol Inflamm 2002;10(3):213–21
5. Balansard B, Bodaghi B, Cassoux N, et al. (2005) Necrotising retinopathies simulating acute retinal necrosis syndrome. Br J Ophthalmol 2005;89(1):96–101
6. Benson WE, Chan P, Sharma S, et al. (1999) Current popularity of pneumatic retinopexy. Retina 1999;19(3):238–41
7. Blumenkranz M, Clarkson J, Culbertson WW, et al. (1989) Visual results and complications after retinal reattachment in the acute retinal necrosis syndrome. The influence of operative technique. Retina 1989;9(3):170–4

8. Bonfioli AA, Eller AW (2005) Acute retinal necrosis. Semin Ophthalmol 2005;20(3):155–60
9. Bonfioli AA, Damico FM, Curi AL, et al. (2005) Intermediate uveitis. Semin Ophthalmol 2005;20(3):147–54
10. Canzano JC, Morse LS, Wendel RT (1999) Surgical repair of cytomegalovirus-related retinal detachment without silicone oil in patients with AIDS. Retina 1999;19(4):274–80
11. Chang PY, Yang CM, Yang CH, et al. (2005) Clinical characteristics and surgical outcomes of pediatric rhegmatogenous retinal detachment in Taiwan. Am J Ophthalmol 2005;139(6):1067–72
12. Chang S (2006) LXII Edward Jackson lecture: open angle glaucoma after vitrectomy. Am J Ophthalmol 2006;141(6):1033–43
13. Charteris DG, Aylward GW, Wong D, et al. (2004) A randomized controlled trial of combined 5-fluorouracil and low-molecular-weight heparin in management of established proliferative vitreoretinopathy. Ophthalmology 2004;111(12):2240–5
14. Davis JL, Hummer J, Feuer WJ (1997) Laser photocoagulation for retinal detachments and retinal tears in cytomegalovirus retinitis. Ophthalmology 1997;104(12):2053–60; discussion 60–1
15. Doft BM, Kelsey SF, Wisniewski SR (2000) Retinal detachment in the endophthalmitis vitrectomy study. Arch Ophthalmol 2000;118(12):1661–5
16. El-Asrar AM, Al-Kharashi SA (2002) Full panretinal photocoagulation and early vitrectomy improve prognosis of retinal vasculitis associated with tuberculoprotein hypersensitivity (Eales' disease). Br J Ophthalmol 2002;86(11):1248–51
17. Feltgen N, Weiss C, Wolf S, et al. (2007) Scleral buckling versus primary vitrectomy in rhegmatogenous retinal detachment study (SPR study): recruitment list evaluation. Study report no. 2. Graefes Arch Clin Exp Ophthalmol 2007;245(6):803–9
18. Geier SA, Klauss V, Bogner JR, et al. (1994) Retinal detachment in patients with acquired immunodeficiency syndrome. Ger J Ophthalmol 1994;3(1):9–14
19. Heimann H, Hellmich M, Bornfeld N, et al. (2001) Scleral buckling versus primary vitrectomy in rhegmatogenous retinal detachment (SPR study): design issues and implications. Study report no. 1. Graefes Arch Clin Exp Ophthalmol 2001;239(8):567–74
20. Heimann H, Bartz-Schmidt K, Bornfeld N, et al. (2007) Scleral buckling versus primary vitrectomy in rhegmatogenous retinal detachment – a prospective randomized multicenter clinical study (SPR study). Ophthalmology 2007; 114(12):2142–54
21. Heimann H, Zou X, Jandeck C, et al. (2006) Primary vitrectomy for rhegmatogenous retinal detachment: an analysis of 512 cases. Graefes Arch Clin Exp Ophthalmol 2006;244(1):69–78
22. Hikichi T, Ueno N, Chakrabarti B, et al. (1996) Evidence of cross-link formation of vitreous collagen during experimental ocular inflammation. Graefes Arch Clin Exp Ophthalmol 1996;234(1):47–54
23. Holland GN (1994) The progressive outer retinal necrosis syndrome. Int Ophthalmol 1994;18(3):163–5
24. Hudde T, Althaus C, Sundmacher R (1998) [Acute retinal necrosis syndrome. argon laser coagulation for prevention of rhegmatogenic retinal detachment]. Ophthalmologe 1998;95(7):473–7
25. Kakehashi A, Kado M, Akiba J, et al. (1997) Variations of posterior vitreous detachment. Br J Ophthalmol 1997;81(7):527–32
26. Karavellas MP, Song M, Macdonald JC, et al. (2000) Long-term posterior and anterior segment complications of immune recovery uveitis associated with cytomegalovirus retinitis. Am J Ophthalmol 2000;130(1):57–64
27. Kempen JH, Jabs DA, Dunn JP, et al. (2001) Retinal detachment risk in cytomegalovirus retinitis related to the acquired immunodeficiency syndrome. Arch Ophthalmol 2001;119(1):33–40
28. Kerkhoff FT, Lamberts QJ, van den Biesen PR, et al. (2003) Rhegmatogenous retinal detachment and uveitis. Ophthalmology 2003;110(2):427–31
29. Kosobucki BR, Freeman WR (2006) Retinal disease in HIV-infected patients. In: Ryan SJ, ed. Retina. Philadelphia: Mosby, 2006; v. 1
30. Kreiger AE, Gonzales CR (2006) Management of combined inflammatory and rhegmatogenous retinal detachments (AIDS and ARN). In: Ryan SJ, ed. Retina. Philadelphia: Mosby, 2006; v. 2
31. Laqua H, Honnicke K (2001) [Is scleral buckling still current?] Ophthalmologe 2001;98(9):881–5
32. Lieb DF, Scott IU, Flynn HW Jr, et al. (2003) Open globe injuries with positive intraocular cultures: factors influencing final visual acuity outcomes. Ophthalmology 2003;110(8):1560–6
33. Lim WK, Chee SP (2004) Retinal detachment in atopic dermatitis can masquerade as acute panuveitis with rapidly progressive cataract. Retina 2004;24(6):953–6
34. McDonald HR, Lewis H, Kreiger AE, et al. (1991) Surgical management of retinal detachment associated with the acute retinal necrosis syndrome. Br J Ophthalmol 1991;75(8):455–8
35. Morrison VL, Labree LD, Azen SP, et al. (2005) Results of silicone oil removal in patients with cytomegalovirus retinitis related retinal detachments. Am J Ophthalmol 2005;140(5):786–93
36. Nagpal A, Biswas J (2006) Pseudouveitis—analysis of cases misdiagnosed as posterior uveitis. Ocul Immunol Inflamm 2006;14(1):13–20
37. Natkunarajah M, Goldsmith C, Goble R (2003) Diagnostic effectiveness of noncontact slitlamp examination in the identification of retinal tears. Eye 2003;17(5):607–9
38. Pastor JC, de la Rua ER, Martin F (2002) Proliferative vitreoretinopathy: risk factors and pathobiology. Prog Retin Eye Res 2002;21(1):127–44

39. Saw SM, Gazzard G, Wagle AM, et al. (2006) An evidence-based analysis of surgical interventions for uncomplicated rhegmatogenous retinal detachment. Acta Ophthalmol Scand 2006;84(5):606–12
40. Schubert HD (1996) Postsurgical hypotony: relationship to fistulization, inflammation, chorioretinal lesions, and the vitreous. Surv Ophthalmol 1996;41(2):97–125
41. Scott IU, Smiddy WE, Feuer WJ, et al. (2004) The impact of echography on evaluation and management of posterior segment disorders. Am J Ophthalmol 2004;137(1):24–9
42. Shanmugam MP, Badrinath SS, Gopal L, et al. (1998) Long term visual results of vitrectomy for Eales disease complications. Int Ophthalmol 1998;22(1):61–4
43. Sidikaro Y, Silver L, Holland GN, et al. (1991) Rhegmatogenous retinal detachments in patients with AIDS and necrotizing retinal infections. Ophthalmology 1991;98(2):129–35
44. Sternberg P Jr, Han DP, Yeo JH, et al. (1988) Photocoagulation to prevent retinal detachment in acute retinal necrosis. Ophthalmology 1988;95(10):1389–93
45. Thorne JE, Jabs DA, Kempen JH, et al. (2006) Causes of visual acuity loss among patients with AIDS and cytomegalovirus retinitis in the era of highly active antiretroviral therapy. Ophthalmology 2006;113(8):1441–5

46. Tran TH, Bodaghi B, Rozenberg F, et al. (2004) [Viral cause and management of necrotizing herpetic retinopathies]. J Fr Ophtalmol 2004;27(3):223–36
47. Ung T, Comer MB, Ang AJ, et al. (2005) Clinical features and surgical management of retinal detachment secondary to round retinal holes. Eye 2005;19(6):665–9
48. Veckeneer M, Van Overdam K, Bouwens D, et al. (2001) Randomized clinical trial of cryotherapy versus laser photocoagulation for retinopexy in conventional retinal detachment surgery. Am J Ophthalmol 2001;132(3):343–7
49. Vrabec TR (1997) Laser photocoagulation repair of macula-sparing cytomegalovirus-related retinal detachment. Ophthalmology 1997;104(12):2062–7
50. Weinberg DV, Lyon AT, Greenwald MJ, et al. (2003) Rhegmatogenous retinal detachments in children: risk factors and surgical outcomes. Ophthalmology 2003;110(9):1708–13
51. Wilkinson CP (2000) Evidence-based analysis of prophylactic treatment of asymptomatic retinal breaks and lattice degeneration. Ophthalmology 2000;107(1):12–5; discussion 15–8

Chapter 22

Surgical Management of Ocular Hypotony

Mark Hammer, W. Sanderson Grizzard

Core Messages

- Many types of chronic uveitis can lead to chronic hypotony.
- Chronic hypotony should be diagnostically evaluated to eliminate nonuveitic causes of hypotony.
- If the ultrasound biomicroscopy (UBM) indicates fibrous traction in the region of the ciliary body, surgical dissection of the ciliary body can be effective in restoring intraocular pressure.
- Visualization with the vitreoretinal endoscope can improve dissection of the ciliary body.
- Silicone oil is usually used to fill uveitic hypotonous eyes when there is zero pressure and scleral infolding.
- Good visual acuities and large improvements in visual acuity are rarely achieved.

Contents

22.1	Introduction 231	22.6	What Are the Preferred Surgical Instruments and Machines for These Procedures? 234
22.2	Which Patients Get Hypotony? 232		
22.3	What Are the Anatomic Mechanisms of Hypotony? 232	22.7	How Can Postoperative Complications Be Avoided? 235
22.5	What Are the Absolute and Relative Indications and Contraindications for the Procedure? 233	References 235	

This chapter contains the following video clips on DVD: Video 37 shows Further applications of Videoendoscopy for VR-surgery (Surgeons: Mark Hammer, W. Sanderson), Video 38 shows Videoendoscopy for VR-surgery – Presumptive sarcoid uveitis and Video 39 shows Videoendoscopy for VR-surgery – Chronic non-rheumatoid arthritic uveitis (Surgeon: Mark Hammer).

22.1 Introduction

Hypotony associated with chronic uveitis occurs infrequently but is a disturbing finding. When the intraocular pressure is below 5 mmHg, the patient's vision may be compromised by hypotony-maculopathy or astigmatic distortions due to the globe's loss of turgor. The lowest pressure ranges of hypotony are often regarded as prephthisical since shrinkage and eventual disorganization of the entire globe frequently ensue. Severe hypotony is usually encountered after extensive and often prolonged surgical and medical management of ocular trauma, glaucoma, retinal disease, or uveitis. Often hypotony is just one of a number of apparently overwhelming problems of end-stage ocular disease. However, many times every other condition is resolved, stabilized, or manageable. This is particularly likely to be the case for uveitic hypotony because of recent and continuing advances in medical and surgical treatment of uveitis as exhibited in this book. The physician and patient have usually invested enormously in time, money, effort, and hope when severe uveitic hypotony is first encountered. It is therefore poignantly asked, "What can be done for hypotony?"

22.2 Which Patients Get Hypotony?

Uveitic hypotony is most frequently reported for chronic granulomatous uveitis and chronic autoimmune uveitis. The reported autoimmune diseases associated with hypotony-uveitis are systemic lupus erythematosis, psoriatic arthritis, juvenile rheumatoid arthritis, juvenile onset chronic iridocyclitis, Reiter's syndrome related uveitis, intermediate uveitis, and severe episodic anterior uveitis [1, 2]. The associated granulomatous diseases are sarcoidosis, Vogt-Koyanagi-Harada's disease, and toxoplasmosis uveitis [3].

Hypotony after failed vitrectomy for retinal detachment with proliferative vitreoretinopathy is a frequent complication. In the "Silicone oil study: report number 4," 31% of patients tamponaded with perfluoropropane and 18% of patients tamponaded with silicone oil had postoperative intraocular pressures of 5 mmHg or less [4]. Additionally, hypotony is a frequent complication of many glaucoma procedures since lowering the intraocular pressure is the specific goal of the glaucoma surgeon.

22.3 What Are the Anatomic Mechanisms of Hypotony?

The general categories of mechanisms of chronic hypotony are external wound leakage, external fistula, cyclodialysis cleft, ciliary body detachment, ciliary body ablation, ciliary body traction detachment, and primary ciliary body failure (Table 22.1) [5].

External leakage arises from penetrating injury or inadequate closure after a prior surgery. An external fistula is the intentional result of glaucoma-filtering surgery. A cyclodialysis cleft is a tear or surgical incision into the iris root. Diagnosis of an occult dialysis cleft may be difficult with a gonioscopic evaluation alone (Table 22.2).

The ultrasonic biomicroscope (UBM) can be helpful in visualizing an occult dialysis cleft as well as shallow or more obvious ciliary body detachment [7]. Ciliary body detachment is often associated with choroidal detachment, especially choroidal effusion. Ordinary B-scan ultrasonography can be useful in visualizing posterior segment choroidal detachments and effusions. Ciliary body ablation can be seen after cryo or laser

Table 22.1 Mechanisms of hypotony

Mechanism	Example
External leakage	Wound leak
External fistula	Glaucoma fistula
Occult cyclodialysis cleft	After injury or surgery
Ciliary body detachment	Associated with choroidal detachment
Ciliary body ablation	After laser or cryopexy for glaucoma
Ciliary body traction detachment	Associated with PVR
Primary or secondary ciliary body failure	Chronic uveitis, cidofovir [6], mitomycin

Table 22.2 Diagnostic techniques

Technique	Notes
Ocular examination with IOP	10–5 mmHg = hypotonous; 5–0 mmHg = prephthisical, also hypotonous
Gonioscopy	Evaluate for cyclodialysis cleft
B-scan ultrasonography	Evaluate for choroidal detachment
UBM (ultrasonic biomicroscopy)	Evaluate for ciliary body traction, ablation

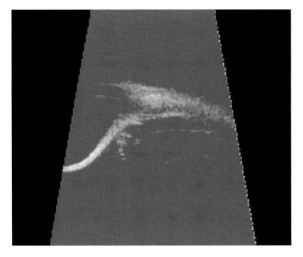

Fig. 22.1 Ultrasonic biomicroscopy demonstrating iris root being pulled posteriorly by fibrous strands over the ciliary body

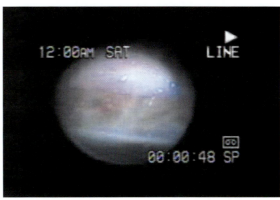

Fig. 22.2 The ciliary processes in this endoscopic video frame are encased in a thick fibrotic membrane, although they are distinguishable through the translucent fibrous tissue

ablation of the ciliary processes. Ciliary body traction detachment occurs when there is fibrous proliferation and contraction of collagen fibers of the anterior vitreous extending around the ciliary processes. Traction distortion and detachment of the ciliary processes is easily demonstrated with the UBM (Fig. 22.1). Primary ciliary body failure occurs when the ciliary processes no longer secrete aqueous, but are otherwise anatomically intact.

22.4 What Role Does Medical and Pharmacological Therapy Play in the Treatment of Uveitic Hypotony?

Topical, periocular, and intravitreal steroids are usually given to further decrease inflammation of the ciliary body. The intent is also to take advantage of decreased outflow facility induced by ocular steroid use in many individuals. The inflammatory component of the uveitis should be optimally controlled with systemic anti-inflammatory, antiproliferative, antimetabolite, and the newer biological anti-tumor-necrosis-factor agents as required. The use of implantable ocular steroid slow-release devices, e.g., Retisert, is a promising avenue of further development. The slow, steady release of a steroid implant should prevent the accumulation of inflammatory debris and subsequent scar tissue formation around the ciliary processes, favoring long-term maintenance of favorable results from surgery for hypotony.

22.5 What Are the Absolute and Relative Indications and Contraindications for the Procedure?

The most important first step is to eliminate all of the nonuveitic causes of hypotony noted in Table 22.1. The absolute indication for surgery is an eye with chronic, not acute, uveitis with zero or almost zero intraocular pressure and at least light-perception visual acuity [8]. These eyes usually show scleral infolding without choroidal detachment. The eye should not have progressed to shrinkage of the globe with other signs of prolonged phthisis. Eyes with signs of prolonged phthisis often have ciliary processes that are encased in thick fibrotic tissue or have been completely replaced by scar tissue (Fig. 22.2).

Relative indications for surgery are characterized by hypotony-maculopathy often with associated choroidal detachments. Since choroidal detachments can also be associated with hypotony by themselves, it is especially important to exhaust anti-inflammatory treatment, including systemic steroids where feasible. Another relative indication is a patient who has already lost an eye to phthisis and now has ominously progressive hypotony in the remaining eye.

Table 22.3 Surgical techniques

Technique	Notes
Intravitreal triamcinolone injection	Helps control noninfectious uveitis
Intravitreal sodium hyaluronate injection [9]	Lasts 3 months, probably temporary
Repair leak, fistula, or dialysis cleft if present	Suture wound leak or dialysis cleft
Vitrectomy for ciliary body traction	Variable-quality view requiring scleral depression
Vitreoretinal videoendoscopic-assisted vitrectomy	Allows evaluation, video documentation, and surgical visualization without scleral depression
Silicone oil filling	For prephthisical eyes, decreases posterior filtration

22.6 What Are the Preferred Surgical Instruments and Machines for These Procedures?

The preferred instruments and machines will depend on what is causing the hypotony and which procedure is preferred (Table 22.3).

Injections of triamcinolone or sodium hyaluronate can be done in the office or clinic setting. Prepping the cornea and conjunctiva with iodine–povidone solution 5–10% and use of a lid retractor is essential to minimize the risk of endophthalmitis. Pre- and postoperative antibiotic drops and a "clean" if not completely sterile technique is also recommended. Due to the particulate nature of triamcinolone injectibles, a 27-gauge needle is recommended to prevent clogging that can occur at smaller gauges.

Standard anterior segment techniques are used to repair a wound leak, fistula, or dialysis cleft [5]. Laser cautery or cryopexy has also been used to treat dialysis clefts without the use of incisions or sutures. Limbal incisions or flaps can also be used to approach the closure of leaks and fistulas. Removal of an intraocular lens and all capsular remnants through the limbus is usually performed when the IOL has become involved by a cyclitic membrane or capsular fibrosis and contraction.

Pars plana vitrectomy is required for surgery of the ciliary body. Either the fiber-optic or gradient index of refraction (GRIN) glass rod vitreoretinal endoscope can be used. The GRIN endoscope gives a higher resolution view of the ciliary processes, has an imbedded light channel, an empty channel through which a laser fiber may be threaded, and an adjustable focus which is effective over a wide range (Fig. 22.3) [10]. The fiber-op-

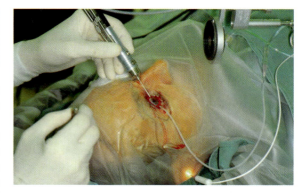

Fig. 22.3 The GRIN-rod endoscope handpiece is fairly large but allows high resolution and has an adjustment for focus valuable when high magnification is desired

tic endoscope has a higher light transmission, a smaller handpiece, an imbedded laser and light fiber, and is less likely to be damaged. Since the endoscopes are 20-gauge, a vitrectomy system that is 20-gauge is usually selected.

The vitreoretinal endoscope is used to assess the location, severity, and type of ciliary process involvement by the uveitic and secondary or associated inflammatory and fibrotic response. The kind of abnormal findings that are frequently described include ciliary processes that are slightly grayish, are distorted by traction membranes, have "white caps" on their crests, are depigmented with a visible blood vessel, or are atrophic and shrunken [10].

Distorted ciliary processes under traction by fibrous "anterior loop" membranes are those most likely to benefit from surgical dissection by relieving the fibrous traction. The dissection is performed with intraocular scissors, knives, and forceps. When these instruments are unable to dissect especially dense fibrous tissue without damaging the underlying ciliary processes, segmentation of the fibrous tissue is performed to release the circumferential contraction. Visualization with a surgical microscope is frequently chosen for dissection because the operator is familiar with this system. The surgical microscope has the advantages of a wide, well-lighted field of view and stereopsis due to the binocular view [11]. Visualization using the endoscope to direct the dissection is possible but there is a "learning curve." As with all endoscopy, (1) there is no stereopsis, (2) the view changes radically with slight translations and rotations of the endoscope, (3) the illumination and laser system move with the view, and (4) one hand and a great deal of the surgeon's attention is required by the "viewing" system.

Nevertheless, other surgical specialties have overcome these difficulties with training and experience. Due to the limited space outside the eye, it is difficult to delegate the management of the endoscope to an assistant. The close confinement and delicate structures inside the eye also leave a smaller and more perilous volume for surgical maneuvers than in other surgical specialties. Surgery with endoscopic visualization has the advantage of not requiring scleral depression, which is usually necessary to view the ciliary processes with surgical microscopic visualization. Scleral depression often relaxes the traction and always compresses the surgical planes, making surgical dissection more difficult and increasing the risk of damaging the ciliary processes. Reevaluation of the ciliary body with the endoscope after surgical dissection is valuable even if the dissection is done with the surgical microscope because it gives a much better view than scleral depression.

If the eye has zero pressure with scleral infolding from uveitis with all other causes of hypotony treated or ruled out, filling the vitreous cavity with silicone oil is recommended even after ciliary body dissection [12]. In a few eyes, ciliary body dissection may restore normal pressure. However, about 50% of eyes with fibrous traction involving the ciliary processes, and most of the other eyes without traction, will show limited response to surgery. Filling the vitreous cavity with silicone oil may leverage a small increase in aqueous secretion to a higher intraocular pressure by "waterproofing" the posterior segment, thus reducing any posterior segment contribution to aqueous outflow. Highly refined silicone with a higher viscosity, 5,000 centistoke in the United States, is preferred because it has a better chance of being tolerated by the eye for the long term. If normal aqueous inflow truly seems to be restored, the silicone oil can always be removed.

22.7 How Can Postoperative Complications Be Avoided?

One intraoperative complication is the production of unintended iridotomies when working near the zonule and anterior ciliary body. Trauma to the ciliary processes including hemorrhage, tearing, or detachment can occur especially if vigorous dissection is required with reoperation or dense scar tissue.

Overfilling of the eye with silicone oil can result in oil touching the cornea and loss of the endothelium over time. This is, of course, inevitable if the pressure remains or falls to zero after the surgery. A 6-o'clock peripheral iridectomy (Ando iridectomy) can minimize the corneal touch if there is any remaining aqueous production. Vigilance to the underlying uveitis should be maintained. Increased amounts of anti-inflammatory medication are usually warranted in the immediate postoperative period. Surgical treatment of uveitic hypotony is usually successful at preventing loss of the globe, often maintains at least low levels of intraocular pressure, and often maintains reduced visual acuities. Good visual acuities and large improvements in visual acuity are rarely achieved.

Take Home Pearls

- Despite medical treatment, a variety of chronic uveitic diseases can lead to chronic hypotony.
- After eliminating and or treating nonuveitic causes of hypotony, ciliary body dissection and filling the vitreous cavity with silicone oil can stabilize and sometimes improve the intraocular pressure.
- Using a vitreoretinal endoscope, either the fiber-optic or GRIN-rod version, can improve the surgical evaluation and control of ciliary body dissection.
- Highly refined 5,000 centistoke silicone oil is preferred for filling the vitreous cavity because it is better tolerated in the long term.

References

1. Yu EN, Paredes I, Foster CS, Surgery for hypotony in patients with juvenile idiopathic arthritis-associated uveitis, Ocul Immunol and Inflamm 15:11–17, 2007

2. Fox GM, Flynn HW, Davis JL, Culbertson W, Causes of reduced visual acuity on long-term follow-up after cataract extraction in patients with uveitis and juvenile rheumatoid arthritis, Am J Ophthalmol 114:708–714, 1992
3. De Smet MD, Gunning F, Feenstra R, The surgical management of chronic hypotony due to uveitis, Eye 19:60–64, 2005
4. Barr CC, Lai MY, Lean JS, et al., Postoperative intraocular pressure abnormalities in the silicone oil study: silicone study report 4, Ophthalmology 100:1629–1635, 1993
5. Schubert HD, Major review: postsurgical hypotony: relationship to fistulization, inflammation, chorioretinal lesions, and the vitreous, Surv Ophthalmol 41:97–125, 1996
6. Banker AS, Arevalo JF, Munguia D, et al., Intraocular pressure and aqueous humor, dynamics in patients with AIDS treated with intravitreal cidofovir (HPMPC. for cytomegalovirus retinitis, Am J Ophthalmol 124:168–180, 1997
7. Roters S, Szurman P, Engels BF, et al., Ultrasound biomicroscopy in chronic ocular hypotony: its impact on diagnosis and management, Retina 22:581–588, 2002
8. Hammer ME, Grizzard WS, Davis JL, Endoscopic evaluation and surgery for sever uveitic hypotony, presented at the annual meeting of the American Uveitis Society, Chicago, October 2005
9. Tosi GM, Schiff W, Barile G, et al., Management of severe hypotony with intravitreal injection of viscoelastic, Am J Ophthalmol 140:952–954, 2005
10. Hammer ME, Grizzard WS, Endoscopy for evaluation and treatment of the ciliary body in hypotony, Retina 23:30–36, 2003
11. O'Connell SR, Majji AB, Humayan MS, deJuan E, The surgical management of hypotony, Ophthalmology 107:318–323, 2000
12. Morse LS, McCuen BW, The use of silicone oil in uveitis and hypotony, Retina 11:399–404, 1991

Part C
Surgery for Diagnosis of Uveitis

Chapter 23

Anterior Chamber Tap and Aqueous Humor Analysis

Uwe Pleyer, Justus G. Garweg

Core Messages

- Differentiation between infectious and noninfectious uveitis is often of crucial value for accurate management of patients with intraocular inflammation.
- Aqueous humor analysis may provide useful information to establish a specific diagnosis of intraocular inflammation in order to confirm or exclude a suspected specific etiology.
- Analysis of aqueous humor yields more relevant information about the local process than those performed in serum.
- Specific analysis, e.g., in suspected masquerade syndromes, should be performed in specialized centers.

Contents

23.1	Introduction 239	23.4	Diagnostic Procedure 240
23.2	Background on Immune Responses Within the Eye—Intraocular Antibody Production 239	23.4.1	General Considerations 240
		23.4.2	Indication for Anterior Chamber Puncture 241
23.3	General Aspects on Anterior Chamber Puncture in Uveitis 240	23.4.3	Diagnostic Techniques 241
23.3.1	Patient Selection 240	23.4.3.1	PCR 242
23.3.2	Timing of Diagnostic Tap 240	23.4.3.2	Local Antibody Formation 242
23.3.3	Preparation and Anesthesia 240	23.4.3.3	Cytology 242
23.3.4	Technique 240	23.5	Postoperative Complications 242
		References 242

23.1 Introduction

The underlying cause of intraocular inflammation is often difficult to establish but particularly important in infectious uveitis or a masquerade syndrome that will benefit from subsequent, specific therapy. Some of the most common causes of uveitis (e.g., herpetic keratouveitis and toxoplasmic retinochoroiditis) are not diagnosable using serology because of the high rate of seropositive individuals in the general population. Investigations using molecular biological techniques and antibody testing with the analysis of specific antibody formation within the eye provide useful information.

23.2 Background on Immune Responses Within the Eye—Intraocular Antibody Production

For decades the humoral immune response in the eye has been used to confirm the clinical diagnosis of intraocular infection by pathogens such as *Toxoplasma gondii* and the herpes family viruses, namely herpes simplex (HSV-1, HSV-2), cytomegalovirus and varicella zoster virus.

Early studies demonstrated that B-lymphocytes and/or plasma cells can be detected in the vitreous during infections with pathogens [2, 11]. Subsequent studies confirmed that B cells do occur intraocularly but form a minor component of the infiltrating lymphocytes [4]. The portion of B cells among infiltrating lymphocytes is increased in samples obtained from eyes graded as having active inflammation. So far, limited information is available on the specificity of intraocular antibodies. However, recent information indicates that a dissociated immune response may occur that confirms a compartmentalized, specific intraocular immune response following intraocular infection by *T. gondii* and HSV-1 [14]. Further evidence indicates that local antibody production is highly specific for the underlying pathologic mechanism. The detection of local antibody production may thus have a high positive predictive value, whereas its negative predictive meaning varies widely depending on the underlying diagnosis.

23.3 General Aspects on Anterior Chamber Puncture in Uveitis

23.3.1 Patient Selection

An anterior chamber puncture may be considered in case of acute and chronic endophthalmitis, progressive inflammatory eye disease, severe bilateral uveitis and uveitis unresponsive to the previous treatment in order to establish or exclude a specific diagnosis. Anterior chamber puncture in inflammatory disease is performed mainly for diagnostic purposes.

23.3.2 Timing of Diagnostic Tap

In general, intraocular fluid from a patient with suspected infection has to be examined in the active state in order to prove a specific origin of the inflammation. Several studies have shown that, depending on the diagnostic testing that is applied, specimen acquisition between 1 and 6 weeks after onset is critical for detection of local antibody formation [9]. Little information is available on the time frame of B-cell activation in humans. However, experimental data suggests that activation may occur as early as 3 days after onset in recurrent disease [23].

23.3.3 Preparation and Anesthesia

Since the procedure itself is straightforward, there are no major contraindications for an anterior chamber tap. As it is an elective intraocular procedure, certain precautions can minimize risk. Particular concerns are:

- Inoculation of the eye with infectious organisms
- Damage to intraocular structures
- Trauma to the lens and induction of cataract

In almost all patients, topical anesthesia is appropriate. Lidocaine gel or repeated procaine or other anesthetic eyedrops applied before the procedure are adequate. Concomitant sedatives are not necessary. It is our experience that even in cooperative children, anterior chamber tap is a safe procedure. In rare instances in uncooperative individuals such as younger children and developmentally-delayed patients, mask anesthesia might be preferred.

23.3.4 Technique

Anterior chamber tap is performed as an outpatient procedure. Precautions must be taken to provide the highest standard of care for this elective procedure. Performance of anterior chamber paracenthesis at the slit lamp utilizing polyvidone iodine preparation and postoperative topical antibiotics has been reported to be a safe procedure without adverse reactions [3]. We prefer preparing the patient as for any intraocular surgery. After informed consent has been obtained, the patient is prepped with polyvidone iodine and draped utilizing sterile technique. After application of one drop of polyvidone iodine 5% to the ocular surface, a speculum retracts the eyelids, and either a sponge or small-toothed forceps are used to stabilize the eye. We use a 30-gauge needle (bevel up) placed through the clear cornea in the temporal inferior quadrant over the iris stroma to aspirate approximately 100–250 µl of aqueous humor. After puncture, prophylactic local antibiotics are given for 3 days.

23.4 Diagnostic Procedure

23.4.1 General Considerations

Consideration of the underlying pathob biology is a prerequisite for a successful diagnostic strategy. Since the aqueous humor sample volume is limited to no more than 250 µl, only two to three tests can be performed. Therefore, a working diagnosis and a diagnostic strategy need to be specified in advance. As anterior chamber puncture is considered namely in unclear diagnostic situations after serologic tests have failed to establish a diagnosis, this is a critical point regarding the sensitivity of aqueous humor analysis. Whereas aqueous humor analysis without parallel serologic testing may be helpful in the detection of a localized infection or malignancy by microbial culture, antigen detection, PCR and cytokine assays, the meaning of intraocular antibodies without parallel testing of serum is less certain. Therefore, assays of the intraocular humoral immune response should be also performed in a simultaneous blood sample (2–5 ml). Both samples are apportioned according to the minimum volume requirements for the tests to be done and forwarded after personally contacting the corresponding laboratories.

In patients requiring cytology or culture of intraocular organisms, aqueous is transported at room temperature overnight. Specimens for PCR and antibodies may be refrigerated, depending upon the time to assay. Freezing may result in a 10% loss of antibodies and should be restricted to samples that will not be assayed within 7–10 days. Coordination with the laboratory prior to analysis is necessary to avoid waste or damage to the specimen.

23.4.2 Indication for Anterior Chamber Puncture

Diagnostic aqueous humor analysis is usually performed in intraocular inflammation with an atypical presentation that threatens visual acuity and does not adequately respond to therapy. The intent is to confirm or exclude an infectious etiology or masquerade syndrome such as intraocular lymphoma (Table 23.1). So far, there is no assay of aqueous humor to confirm a diagnosis of chronic noninfectious immunologically mediated intraocular inflammation.

23.4.3 Diagnostic Techniques

None of the commercially available tests is designed for aqueous humor analysis. This is important to mention since intraocular antibody synthesis is often well below the established detection limit of these tests. Quantitative analysis may be achieved if the sample is analyzed

Table 23.1 Indications for anterior chamber puncture

Suspected disorder	Timing of puncture	Preferred method of analysis	Comments	References
HSV keratouveitis	Active disease	PCR and AB	Sensitivity of combined analysis nearly 40%	19, 25, 27
Heterochromic cyclitis	Any time	AB and PCR	Rubella virus	24
Acute retinal necrosis syndrome	Active disease, no more than 48 h after start of antiviral therapy	PCR (+ AB)	Emergency situation	5, 8, 16, 20, 29
Toxoplasmosis retinochoroiditis	Active disease	AB; PCR in atypical and severe cases	Mainly in atypical clinical presentations	9, 13, 28
CMV retinitis	Active disease	PCR (+ AB)	Local antibody synthesis might be impaired in HIV+ patients	6
Masquerade syndrome	Any time	Cytology with or without immunocytochemistry; interleukin 6 and 10 levels	Analysis in specialized centers	7

AB antibody synthesis, *PCR* polymerase chain reaction

other than routinely, using a higher sensitivity assay or if it is individually diluted, tenfold to one hundredfold less than the standard dilution factor for testing, depending on the volume requirements of the test.

Progress in molecular biology has allowed novel diagnostic approaches to investigate intraocular infection. A close collaboration with a microbiology department with sufficient expertise to analyze infectious agents in intraocular specimen as well as an immediate transfer of material to a cytopathology department is essential. Besides classical culture techniques, detection of DNA by polymerase chain reaction (PCR), antibodies by ELISA or immunoblots are the most frequently applied techniques [22].

23.4.3.1 PCR

PCR is a highly sensitive and specific method to detect DNA from small sample volumes. However, the limitations and possibilities of this technique have to be kept in mind. Yield is largely dependent on sample processing and the skills of the investigator. The application of molecular biologic methods has greatly facilitated the identification of a causative organism. Amplification of a common bacterial sequence, 16S ribosomal RNA, can rapidly identify a bacterial cause of severe intraocular inflammation and postoperative endophthalmitis [15, 16, 20, 21]. Subsequent amplification with specific primers can be used for speciation. Panviral and panfungal PCR techniques also exist. However, these laboratory tests may contribute little if they are not based on clinical grounds. Furthermore, the detection of microorganisms by means of microbiological or molecular techniques does not necessarily confirm their active contribution. Especially in PCR, detection of microbial presence may be due to sample contamination. Finally, the negative predictive value of testing varies depending on the target DNA to be detected and the laboratory's proficiency. Therefore, the information obtained has to be interpreted in the clinical context considering sensitivity and specificity of the tests in the particular laboratory.

23.4.3.2 Local Antibody Formation

Local production of antibodies is confirmed by the Goldmann–Witmer coefficient (GWc), which is the ratio of the local pathogen-specific titer × total systemic antibody titer divided by the systemic specific × total local antibody titer. An index of over 3 is considered proof of a specific intraocular infection [10, 13, 29]. In intraocular infection affecting the posterior segment, calculation of the GWc may be the only reliable way of confirming or establishing a specific clinical diagnosis.

23.4.3.3 Cytology

Generally, information obtained from cytology is of limited value due to the low total cell count even with significant cellular infiltration of the anterior chamber. However, cytopathology may uncover an underlying fungal, mycobacterial or lymphomatous etiology [18]. The major diagnostic challenge lies in the distinction between inflammatory lymphoid infiltrates and intraocular lymphoma, especially when only a few cells are intact [12]. Nevertheless, cytological determination of cell surface markers and cytokine levels yield sufficiently sensitive results to provide valuable information in the diagnosis of intraocular lymphoma [7].

23.5 Postoperative Complications

According to published evidence and personal experience, anterior chamber puncture is a sufficiently safe procedure to recommend it if a specific diagnosis needs to be confirmed or excluded [3]. In a retrospective study of 361 patients with uveitis who underwent a diagnostic anterior chamber paracentesis, no severe intra- or postoperative complications were reported. Within a follow-up of at least 6 months, no serious side effects such as cataract, keratitis, or endophthalmitis were observed [29]. A small hyphema may occur during the procedure or in the early postoperative course (Amsler's sign), especially in patients with heterochromic iridocyclitis and viral anterior uveitis, occurring in 5–7% of cases [29]. Rarely, particularly in the case of longer preexisting secondary glaucoma, significant retinal hemorrhage may be observed from the induced hypotony [17]. Occasionally, minor leakage from the paracentesis might temporarily reduce intraocular pressure. Infectious complications have rarely been observed [1].

References

1. Azuara-Blanco A, Katz LJ. Infectious keratitis in a paracentesis tract. Ophthalmic Surg Lasers 1997; 28: 332–3
2. Belfort R, Moura NC, Mendes NF. T and B lymphocytes in the aqueous humor of patients with uveitis. Arch Ophthalmol 1982; 100: 465–467
3. Cheung CM, Durrani OM, Murray PI. Safety of anterior chamber puncture. Br J Ophthalmol 2004; 88: 582–3
4. Davis JL, Solomon D, Nussenblatt RB, Palestine AG, Chan CC. Immunocytochemical staining of vitreous cells. Indications, techniques, and results. Ophthalmology 1992; 99: 250–256

5. de Boer JH, Luyendijk L, Rothova A, Baarsma GS, de Jong PT, Bollemeijer JG, Rademakers AJ, Van der Zaal MJ, Kijlstra A. Detection of intraocular antibody production to herpesviruses in acute retinal necrosis syndrome. Am J Ophthalmol 1994; 117: 201–210
6. Fenner T, Garweg JG, Hufert FT, Böhnke M, Schmitz H. Diagnosis of human cytomegalovirus-induced retinitis in human immunodeficiency virus type infected subjects using the polymerase chain reaction. J Clin Microbiol 1991; 29: 2621–2622
7. Finger PT, Papp C, Latkany P, Kurli M, Iacob CE. Anterior chamber paracentesis cytology (cytospin technology) for the diagnosis of intraocular lymphoma. Br J Ophthalmol 2006; 90: 690–2
8. Garweg JG, Böhnke M. Varicella-zoster virus is strongly associated with atypical necrotizing herpetic retinopathies. Clin Infect Dis 1997; 24: 603–608
9. Garweg JG, Jacquier P, Böhnke M. Early aqueous humor analysis in patients with human ocular toxoplasmosis. J Clin Microbiol 2000; 38: 996–1001
10. Goldmann H, Witmer R. Antibodies in the aqueous humor. Ophthalmologica 1954; 127: 323–30
11. Kaplan HJ, Waldrep JC, Nicholson JK, Gordon D. Immunologic analysis of intraocular mononuclear cell infiltrates in uveitis. Arch Ophthalmol 1984; 102: 572–575
12. Karikehalli S, Nazeer T, Lee CY. Intraocular large B-cell lymphoma. A case report. Acta Cytol 2004; 48: 207–210
13. Kijlstra A, Luyendijk L, Baarsma GS, Rothova A, Schweitzer CM, Timmerman Z, de Vries J, Breebaart AC. Aqueous humor analysis as a diagnostic tool in toxoplasma uveitis. Int Ophthalmol 1989; 13: 383–386
14. Klaren VN, Peek R. Evidence for a compartmentalized B cell response as characterized by IgG epitope specificity in human ocular toxoplasmosis. J Immunol 2001; 167: 6263–6269
15. Knox CM, Cevallos V, Margolis TP. Identification of bacterial pathogens in patients with endophthalmitis by 16S ribosomal DNA typing. Am J Ophthalmol 1999; 128: 511–512
16. Kumano Y, Manabe J, Hamamoto M, Kawano Y, Minagawa H, Fukumaki Y, Inomata H. Detection of varicella-zoster virus genome having a PstI site in the ocular sample from a patient with acute retinal necrosis. Ophthalmic Res 1995; 27: 310–316
17. Lee SJ, Lee JJ, Kim SD. Multiple retinal hemorrhage following anterior chamber paracentesis in uveitic glaucoma. Korean J Ophthalmol 2006; 20: 128–30
18. Liu K, Klintworth GK, Dodd LG. Cytologic findings in vitreous fluids. Analysis of 74 specimens. Acta Cytol 1999; 43: 201–206
19. Liekfeld A, Schweig F, Jaeckel C, Wernecke K-D, Hartmann C, Pleyer U. Intraocular antibody production in intraocular inflammation. Graefes Arch Clin Exp Ophthalmol 2000; 238: 222–227
20. Müller B, Velhagen KH, Pleyer U. Akute Retina Nekrose: Analyse, Therapie und Langzeitbeobachtung an 14 Augen. Klin Monatsbl Augenheilkd 2000; 217: 345–350
21. Okhravi N, Adamson P, Matheson MM. PCR-RFLP-mediated detection and speciation of bacterial species causing endophthalmitis. Invest Ophthalmol Vis Sci 2000; 41: 1438–1447
22. Otasevic L, Walduck A, Meyer TF, Aebischer T, Hartmann C, Orlic N, Pleyer U. Helicobacter pylori infection: a possible risk factor for anterior uveitis? Infection 2005; 33: 82–85
23. Pleyer U, Mondino BJ, Adamu S, Halabi H. Immune response to staphylococcus epidermidis induced endophthalmitis in a rabbit model. Invest Ophthalmol Vis Sci 1992; 33: 2650–2663
24. Quentin CD, Reiber H. Fuchs heterochromic cyclitis: rubella virus antibodies and genome in aqueous humor. Am J Ophthalmol 2004; 138: 46–54
25. Robert PY, Liekfeld A, Jaeckel C, Ranger-Rogez S, Adenis JP, Hartmann C, Pleyer U. Specific antibody production in herpes keratitis: intraocular inflammation and corneal neovascularisation as predicting factors. Graefes Arch Clin Exp Ophthalmol 2005; 26: 1–6
26. Santos LM, Marcos MC, Gallardo GJM, Gomez VMA, Collantes EE, Ramirez CR, Omar M. Aqueous humor and serum tumor necrosis factor-alpha in clinical uveitis. Ophthalmic Res 2001; 33: 251–255
27. Schacher S, Garweg JG, Böhnke M. Die Diagnostik der herpetischen uveitis und keratouveitis. Klin Mbl Augenheilk 1998; 212: 359–362
28. Torun N, Liekfeld A, Hartmann C, Metzner S, Pleyer U. Okuläre Toxoplasmose-Antikörper in Kammerwasser und Serum. Ophthalmologe 2002; 99: 109–112
29. Van Gelder RN, Willig JL, Holland GN, Kaplan HJ. Herpes simplex virus type 2 as a cause of acute retinal necrosis syndrome in young patients. Ophthalmology 2001; 108: 869–876

Chapter 24

Surgery for the Diagnosis of Uveitis – Anterior Segment Biopsy

Bahram Bodaghi

Core Messages

- Surgery for the diagnosis of uveitis is rarely performed since the development of less invasive techniques, such as PCR, can be applied to ocular fluids.
- In some specific and challenging situations, tissue biopsy is a highly valuable tool.
- Biopsy should be considered if a directed workup does not yield positive results.
- Infectious and malignant conditions should be excluded in atypical cases that do not respond to corticosteroids and/or antimicrobial agents.
- Scleral biopsy is usually noncontributory in autoimmune conditions.
- Orbital lymphoma, infections, granulomatous disorders and sarcoidosis are the major indications for tissue biopsy.
- Surgical techniques are usually easy to perform, but final diagnosis depends on the quality of histopathological analysis.

Contents

24.1	Introduction	245
24.2	Patient Selection	246
24.3	Technical Considerations	246
24.3.1	Corneal Biopsy	246
24.3.2	Conjunctival and Scleral Biopsies	246
24.3.3	Iris Biopsy	246
24.4	Principle Indications	247
24.4.1	Infectious Necrotizing Scleritis, Keratitis and Uveitis	247
24.4.1.1	Bacterial Infections	247
24.4.1.2	Viral Infections	247
24.4.2	Masquerade Syndromes	248
24.4.2.1	Juvenile Xanthogranuloma	248
24.4.2.2	MALT Lymphoma and Uveal Lymphoid Infiltration	249
24.4.2.3	Primary Intraocular Lymphoma	250
24.4.2.4	Hodgkin's Lymphoma-Associated Posterior Scleritis and Uveitis	250
24.4.2.5	Conjunctival and Corneal Intraepithelial Neoplasia	251
24.4.2.6	Immune-Mediated Entities—Sarcoidosis	251
References		252

24.1 Introduction

Presuming that all undiagnosed ocular inflammation is idiopathic is not advised. Ophthalmologists must reconsider the etiology of primary inflammatory conditions when the clinical examination does not yield a definitive diagnosis or when the course of the disease on corticosteroids is atypical. Despite substantial recent progress, laboratory tests based on the analysis of serum have limited value, especially when ocular inflammation occurs in the absence of the involvement of other organs.

Diagnostic management has been greatly improved by the use of molecular techniques applied to ocular fluids and tissues [1]. Ocular fluid sampling and analysis can be very informative and should be proposed in uveitis of uncertain, but potentially infectious, origin. Polymerase chain reaction and its variants have changed our practical approach to intraocular inflammatory disorders. Tests are now available for almost all pathogens. Yield of a technique may depend on the type of sample. This technology is also applied in selected cases to ocular tissues, such as sclera, cornea conjunctiva and iris. Prompt administration of specific antimicrobial, antiviral or antiparasitic therapy will control the inciting factor of the inflammation and eventually reduce the duration of corticosteroid administration.

24.2 Patient Selection

Anterior segment biopsy may be proposed in all atypical cases of ocular inflammation in order to exclude masquerade syndromes of infectious or tumoral origin. However, biopsy may be unnecessary if minimally invasive techniques, based on the analysis of ocular fluids, can be used. Nevertheless, final diagnosis is sometimes obtained only after enucleation.

24.3 Technical Considerations

24.3.1 Corneal Biopsy

Inflammatory conditions requiring a corneal biopsy are rare [2]. Corneal infections remain the major indication. Most corneal samples are obtained by scraping using a sterile needle or a mini spatula. New imaging techniques, such as confocal microscopy, help specify the best sampling technique. Deep stromal infiltrates and lesions with initially negative culture that continue to progress may require corneal biopsy for further microbial identification. Lamellar excisions of different depths can be performed in order to reach a corneal abscess. A 3–5 mm trephine set to a depth of 0.2–0.3 mm can be used to initiate the biopsy. The edge of the specimen is then dissected. The tissue is used for histopathology and culture. Furthermore, the base of the dissection should be scraped for additional cultures. If the infiltrate is isolated, small and located in the mid stroma, a corneal flap can be dissected followed by lamellar excision. In other exceptional situations, where lesions are close to Descemet's membrane, a full-thickness corneal biopsy may be performed using a small corneal trephine.

24.3.2 Conjunctival and Scleral Biopsies

Tissue sampling is not routinely performed in patients with scleritis, even though anterior scleral nodules seem easy to biopsy [3]. The majority of these nodules contain fluid, easily detectable by ultrasound biomicroscopy scanning. In these cases, biopsy will lead to fluid leakage without yielding any tissue for further histopathological analysis. Even when biopsy specimens are obtained, pathology often reveals nonspecific results, such as degenerated collagen infiltrated with lymphocytes and polymorphonuclear cells. The sclera may fail to heal after biopsy without it having confirmed a definite etiology. Biopsy is also contraindicated in patients with scleromalacia, so as to avoid perforation.

Conjunctival, episcleral and scleral biopsies may be performed. Conjunctival and episcleral tissue is quite easy to obtain after conjunctival reflection and appropriate dissection. There is no standard, recommended technique for scleral biopsy.

A deep, sub-Tenon injection of 0.5–1 ml of bupivacaine 0.5% anesthetic is performed. Conjunctiva is reflected. Light diathermy is applied to bleeding vessels, avoiding the conjunctival or scleral area to be dissected if possible. Conjunctival biopsy is performed directly at the lesion site. There is usually no indication for a conjunctival autograft. However, this may be necessary if there is a suspicion of malignancy. Alternatively, if the conjunctiva is uninvolved, it can be dissected free from the underlying lesion and used to cover the biopsy site, a technique described by Shields for conjunctival lymphoma [42].

For scleral biopsy, the site should include the area spanning normal and necrotic zones. In some cases, especially when scleral or conjunctival lymphoma is suspected, biopsies should also include conjunctiva and extraocular muscles. Superficial nodules may be dissected from the sclera by a crescent knife. Deeper lesions need a more appropriate intrascleral dissection. The technique is similar to that used during trabeculectomy or deep sclerectomy. A scleral incision, to 33% depth, is created. A crescent-shaped knife is then introduced through the scleral incision, which completes the dissection. The tunnel is then widened laterally and the biopsy is taken. Biopsy specimens are divided into two halves: one is placed in formalin for histology and the other is immediately frozen at −25°C for immunohistochemistry. There is usually no scleral defect after scleral biopsy. However, an appropriate graft may be necessary. In some cases, replacing the conjunctiva with the underlying episclera will ensure the formation of a solid scar.

24.3.3 Iris Biopsy

Excisional iris biopsy is usually performed as a sector iridectomy. However, in very rare situations, a deliberate en bloc excision may be carefully performed through a scleral groove. Dissection is performed with forceps and Vannas scissors. It is highly important to dissect the lesion from the surrounding normal iris tissue and the ciliary body.

24.4 Principle Indications

24.4.1 Infectious Necrotizing Scleritis, Keratitis and Uveitis

24.4.1.1 Bacterial Infections

Tuberculosis

Ocular tuberculosis may have various clinical presentations, including retinal vasculitis, choroidal granuloma, optic nerve infiltration and iris tuberculoma [4]. Iris and scleral biopsy are rarely necessary in these cases, but they may provide valuable information [5]. In some cases of anterior involvement with pseudotumoral tuberculosis, eye wall resection associated with donor scleral grafting and antimicrobial therapy may be helpful. This technique is similar to that described in the management of uveal tumors [6].

Lyme Disease

Despite the wide spectrum of clinical entities, eye involvement remains a rare event in patients with Lyme borreliosis. Most ocular manifestations occur during the late phase of the disease. The infection needs to be considered along with more conventional causes of ocular inflammation, particularly in areas where Lyme disease is common. The pathogenesis of this condition remains controversial. Direct ocular infection and a delayed hypersensitivity mechanism may be involved at different times during the disease. Uveitis and optic neuritis are the most common types of ocular complications. Serological testing lacks sensitivity and specificity. In atypical cases, ocular fluid sampling and analysis may be proposed. PCR is a potential diagnostic tool, allowing genotype analysis. Isolation of bacterial agents after tissue biopsy remains exceptional in Lyme disease, even though it has been reported previously [7].

Lepromatous Uveitis

Leprosy should be considered in the differential diagnosis of uveitis and keratitis. *Mycobacterium leprae* may be localized in the conjunctiva, sclera, iris, ciliary body, vitreous and retina [8]. Diagnosis is usually based on skin biopsy, but in some rare cases, iris specimens may contribute information [9]. Peripheral iridectomy may include a portion of the ciliary body. Histopathological features are similar to that of skin lesions [10]. Iris dysfunction in these cases seems to be related to autonomic nerve destruction.

24.4.1.2 Viral Infections

Herpetic Keratitis

Clinical diagnosis of herpetic keratitis is usually straightforward, and the need for corneal biopsy is rare. Inflammation following herpes simplex virus type 1 infection may lead to severe complications in immunocompromised patients, especially in the late stages of AIDS. In these cases, antiviral drug resistance may occur and reduce the efficacy of specific antiviral therapy. Clinical presentations are then sometimes difficult to analyze. Diagnosis and subsequent therapeutic management may be delayed, leading to dramatic visual loss. Viral identification may be difficult. In the case of unsuccessful isolation of the viral strain by standard virological methods, immunohistochemistry, molecular diagnosis using in situ hybridization, PCR and in situ PCR may provide precise evidence of HSV infection and allow further nucleotide sequencing of other antiviral targets, such as viral thymidine kinase or DNA polymerase with relevance for drug resistance.

We have previously reported a case of bilateral severe, active keratitis of 6-months duration in a 31-year-old HIV-positive patient, which was resistant to acyclovir [11]. After corneal biopsy, samples analyzed by standard virological procedures were inconclusive. However, in situ hybridization and PCR confirmed the viral etiology. Furthermore, the thymidine kinase gene was cloned and subsequently sequenced, revealing the presence of five variations previously described in two reference strains, as well as a new point mutation. This change supported the hypothesis of a putatively altered functional form of the enzyme. Intravenous foscarnet, which does not rely on thymidine kinase for activation, was rapidly efficacious.

Three other rare situations in which intraocular inflammation is associated with conjunctival and scleral involvement should be considered.

Ocular Posttransplant Lymphoproliferative Disorder

This rare condition has mainly been reported in children after organ transplantation [12]. No more than 11 cases have been described to date, but the frequency may increase in the future. Al-Attar et al. used anterior chamber paracentesis and iris biopsy in a case of papillitis and hypopyon uveitis, occurring 8 months after an infectious mononucleosis in an 11-year-old girl who was 15-months status post-renal transplantation and under immunosuppressive therapy [13]. Diagnosis of ocular posttransplant lymphoproliferative disorder associated with Epstein-Barr virus infection was confirmed by PCR, and histopathology disclosed virus-infected lymphocytic infiltrates in the iris specimen. Resolution of iris nodules was achieved after reduction of immunosuppressive medication. A similar case was reported in a 7-year-old child after heart transplantation [14].

Kaposi Sarcoma Herpes Virus-Associated Uveitis

Ocular lesions associated with Kaposi sarcoma (KS) usually involve the orbit and the conjunctiva (Fig. 24.1). In 1994, a new human herpes virus, designated HHV-8, was found to be present in almost 100% of KS lesions. In 2005, we reported the case of a 77-year-old Italian woman presenting with a 2-year history of bilateral panuveitis treated with sustained corticotherapy [15]. She had a past medical history of multifocal conjunctival KS diagnosed in 2000. There were no systemic symptoms of KS. Visual acuity was 20/200 OD and 20/40 OS, and slit lamp biomicroscopy confirmed conjunctival involvement and mild, chronic anterior uveitis with posterior synechiae. Bilateral macular edema with visual loss complicated the ocular inflammation. HHV-8 serology was positive. A conjunctival biopsy was performed. Pathological analysis was contributive. Furthermore, molecular detection of HHV-8 in the biopsy specimen was performed with PCR and confirmed the viral diagnosis. IFN-α2a was introduced as an antiviral and immunomodulatory agent, and control of ocular inflammation was achieved, allowing corticosteroid tapering.

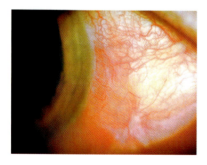

Fig. 24.1 Kaposi's sarcoma-associated conjunctivitis and uveitis in an HIV-negative patient. Diagnostic confirmation after conjunctival biopsy (Bodaghi B, Am J Opthalmol, 2005)

Catastrophic Acute Retinal Necrosis Syndrome

A consensus statement of the American Uveitis Society defines acute retinal necrosis syndrome (ARNS) as peripheral necrotizing retinitis, occlusive vasculopathy, with a prominent inflammatory reaction in the vitreous and anterior chamber [43]. We have recently reported the case of a patient presenting with acute retinal necrosis syndrome masquerading as endogenous endophthalmitis and orbital cellulitis or a lymphomatous process [16]. In this case, despite typical retinal necrosis, hypopyon and proptosis were confounding findings. Therefore, diagnostic confirmation of HSV-2 retinitis based on PCR analysis of ocular fluids was complemented by conjunctival and orbital biopsies. Pathological and immunohistological findings disclosed nonspecific inflammation in those tissues without viral replication. This rare presentation shows that ARNS may be associated with a major orbital inflammatory reaction (Fig. 24.2a–c) with a poor final visual prognosis despite rapid diagnostic confirmation and aggressive antiviral therapy.

24.4.2 Masquerade Syndromes

24.4.2.1 Juvenile Xanthogranuloma

Juvenile xanthogranuloma (JXG) is a cutaneous disease, occurring mainly in children less than 1 year old and rarely in older children and adults [17, 18]. Cutaneous lesions appear predominantly over the face, neck and upper trunk of the patient and may resolve spontaneously over a period of 1–5 years. Approximately 10% of cases may develop ocular or adnexal involvement, most commonly in the iris.

The first case of JXG was described in 1949 in a 4-month-old child with an iris mass and secondary glaucoma. Because of a suspicion of ocular sarcoma, the eye was enucleated, and skin lesions appeared later. Histological features were similar to the eye lesion. In the series of 20 cases reported by Sanders in 1960, 19 cases were histopathologically confirmed [19]. Of these, 15 were diagnosed after enucleation. The majority of cases involve the iris and eyelids. The workup should include ultrasound biomicroscopy in case of iris involvement [20]. Diffuse involvement and recurrent hemorrhage can result in heterochromia. Other more rarely involved sites include the cornea, conjunctiva, episclera, retina, choroid and optic nerve and orbit. To the best of our knowledge, only 19 cases of limbal JXG have been reported in the literature. The majority of lesions are uni-

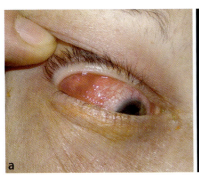 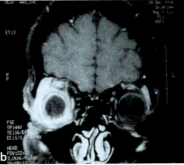 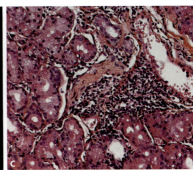

Fig. 24.2 Catastrophic acute retinal necrosis. **a** Acute orbital inflammation of the right eye masquerading as pseudo-cellulitis. **b** Orbital MRI revealing diffuse orbital involvement. **c** Histopathological analysis of an orbital specimen showing a lymphocytic reaction without active herpetic replication (original magnification × 200)

lateral and usually dissected free from the surface of the cornea.

Diagnosis and treatment of juvenile xanthogranuloma may be straightforward, particularly in cases when ocular lesions respond well to topical steroids and when there is no hyphema. However, in other circumstances, this entity may be difficult to manage and may necessitate iris or limbal biopsy for diagnosis and occasionally radiation therapy. Histopathologically, the disease is a non-Langerhans cell histiocytic inflammatory disorder with a mixture of foamy and epithelioid histiocytes associated with lymphocytes, eosinophils and scattered plasma cells. Touton giant cell with its ring of nuclei is often a diagnostic feature, especially in mature lesions.

Shields et al. reported the case of a 19-month-old child with a large solitary iris mass without intraocular inflammation and hyphema, which was removed by iridocyclectomy and studied by light microscopy, immunohistochemistry, and flow cytometry [21]. The excised mass consisted of granulomatous inflammation with numerous osteoclast-like giant cells and scattered atypical Touton giant cells. Immunohistochemical studies showed that the cells were most consistent with mononuclear histiocytes. Flow cytometry showed that 90% of the sampled cells were T-lymphocytes, with a predominance of T-suppressor cytotoxic cells.

24.4.2.2 MALT Lymphoma and Uveal Lymphoid Infiltration

Lymphoma deriving from mucosa-associated lymphoid tissue (MALT) is the most common type of orbital lymphoma (Fig. 24.3). Patients presenting with this particular feature are usually referred for management of a corticosteroid-resistant form of scleritis or posterior uveitis [22, 23].

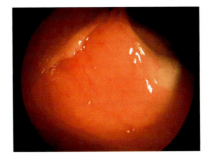

Fig. 24.3 MALT lymphoma infiltrating the conjunctiva

The use of nonsteroidal anti-inflammatory drugs is also ineffective in these cases. Therefore, in atypical forms of scleritis, it is important to exclude the diagnosis of low-grade non-Hodgkin's B-lymphocytic lymphoma. Biopsy must be considered when the mass is elevated and solid with a salmon-pink color. Posterior segment involvement may also masquerade as an atypical form of birdshot retinochoroidopathy with diffuse yellow dots (Fig. 24.4a–d). However, orbital CT-scan and MRI are valuable tools to identify other lesions, especially close to the optic nerve.

Hoang-Xuan et al. reported a challenging case of scleritis associated with choroidal white dots, such as those observed in patients with birdshot retinochoroidopathy [24]. The initial diagnosis of nonspecific scleritis was confirmed after scleral biopsy, but because of clinical resistance to treatment with corticosteroids and cyclophosphamide, a conjunctival biopsy was performed. Interestingly, analysis of the new specimen disclosed a morphologically and immunohistochemically typical mu-kappa immunoglobulin light chain secreting B-cell MALT lymphoma. Diagnostic confirmation led to a rec-

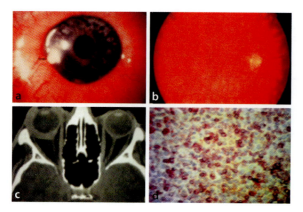

Fig. 24.4 **a** Chemosis associated with a nonnecrotizing scleritis in the right eye. **b** Fundus photograph of the right eye showing yellow-white choroidal infiltrates. **c** CT-scan: diffuse scleral thickening of the right eye. **d** Conjunctival biopsy: lymphoid infiltrate stained for kappa light chains (original magnification ×400), (Bodaghi B, Opthalmology, 1996)

ommendation for radiotherapy, which finally controlled the process.

Biopsy of subconjunctival nodules [42] is usually sufficient to confirm the diagnosis and propose specific therapy, including localized radiotherapy and chemotherapy (Fig. 24.5a, b).

Histopathology shows conjunctiva and fibrous tissue with areas of lymphoid infiltration. Different cell populations are identified, including centrocyte-like cells, small lymphocyte-like cells and plasmocytoid cells. Immunostaining ordinarily shows CD20-positive cells with kappa light chain restriction and CD43 positivity. A diagnosis of extra-nodal marginal zone lymphoma can be made according to the World Health Organization modification of the revised European-American classification

Dorey et al. have also reported two cases of orbital lymphoma, misdiagnosed as scleritis [25]. In rare situations, biopsy should be considered when pain is atypical for scleritis, the color is salmon pink and the mass is elevated and solid. Severe cases of scleritis need aggressive immunosuppressive therapy. Therefore, it is highly important to propose extensive investigations, including orbital imaging and biopsy in order to exclude a malignancy.

Patients with uveal lymphoid infiltration may present with solitary or multiple yellow uveal infiltrates. It is important to carefully analyze the conjunctiva for the presence of small pink lesions. Conjunctival biopsies may contribute to the final diagnosis [26].

24.4.2.3 Primary Intraocular Lymphoma

Non-Hodgkin's lymphoma may involve ocular tissues either as a primary tumor or as secondary metastasis from systemic disease. The diagnosis is usually based on the analysis of vitreous cells obtained after an appropriate vitrectomy. Optic nerve, ciliary body and iris involvement remains rare. However, in a few cases, vitreous infiltration is mild and diagnostic confirmation is made after iris biopsy [27–29].

24.4.2.4 Hodgkin's Lymphoma-Associated Posterior Scleritis and Uveitis

Hodgkin's disease rarely involves the orbit, especially the sclera and/or the uvea, and rarely the conjunctiva. Bilateral granulomatous uveitis has been previously described in association with this malignancy [30]. Other ocular features include vitritis, retinal vasculitis and discrete white chorioretinal lesions (Fig. 24.6) [31]. However, diagnosis of Hodgkin's lymphoma is usually confirmed after mediastinal or cervical lymph node bi-

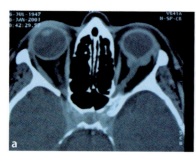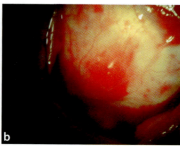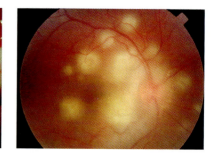

Fig. 24.5 MALT lymphoma associated with uveitis. **a** Orbital CT-scan showing two isolated nodules around the optic nerve. **b** Intraoperative view of specific subconjunctival nodules

Fig. 24.6 Chorioretinitis revealing a Hodgkin's lymphoma with orbital involvement

opsy. Examination of episcleral nodules may reveal a necrotizing granuloma and vasculitis [32].

24.4.2.5 Conjunctival and Corneal Intraepithelial Neoplasia

Ocular surface squamous neoplasia is in a spectrum of malignancy that includes intraepithelial dysplasia, carcinoma in situ of the conjunctiva and cornea, and invasive squamous cell carcinoma (Fig. 24.7) [33]. In some cases, patients are referred for an aggressive form of scleritis resistant to NSAIDs and corticosteroids. Total surgical excision may be associated with cryotherapy and autologous conjunctival-limbal transplantation. Histopathology confirms the malignancy [34, 35].

24.4.2.6 Immune-Mediated Entities—Sarcoidosis

Sarcoidosis is an inflammatory multisystem condition of unknown origin. Presenting as a granulomatous or nongranulomatous uveitis in the majority of cases, it may involve the conjunctiva, the sclera, the lacrimal gland (Fig. 24.8a,b), the orbit, the anterior and posterior segments [36].

Its incidence remains low (6–10/100,000) [37]. The disease affects blacks more frequently than whites and females more than males. The age of onset is usually between 20 and 50 years old, but the disease has been reported in younger and older patients. Ocular involvement is one of the most extrathoracic manifestations, occurring in 25–60% of cases [38, 39]. In the absence of a known causative agent, the diagnosis of sarcoidosis remains a diagnosis by exclusion. Anterior segment biopsy is not usually recommended if sarcoidosis is suspected. However, in some situations, especially in young children (less than 5 years of age), sarcoidosis may present with different manifestations than in adults or older children [40]. In these cases, uveitis is part of a triad, which also includes arthritis and rash. The uveitis is usually granulomatous with iris masses and gradually becomes resistant to corticosteroids. Diagnosis of sarcoidosis can be confirmed by histopathological evaluation disclosing noncaseating epithelioid granulomas.

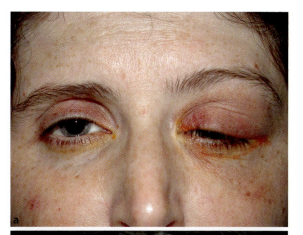
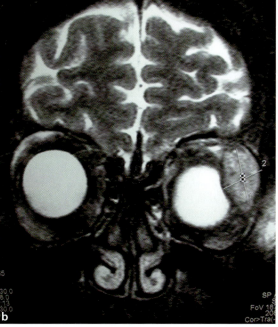

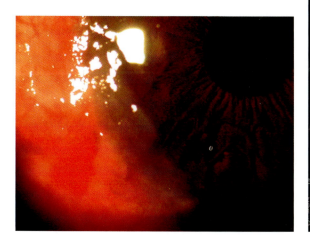

Fig. 24.7 Invasive conjunctival carcinoma masquerading as a scleritis

Fig. 24.8 Orbital sarcoidosis. **a** Left orbit involvement. **b** Orbit MRI showing lacrimal gland involvement

Clinical examination should be performed accurately in order to identify iris nodules or granulomas and localize them. Gonioscopy may disclose nodules within the iridocorneal angle.

An extensive workup is usually recommended, including complete blood count, serum angiotensin-converting enzyme and serum lysozyme. Chest X-ray or CT-scan and gallium scan are also often performed.

Excision of iris granulomas may be crucial in establishing the definite diagnosis of sarcoidosis. Moreover, in some cases, removal of iris nodules may lead to the prolonged remission of the disease [41].

Take Home Pearls

- Diagnostic evaluation of ocular inflammation remains a challenging issue.
- New entities have been described recently, and their confirmation may require molecular techniques and histopathological evaluation.
- Tissue biopsy is a valuable tool in establishing the diagnosis and directing treatment of masquerade syndromes of tumoral or infectious origin.
- Recourse to the biopsy remains limited and is only considered in atypical and difficult cases.
- Conjunctival biopsy is technically easy to perform and may yield valuable diagnostic information.

References

1. Bodaghi B, LeHoang P. Testing ocular fluids in uveitis. Ophthalmol Clin North Am 2002;15(3):271–9
2. Krachmer H, Mannis M, Holland E. In: Mannis M, Holland E, eds. Cornea. New York: Mosby, 2004
3. Watson P. Investigation of scleral disease. In: Watson P, Hazleman B, Pavesio C, eds. Sclera and systemic disorders. Oxford: Butterworth-Heinemann, 2004
4. Rosen PH, Spalton DJ, Graham EM. Intraocular tuberculosis. Eye 1990;4(Pt 3):486–92
5. Gain P, Mosnier JF, Gravelet C, et al. [Iris tuberculosis. A propos of a case diagnosed by iridectomy]. J Fr Ophtalmol 1994;17(8–9):525–8
6. Gopal L, Rao SK, Biswas J, et al. Tuberculous granuloma managed by full thickness eye wall resection. Am J Ophthalmol 2003;135(1):93–4
7. Preac-Mursic V, Pfister HW, Spiegel H, et al. First isolation of Borrelia burgdorferi from an iris biopsy. J Clin Neuroophthalmol 1993;13(3):155–61; discussion 162
8. Orefice F, Miranda D, Boratto LM. Presence of M. leprae in the conjunctiva, vitreous body and retina of a patient having lepromatous leprosy. Indian J Lepr 1998;70(1):97–102
9. Messmer EM, Raizman MB, Foster CS. Lepromatous uveitis diagnosed by iris biopsy. Graefes Arch Clin Exp Ophthalmol 1998;236(9):717–9
10. Job CK, Thompson K. Histopathological features of lepromatous iridocyclitis; a case report. Int J Lepr Other Mycobact Dis 1998;66(1):29–33
11. Bodaghi B, Mougin C, Michelson S, et al. Acyclovir-resistant bilateral keratitis associated with mutations in the HSV-1 thymidine kinase gene. Exp Eye Res 2000;71(4):353–9
12. Clark WL, Scott IU, Murray TG, et al. Primary intraocular posttransplantation lymphoproliferative disorder. Arch Ophthalmol 1998;116(12):1667–9
13. Al-Attar L, Berrocal A, Warman R, et al. Diagnosis by polymerase chain reaction of ocular posttransplant lymphoproliferative disorder after pediatric renal transplantation. Am J Ophthalmol 2004;137(3):569–71
14. Rohrbach JM, Krober SM, Teufel T, et al. EBV-induced polymorphic lymphoproliferative disorder of the iris after heart transplantation. Graefes Arch Clin Exp Ophthalmol 2004;242(1):44–50
15. Brasnu E, Wechsler B, Bron A, et al. Efficacy of interferon-alpha for the treatment of Kaposi's sarcoma herpesvirus-associated uveitis. Am J Ophthalmol 2005;140(4):746–8
16. Rozenbaum O, Rozenberg F, Charlotte F, Bodaghi B. Catastrophic acute retinal necrosis syndrome associated with diffuse orbital cellulitis: a case report. Graefes Arch Clin Exp Ophthalmol 2007;245(1):161–3
17. Harley RD, Romayananda N, Chan GH. Juvenile xanthogranuloma. J Pediatr Ophthalmol Strabismus 1982;19(1):33–9
18. Karcioglu ZA, Mullaney PB. Diagnosis and management of iris juvenile xanthogranuloma. J Pediatr Ophthalmol Strabismus 1997;34(1):44–51
19. Sanders TE. Intraocular juvenile xanthogranuloma (nevoxanthogranuloma): a survey of 20 cases. Trans Am Ophthalmol Soc 1960;58:59–74
20. Lichter H, Yassur Y, Barash D, et al. Ultrasound biomicroscopy in juvenile xanthogranuloma of the iris. Br J Ophthalmol 1999;83(3):375–6
21. Shields JA, Eagle RC Jr, Shields CL, et al. Iris juvenile xanthogranuloma studied by immunohistochemistry and flow cytometry. Ophthalmic Surg Lasers 1997;28(2):140–4
22. Gaucher D, Bodaghi B, Charlotte F, et al. [MALT-type B-cell lymphoma masquerading as scleritis or posterior uveitis]. J Fr Ophtalmol 2005;28(1):31–8

23. Sarraf D, Jain A, Dubovy S, et al. Mucosa-associated lymphoid tissue lymphoma with intraocular involvement. Retina 2005;25(1):94–8
24. Hoang-Xuan T, Bodaghi B, Toublanc M, et al. Scleritis and mucosal-associated lymphoid tissue lymphoma: a new masquerade syndrome. Ophthalmology 1996;103(4):631–5
25. Dorey SE, Clark BJ, Christopoulos VA, Lightman S. Orbital lymphoma misdiagnosed as scleritis. Ophthalmology 2002;109(12):2347–50
26. Grossniklaus HE, Martin DF, Avery R, et al. Uveal lymphoid infiltration. Report of four cases and clinicopathologic review. Ophthalmology 1998;105(7):1265–73
27. Hykin PG, Shields JA, Shields CL, et al. Recurrent systemic B cell lymphoma of the iris. Br J Ophthalmol 1996;80(10):929
28. Velez G, de Smet MD, Whitcup SM, et al. Iris involvement in primary intraocular lymphoma: report of two cases and review of the literature. Surv Ophthalmol 2000;44(6):518–26
29. Verity DH, Graham EM, Carr R, et al. Hypopyon uveitis and iris nodules in non-Hodgkin's lymphoma: ocular relapse during systemic remission. Clin Oncol (R Coll Radiol) 2000;12(5):292–4
30. Mosteller MW, Margo CE, Hesse RJ. Hodgkin's disease and granulomatous uveitis. Ann Ophthalmol 1985;17(12):787–90
31. Towler H, de la Fuente M, Lightman S. Posterior uveitis in Hodgkin's disease. Aust N Z J Ophthalmol 1999;27(5):326–30
32. Thakker MM, Perez VL, Moulin A, et al. Multifocal nodular episcleritis and scleritis with undiagnosed Hodgkin's lymphoma. Ophthalmology 2003;110(5):1057–60
33. Pe'er J. Ocular surface squamous neoplasia. Ophthalmol Clin North Am 2005;18(1):1–13, vii
34. Giaconi JA, Karp CL. Current treatment options for conjunctival and corneal intraepithelial neoplasia. Ocul Surf 2003;1(2):66–73
35. Doganay S, Er H, Tasar A, Gurses I. Surgical excision, cryotherapy, autolimbal transplantation and mitomycin-C in treatment of conjunctival-corneal intraepithelial neoplasia. Int Ophthalmol 2005;26(1–2):53–7
36. Kawaguchi T, Hanada A, Horie S, et al. Evaluation of characteristic ocular signs and systemic investigations in ocular sarcoidosis patients. Jpn J Ophthalmol 2007;51(2):121–6
37. Chan CC, Wetzig RP, Palestine AG, et al. Immunohistopathology of ocular sarcoidosis. Report of a case and discussion of immunopathogenesis. Arch Ophthalmol 1987;105(10):1398–402
38. Jabs DA, Johns CJ. Ocular involvement in chronic sarcoidosis. Am J Ophthalmol 1986;102(3):297–301
39. Obenauf CD, Shaw HE, Sydnor CF, Klintworth GK. Sarcoidosis and its ophthalmic manifestations. Am J Ophthalmol 1978;86(5):648–55
40. Hoover DL, Khan JA, Giangiacomo J. Pediatric ocular sarcoidosis. Surv Ophthalmol 1986;30(4):215–28
41. Ocampo VV Jr, Foster CS, Baltatzis S. Surgical excision of iris nodules in the management of sarcoid uveitis. Ophthalmology 2001;108(7):1296–9
42. Shields CL, Shields JA, Carvalho C, Rundle P, Smith AF. Conjunctival lymphoid tumors: clinical analysis of 117 cases and relationship to systemic lymphoma. Ophthalmology 2001;108(5):979–84
43. Holland GN, Executive Committee of the American Uveitis Society. Standard diagnostic criteria for the acute retinal necrosis syndrome [Perspective]. Am J Ophthalmol 1994;117:663–7

Chapter 25

Diagnostic Vitrectomy

Christoph M.E. Deuter, Sabine Biester, Karl Ulrich Bartz-Schmidt

Core Messages

- Diagnostic vitrectomy should be considered only if the information sought will result in therapeutic and diagnostic consequences for the patient.
- Diagnosis of endophthalmitis, necrotizing viral retinitis and intraocular lymphoma are the most common indications for diagnostic vitrectomy.
- For diagnosis of primary intraocular lymphoma (PIOL), systemic steroids should be discontinued for at least 2 weeks before the vitrectomy.
- Air infusion allows maximal collection of undiluted vitreous.
- Direct communication between the ophthalmic surgeon and the laboratory staff is essential to ensure suitable investigations and to avoid delays in processing the vitreous specimens.

Contents

25.1	Introduction	255
25.2	Indications	255
25.2.1	Endophthalmitis	256
25.2.1.1	Classification and Epidemiology	256
25.2.1.2	Clinical Features	257
25.2.1.3	Diagnosis	258
25.2.1.4	Treatment	258
25.2.2	Necrotizing Viral Retinopathies	259
25.2.2.1	Classification and Epidemiology	259
25.2.2.2	Clinical Features	260
25.2.2.3	Diagnosis	261
25.2.2.4	Treatment	261
25.2.3	Primary Intraocular Lymphoma	262
25.2.3.1	Classification and Epidemiology	262
25.2.3.2	Clinical Features	262
25.2.3.3	Diagnosis	262
25.2.3.4	Treatment	262
25.2.3.5	Special Considerations	263
25.3	Surgical Procedure	263
25.4	Processing of Vitreous Specimens	264
References		265

This chapter contains the following video clips on DVD: Video 40 shows Vitrectomy for Endophthalmitis and Video 41 shows Vitreous biopsy with indentation (Surgeon: Marc de Smet).

25.1 Introduction

Intraocular inflammation comprises a spectrum of entities. Although diagnosis is usually based on medical history, clinical findings and noninvasive testing, it may be necessary in some cases to collect intraocular fluid or tissue samples to confirm a diagnosis and to enable specific therapy. This diagnostic approach has benefitted both from advances in vitreoretinal surgery and from modern laboratory techniques. Microbiological culture and detection of antibodies are traditional techniques to analyze intraocular fluid; polymerase chain reaction (PCR), cytological analyses and measurement of cytokine levels are now also routinely performed [4].

In this chapter we provide an overview on the indications and technique of diagnostic vitrectomy as well as management of vitreous specimens from patients with intraocular inflammatory disorders.

25.2 Indications

Pars plana vitrectomy is a major ocular surgical procedure, and diagnostic vitrectomy should be considered only if the information gained from it may result in therapeutic or diagnostic consequences for the patient [10]. It is assumed that routinely performed ophthalmological examinations, such as biomicroscopy and fundoscopy, other noninvasive diagnostic methods (X-ray, ultrasound, MRI) and conventional laboratory testing from peripheral blood have failed to classify an intraocular inflammation. Diagnostic vitrectomy is usually considered in patients in whom an acute, chronic or progressive course of the disease is threatening vision and in whom empirical medical treatment has failed to control intraocular inflammation [26]. Common indications for diagnostic vitrectomy include severe, persistent infiltration of the vitreous which is not responding to established anti-inflammatory drug regimens with systemic corticosteroids or immunosuppressants in adequate dose and duration, intraocular inflammatory conditions suspicious for bacterial or mycotic endophthalmitis, and necrotizing viral retinopathies. Moreover, diagnostic vitrectomy represents the most important tool in the diagnosis of intraocular lymphoma, which belongs to the so-called masquerade syndromes mimicking uveitis. In the following, some of these entities will be described in more detail with the main focus on intraocular lymphoma as the most diagnostically challenging disease.

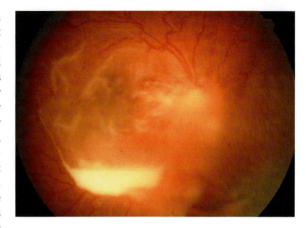

Fig. 25.1 Posttraumatic endophthalmitis [21]

25.2.1 Endophthalmitis

25.2.1.1 Classification and Epidemiology

Infective endophthalmitis is an urgent situation in ophthalmology, since it may result in substantial loss of vision or even in loss of the eye despite medical and surgical treatment. Endophthalmitis is classified as exogenous or endogenous depending on the route of infection.

Acute postoperative endophthalmitis after cataract surgery is the most common type of exogenous endophthalmitis with an estimated incidence of 0.2–0.3%. Whereas acute endophthalmitis following cataract surgery decreased continuously until the early 1990s, an increase in the incidence has been observed during the last decade, perhaps due to sutureless clear corneal incisions in modern cataract surgery [34]. Acute endophthalmitis, which occurs between days 2 and 7 after cataract surgery, is most commonly caused by gram-positive bacteria, especially coagulase-negative staphylococci such as *Staphylococcus epidermidis*, and *Staphylococcus aureus*. Gram-negative organisms like *Pseudomonas aeruginosa* can also cause endophthalmitis after cataract surgery. Postoperative delayed-onset endophthalmitis typically occurs 6 weeks or later after surgery when topical steroid therapy is discontinued and the balance between the immune response of the patient and the mostly low-virulence bacteria becomes disturbed. Posttrabeculectomy endophthalmitis can be delayed for months or years after initial surgery but in other respects behaves as an acute endophthalmitis since it occurs from a new infection through the filtering bleb [21]. *Propionibacterium acnes*, an anaerobic gram-positive organism, is a well-known cause of chronic persistent endophthalmitis, which may occur months to years after extracapsular cataract surgery with implantation of an intraocular lens [6].

Whereas the course of posttraumatic endophthalmitis is similar to that of an acute postoperative endophthalmitis, its visual prognosis is even worse. Eyes with an intraocular foreign body of rural origin are at high risk to develop endophthalmitis (Fig. 25.1). Especially if the foreign body is contaminated with *Bacillus cereus*, a fulminant course with poor prognosis may occur [21].

Endogenous endophthalmitis, which comprises approximately 5–7% of all cases of endophthalmitis, is a result of the hematogenous spread of bacteria or fungi from a remote focus of infection to the eye. Although cases in healthy immunocompetent individuals have been reported, endogenous endophthalmitis usually occurs in patients with predisposing systemic risk factors, such as chronic immune-compromising conditions (e.g., diabetes mellitus), immunosuppressive diseases or therapies (e.g., malignancies, HIV, chemotherapy) or also long-term intravenous catheters. Persons with abuse of intravenous drugs or anabolic steroids are also at a higher risk to develop endogenous endophthalmitis [31, 42]. *Streptococcus* and *Staphylococcus* represent the most common bacterial, and *Candida* the most common fungal, organisms causing endogenous endophthalmitis [21].

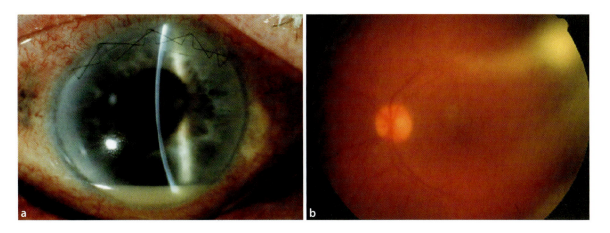

Fig. 25.2 Acute postoperative endophthalmitis with **a** hypopyon and **b** dense infiltration of the vitreous [21]

25.2.1.2 Clinical Features

Major complaints of *acute* postoperative and endogenous bacterial endophthalmitis include ocular and orbital pain, blurred vision or rapid loss of vision, as well as eyelid swelling. Slit lamp examination reveals injected conjunctiva with chemosis, corneal edema, anterior chamber inflammation with or without hypopyon and a reduced or absent red reflex with poor view of the fundus due to dense inflammatory infiltration of the vitreous (Fig. 25.2a,b). So-called Roth spots, intraretinal hemorrhages surrounding a white center, may precede bacterial endogenous endophthalmitis.

In contrast, *chronic persistent* postoperative endophthalmitis, which is often misinterpreted as noninfectious postoperative uveitis, is characterized by only mild complaints with little pain, mild visual impairment, granulomatous retrocorneal precipitates, anterior chamber cells and typical white plaques in the capsular bag containing the microorganisms (Fig. 25.3).

Endogenous fungal endophthalmitis often develops slowly and with fewer symptoms than bacterial infection. Patients suffer from less pain and a slower decrease in vision. Initial findings include yellow-white, round choroidal or retinal infiltrates predominantly at the posterior pole (Fig. 25.4). If the disease is progressive, characteristic snowball or string-of-pearls like vitreal haze occurs. Extensive retinal or subretinal hemorrhages, atypical for Candida endophthalmitis, may indicate Aspergillus as the causative fungus [22].

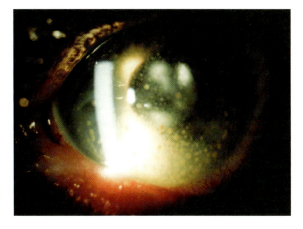

Fig. 25.3 Chronic persistent postoperative endophthalmitis [21]

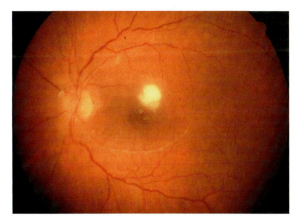

Fig. 25.4 Endogenous endophthalmitis with chorioretinal *Candida* infiltrate [21]

25.2.1.3 Diagnosis

Identification of the causative organism is the best way to ensure effective antimicrobial therapy in endophthalmitis. Pars plana vitrectomy and vitreous tap are common techniques to collect vitreous samples for microbiologic analysis. Pars plana vitrectomy allows simultaneous removal of the reservoir of pathogens and inflammatory mediators from the eye. Regarding visual outcome after postoperative bacterial endophthalmitis, the Endophthalmitis Vitrectomy Study (EVS) indicated a benefit of early vitrectomy over vitreous tap only in those patients with initial vision worse than hand motions [13]. On the other hand, the results of the EVS could be interpreted as demonstrating that pars plana vitrectomy has not shown results inferior to vitreous tap, even in eyes with initial vision better than light perception included [19]. Thus in some cases, pars plana vitrectomy can be recommended before visual acuity drops to light perception. Moreover, subsequent publications of the EVS data have shown that a larger proportion of patients with diabetes achieved 20/40 visual acuity after pars plana vitrectomy than after vitreous tap, although this difference was not statistically significant [11].

Bacterial or fungal culture of vitreous samples is a proven and routinely performed diagnostic technique. A positive result can be expected as soon as after 1 day, whereas the confirmation of a negative result may need 4–7 days. However, in various studies, less than 50% of bacterial or fungal cultures of intraocular fluids from eyes suspicious for endophthalmitis yielded a positive result. Several reasons, such as small sample sizes or prior use of antibiotics, have been postulated [25, 35]. The detection of DNA of sparse or fastidious organisms is one advantage of polymerase chain reaction (PCR), a molecular biologic technique of increasing importance. PCR has been demonstrated to be rapid, with results within 1–2 days, and to have higher sensitivity than bacterial or fungal culture. This high sensitivity makes PCR susceptible to false-positive results due to exogenous contaminations of the samples. Moreover, compared to culture, PCR does not confirm viability of the organism or allow assessment of antibiotic susceptibility [18]. Thus, in routine practice, both techniques are used in parallel. In a first step, universal PCR is performed to detect bacterial DNA in the sample. In a second step, sequencing of DNA could theoretically be used to identify the organism, or more specific primers could be used to identify selected organisms. At the same time, culture media are inoculated. Microbiologic culture still represents the "gold standard" in detecting bacteria or fungi.

To obtain optimal results within a short period of time, undiluted vitreous specimens should be forwarded immediately to an experienced microbiologist. When vitrectomy is performed as an emergency procedure after hours, it may be necessary to inoculate the vitreous samples directly in the operating room on appropriate media, incubate them and pass them to the microbiologist later. The successful use even by less experienced residents of a special "endophthalmitis set" containing all necessary equipment to culture vitreous samples in the operation room has been reported by Ness et al. [24]. Although it is easy to perform, inoculation of blood culture bottles holds the risk that a rapidly growing microorganism may overwhelm others that are growing more slowly in the rare case of polymicrobial infection [24].

In cases of endogenous endophthalmitis with hematogenous spread of organisms, blood culture may additionally be helpful to establish the diagnosis, but it cannot replace culture and PCR testing of intraocular fluids [18].

25.2.1.4 Treatment

Aims of endophthalmitis therapy are the eradication of the infective agent as well as the reduction of immune response. Primary vitrectomy may be beneficial not only to collect enough material for microbiological tests but also because it offers theoretical advantages, including removal of the infectious organisms and their toxins, removal of vitreous membranes potentially leading to retinal detachment, clearing of vitreous opacities and possibly a better distribution of intravitreal antibiotics [13]. To avoid further damage to the eye, medical treatment should start immediately. As the causative organism is usually not identified at this time, broad spectrum antibiotics are used.

For the treatment of exogenous bacterial endophthalmitis, we prefer systemic administration of either imipenem or vancomycin combined with ceftazidime. Ceftazidime is commonly recommended as effective for both gram-positive and gram-negative bacteria. Because the blood–eye barrier reduces penetration of systemic antibiotics into the vitreous, intravitreal antibiotics are the drugs of choice. Nevertheless, we commonly use intravenous application as well as periocular and topical application of antibiotics [21, 22]. Whereas the European Society of Cataract and Refractive Surgeons recommends vancomycin for intravenous use [3], we prefer imipenem because clinical studies suggest that therapeutic drug levels in the vitreous are achieved after intravenous application of imipenem but not after vancomycin [1, 14]. Combining the antibiotic regimen with systemic corticosteroids treats the concomitant intraocular inflammatory response [21].

In chronic persistent postoperative endophthalmitis due to *Propionibacterium acnes*, pars plana vitrectomy

Table 25.1 Therapy regimens for various forms of exogenous bacterial endophthalmitis [21]

	Systemic therapy (for at least 10 days)		Periocular therapy	Intravitreal therapy
	Adults	Children		
Acute postoperative endophthalmitis Postoperative delayed-onset acute endophthalmitis Posttraumatic endophthalmitis	2 × 500 mg imipenem* i.v. + 3 × 2 g ceftazidime i.v. + up to 1 × 5 mg/kg BW methylprednisolone i.v.	60 mg/kg BW (up to 1 g/day) imipenem* i.v. (in 4 daily doses) + 3 × 17–33 mg/kg BW ceftazidime i.v. + up to 1 × 5 mg/kg BW methylprednisolone i.v.	25 mg vancomycin + 100 mg ceftazidime + 12 mg dexamethasone	1 mg vancomycin + 2 mg ceftazidime + 1 mg dexamethasone
Chronic persistent endophthalmitis	2 × 500 mg imipenem* i.v.		25 mg vancomycin + 12 mg dexamethasone	1 mg vancomycin + 1 mg dexamethasone

* 2 × 1 g vancomycin i.v.: in case of intolerance for imipenem. For children, 2 × 20 mg/kg BW per day

with total capsular bag removal, exchange or removal of the intraocular lens and the application of intravitreal antibiotics may be necessary to stop recurrent intraocular inflammation [6]. Table 25.1 provides therapy regimens for various forms of exogenous bacterial endophthalmitis.

Treatment of endogenous endophthalmitis has to be coordinated with other involved specialties depending on the extraocular focus of the infection. Systemic antibiotics are more important in endogenous than exogenous bacterial endophthalmitis, but intravitreal antibiotics are still critically important in most cases.

Systemically administered antimycotic drugs are the mainstay in the therapy of endogenous fungal endophthalmitis. Whereas fluconazole is most commonly used in *Candida* endophthalmitis, amphotericin B remains the first choice for *Aspergillus* endophthalmitis. In the case of intolerance or contraindications for systemic antimycotic treatment or to improve efficacy, amphotericin B may also be injected intravitreally in doses of 5 μg in 0.1 ml. Table 25.2 provides an overview of treatment for fungal endophthalmitis. Intravenous or intravitreal voriconazole is a newer option for the treatment of fungal endophthalmitis and provides broad-spectrum antifungal coverage. The usual intravitreal dose of voriconazole is 50 μg in 0.1 ml.

25.2.2 Necrotizing Viral Retinopathies

25.2.2.1 Classification and Epidemiology

Necrotizing viral retinopathies present acutely and are potentially blinding diseases. Three classic forms caused by viruses of the herpes family are acute retinal necrosis syndrome (ARN), progressive outer retinal necrosis (PORN) and cytomegalovirus (CMV) retinitis.

ARN is characterized by the triad of retinal and choroidal vasculitis, retinal necrosis and vitritis [12, 38]. Varicella zoster virus (VZV) and herpes simplex virus (HSV) types 1 and 2 are major pathogens in both healthy and immunocompromised individuals. However, cytomegalovirus (CMV) has been identified as a

Table 25.2 Treatment regimens for fungal endophthalmitis [21]

***Candida* endophthalmitis:**	
If sensitive for fluconazole: Fluconazole (aqueous humor 80% of serum levels) *Fluconazole: nephrotoxicity*	3 days 1x 400 mg orally, followed by 1x 200 mg orally
If resistant for fluconazole: Amphotericin B (aqueous humor 10% of serum levels)	initially: 1x 0.1 mg/kg BW per day i.v. within 3 days: increase to 1x 0.3 mg/kg +
Flucytosine *Central venous catheter necessary! Amphotericin B: hepato- and nephrotoxicity Flucytosine: hepatotoxicity, dysfunction of hematopoesis*	4x 25–50 mg/kg BW per day i.v. or orally
***Aspergillus* endophthalmitis:**	
Amphotericin B *Central venous catheter necessary! Amphotericin B: hepato- and nephrotoxicity*	initially: 1x 0.1 mg/kg BW per day i.v. within 7 days: increase to 1x 1–1.5 mg/kg
Fungal endophthalmitis of unknown origin:	
Amphotericin B	initially: 1x 0.1 mg/kg BW per day i.v. within 7 days: increase to 1x 1–1.5 mg/kg
or in case of intolerance of systemic application, maximal every second day 0.005–0.01 mg intravitreally. Treatment duration depends on clinical course.	

causative agent of ARN in single cases in immunocompetent patients [12, 33, 37]. Although ARN may affect patients of any age, most of them are between 20 and 60 years of age with two peaks at about 20 and 50 years of age. There might be a slight predilection of the male gender [12].

PORN has been described as a disease with an extremely poor prognosis which is caused by VZV and HSV predominantly in patients with a compromised immune status either due to an underlying disease (e.g., HIV) or immunosuppressive treatment [39].

In the 1980s, CMV retinitis was the most common cause of blindness in patients with AIDS. CMV retinitis usually develops at a late stage of AIDS and is strongly associated with the immune status of the patients which can be assessed by the number of CD4+ cells in peripheral blood. Patients in whom the CD4+ cell number drops below 50–100/mm^3 are at high risk to develop CMV retinitis. With the introduction of highly active antiretroviral therapy (HAART) in AIDS patients, the incidence of CMV retinitis has decreased dramatically. Nevertheless, cases of CMV retinitis still may occur in patients who do not respond to anti-HIV therapy or in non-HIV patients who are under systemic immunosuppressive treatment for other diseases [15].

25.2.2.2 Clinical Features

ARN affects both eyes in approximately one third of patients with a delay of several weeks being not uncommon. Patients may complain of mild to moderate ocular or orbital pain, foreign body sensation, a red eye and decreased vision with floaters [12]. The main clinical characteristics of ARN defined by the American Uveitis Society include focal, well-demarcated areas of retinal necrosis located in the peripheral retina, rapid circumferential progression of necrosis, evidence of occlusive vasculopathy and a prominent inflammatory reaction in the vitreous and anterior chamber. Optic atrophy, scleritis and pain are supportive but not required for the diagnosis [16]. At a later stage of the disease, retinitis typically spreads to the posterior pole. Retinal holes that in combination with vitreous traction lead to rhegmatogenous retinal detachment are frequently seen as a complication of ARN [38].

PORN is characterized by multifocal lesions of deep retinal opacification without granular borders. Lesions are located in the peripheral retina with or without macular involvement and tend to progress to confluence rapidly. In contrast to ARN, there is no or only mild intraocular inflammation and no vasculitis is present [39].

CMV retinitis can occur with two distinct clinical pictures. Fluffy, dense, white confluent opacifications of the retina with no central atrophic zone and multiple retinal hemorrhages with perivasculitis characterize the first type. Lesions are commonly located closer to the posterior pole and follow the nerve fiber layer in an arcuate distribution (Fig. 25.5). The second form presents with more granular, less opaque-appearing lesions with a central atrophic zone as well as fewer hemorrhages and perivasculitis. In both forms the retinal lesions are not sharply edged and only a mild vitritis and anterior chamber reaction occur. Although the retinal infiltrations usually proceed slowly, without treatment, destruction and necrosis of the entire retina will develop within 3–6 months [15].

25.2.2.3 Diagnosis

Necrotizing viral retinopathies often present with an atypical clinical picture or with dense vitreous infiltration which can make clinical diagnosis difficult. Measurement of serologic antibody levels may be of limited diagnostic value due to the normally high seroprevalence of antibodies against herpes viruses in the normal population, and because an infection located in the eye may not induce a detectable increase of antibodies in peripheral blood. Thus, sampling of intraocular fluid may be necessary to identify the causative virus and to enable specific antiviral therapy. Harvested aqueous or vitreous can be analyzed for local antibody production against herpes virus antigens. However, the presence of intraocular specific antibodies is not necessarily the result of a local antibody production, as a breakdown of the blood–eye barrier due to inflammation may lead to a passive antibody passage into the eye. Confirmation of local antibody synthesis is determined by calculating the Goldmann-Witmer coefficient, which compares antibody titers in serum and vitreous while adjusting for total immunoglobulin levels:

A value of 3 or higher is usually assumed as positive [36].

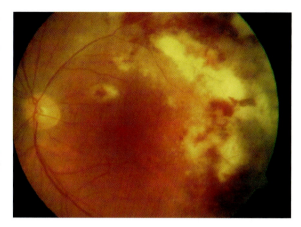

Fig. 25.5 CMV retinitis

Currently, polymerase chain reaction (PCR), a highly sensitive method to detect infectious DNA in small fluid samples, has been established as a means to identify the causative virus in necrotizing retinopathies. Because PCR may become negative due to prior antiviral treatment, concomitant determination of the Goldmann-Witmer coefficient may be useful [5].

25.2.2.4 Treatment

Intravenous acyclovir, which is effective for HSV and VZV, represents the mainstay of therapy in ARN. In resistant cases, a switch to more aggressive antiviral treatment with ganciclovir or foscarnet, or combination antiviral therapy, can be considered. After intravenous administration for 7–10 days, antiviral therapy should be continued orally for a period of 3 months or longer. In addition, intravitreal instillation of ganciclovir or foscarnet can be performed. Laser photocoagulation of retinal holes may be necessary to prevent retinal detachment [5]. There is a trend toward the use of oral rather than intravenous antivirals initially in the treatment of ARN, especially when combined with intravitreal injections.

Ganciclovir intravenously followed by oral administration as well as supplementary intravitreal application is the classic approach to treat CMV retinitis. Valganciclovir, foscarnet and cidofovir represent alternative anti-CMV drugs for systemic use. Additionally, etoposide, a topoisomerase II inhibitor, has been experimentally used for severe and refractory CMV infections [17,

$$\text{Goldmann-Witmer coefficient} = \frac{\text{Antibody titer against herpes antigens in the vitreous} \times \text{IgG amount in the serum}}{\text{Antibody titer against herpes antigens in the serum} \times \text{IgG amount in the vitreous}}$$

20]. A major goal of treatment in patients with AIDS is the prevention of opportunistic infections such as CMV retinitis by recovery of immune status through the use of highly active antiretroviral therapy (HAART) [5].

25.2.3 Primary Intraocular Lymphoma

25.2.3.1 Classification and Epidemiology

Primary intraocular lymphoma (PIOL) is the most common of the neoplastic masquerade syndromes. These are defined as disease entities that mimic uveitis [29]. PIOL generally signifies a primary central nervous system lymphoma (PCNSL) (a highly malignant non-Hodgkin lymphoma) that presents with involvement of retina–choroid, the vitreous and rarely the optic nerve. If both eyes and the CNS are affected, the disease is called "oculocerebral lymphoma". Only half of the patients with ocular presentation are found to have CNS lesions on neuroradiologic examination at the time of diagnosis of intraocular lymphoma. Most PIOL are diffuse large cell B-cell lymphomas, typically affecting elderly patients in their fifth to seventh life decade with a clear preference for females. The prognosis is poor: PIOL is the ocular disorder with the highest five-year mortality [8, 41, 43]. Although there are no exact data available, PIOL shows an increasing incidence in both immunocompetent and immunocompromised populations. This may be due to the incidence of PCNSL, which has increased slowly since 1960, and which has tripled over the past 15 years [27, 28].

25.2.3.2 Clinical Features

Whereas PIOL may be unilateral or bilateral at onset, both eyes will ultimately be involved in the majority of patients.

Blurred vision and floaters are the most common symptoms of patients with PIOL; pain and redness of the eye rarely occur [40]. About 20% of patients may be asymptomatic [27].

The clinical picture of PIOL is diverse. Slit lamp examination may reveal an anterior uveitis with granulomatous keratic precipitates. However, more typical presentations of PIOL are cellular infiltration of the vitreous often mimicking intermediate uveitis, as well as characteristic creamy orange-yellow chorioretinal infiltrations. Glaucoma, neovascularization and optic neuropathy are rare findings in PIOL [8, 43].

25.2.3.3 Diagnosis

The variability in the clinical picture and, often, an initial, moderate response to systemic corticosteroids frequently leads to a delay in the diagnosis of PIOL. However, an early diagnosis of PIOL is crucial both to prevent blindness and to allow early treatment. If there is clinical suspicion of PIOL, the diagnostic program usually includes ultrasound, fluorescein angiography and MRI of the brain. To confirm PCNSL, cytological analysis of the cerebrospinal fluid and occasionally brain biopsy may be indicated; however, vitreous biopsy is the mainstay of diagnosis of intraocular lymphoma.

Vitreous specimens are usually sent as rapidly as possible in nonfixed (fresh) state to a pathology laboratory. A delay during transportation may diminish the quality of the fragile samples. Recently, HOPE fixative (HEPES-glutamic acid buffer mediated organic solvent protection effect) has been demonstrated as a promising conservation medium for vitreous specimens, enabling preservation of cytomorphology and immunoreactivity. Fixation facilitates sending vitreous samples to external reference laboratories in good quality [9].

A wide range of laboratory investigations are in use to analyze vitreous specimens for lymphoma cells.

For cytomorphological evaluation, the unfixed or fixed vitreous specimens are best prepared by the Cytospin preparation technique, at 500 rpm for 5 minutes to concentrate the cells onto glass slides. Subsequently, the slides are air-dried and stained conventionally (May-Gruenwald-Giemsa, hematoxylin-eosin; Fig. 25.6a) and immunocytologically. *Cytological analysis* of PIOL samples usually reveals a mixture of mature inflammatory cells, large neoplastic lymphocytes and necrotic debris. As nearly all PIOL are B-cell lymphomas, *immunocytology* looks for the expression of B-cell surface antigens, such as CD20, CD79a or PAX5, and light immunoglobulin chains (Fig. 25.6b). *Flow cytometry* is used for immunophenotyping and quantitating monoclonal populations of cells in the vitreous specimens. Gene rearrangements detected by polymerase chain reaction (PCR) are indicative of monoclonality [8, 43]. *Cytokine analysis* uses the fact that B-lymphocytes produce interleukin (IL)-10 whereas T-lymphocytes produce IL-6. Therefore, elevated levels of IL-10 and an IL-10/IL-6 ratio larger than 1 in the vitreous have been reported to be supportive but not conclusive for the diagnosis of PIOL [2, 23].

25.2.3.4 Treatment

So far, no uniform recommendations for the treatment of PIOL with or without CNS involvement exist. Treatment strategies include radiation therapy of the CNS and the

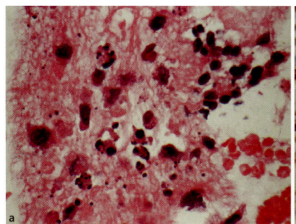 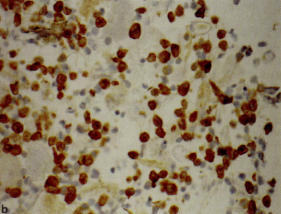

Fig. 25.6 Microphotographs of a vitreous specimen of PIOL. **a** Hematoxylin-eosin stain, showing atypical cells with large pleomorphic nuclei, as well as deteriorated cells in the background (×1,000, oil immersion). **b** CD20 stain demonstrating that the large majority of the vital cells are B-lymphocytes. There are some negative-staining cells, which are probably either reactive T-cells or macrophages (×400). (Courtesy of Dr. S. Coupland, Dept. of Cellular and Molecular Pathology, University of Liverpool)

eyes alone or in combination with systemic chemotherapy with or without intrathecal chemotherapy. Recent promising data suggest that monotherapy with six cycles of high-dose methotrexate intravenously, which has been shown to induce complete remission in 40–89% of patients with PCNSL, may also lead to a dramatic reduction of 5-year mortality in patients with PIOL [32, 43].

25.2.3.5 Special Considerations

Diagnosis of PIOL is challenging. To obtain reliable results from diagnostic vitrectomy, vitreous specimens have to contain an adequate number of evaluable cells, which necessitates a suitable surgical technique. Moreover, the preoperative preparation of the patients is highly important. Because prior steroid therapy will increase the fragility of tumor cells, diagnostic vitrectomy to confirm PIOL should be performed only at a time when patients are on the lowest dose of corticosteroids as possible; a completely corticosteroid-free interval of at least 2 weeks prior to diagnostic vitrectomy is preferred [27, 28]. Even with these precautions, false-negative results of diagnostic vitrectomy are not uncommon. If the suspicion of PIOL persists, diagnostic vitrectomy can be repeated, on the contralateral eye if necessary. If repeated vitrectomies remain negative and a subretinal infiltration is present, a choroidal biopsy can be considered. In rare cases, when vision has been lost or a definitive diagnosis cannot be reached, enucleation may be a further diagnostic option [7, 30].

25.3 Surgical Procedure

Vitreous biopsy can be obtained by vitreous tap (according to the guidelines of the EVS Study [13]) or during complete vitrectomy with a 20-G, 23-G or 25-G pars plana approach. The main disadvantage of vitreous tap is the small amount of harvested volume for microbiological, virological, pathological and immunological laboratory investigations. This disadvantage can be overcome by an approach via pars plana. However, using the standard procedure, diluting the removed vitreous volume with balanced salt solutions would interfere with testing for which undiluted specimens are preferred, such as PCR, antibodies, and cytokine determinations. For that reason, the "air vitrectomy" has been introduced in the armamentarium of vitrectomy techniques. Only two steps of the standard approach need to be modified:

1. Aspiration of the vitrectomized fluid must be performed manually using a 10-ml syringe connected to the aspiration line of the vitreous cutter by an adaptor.
2. To exchange the aspirated volume by air, the automatic air pump of the vitrectomy machine is used. The pressure should be adjusted to 30–40 mmHg to avoid globe collapse by manual aspiration.

Table 25.3 Processing the vitreous specimens

Laboratory	Investigation	Specimen size
Microbiology	Culture and PCR for bacteria and fungi	Culture: 0.5 ml of undiluted vitreous PCR: 0.1 ml of undiluted vitreous
Virology	PCR and antibody detection for viruses of the herpes family (HSV 1 and 2, VZV, CMV, EBV)	Minimum 0.3 ml of undiluted vitreous
Immunology	IL-10 and IL-6 levels	Minimum 0.5 ml, better 0.8 ml of undiluted vitreous
Pathology	Detection of lymphoma cells	Local lab: Minimum 0.5 ml of undiluted vitreous Transport to external reference lab: Minimum 0.5 ml of undiluted vitreous in equivalent amount of HOPE fixative (HOPE by DCS Innovative Diagnostik-Systeme, Hamburg, Germany; www.dcs-diagnostics.de)

By this approach, it is possible to extract a volume of at least 2 ml of undiluted vitreous, which can be divided into several portions for laboratory investigations. Rapid processing of the obtained samples is important.

After aspiration of the vitreous core, the air-filled globe will be diluted by balanced salt solution, and vitrectomy can be completed by manual syringe aspiration performing a posterior vitreous separation and complete anterior vitrectomy to harvest cell-rich material for cytological investigation, which can then be performed after centrifugation of the whole volume.

Two remarks must be made:

1. In eyes following severe ocular trauma with ruptured choroid, air vitrectomy is contraindicated because of the risk of fatal air embolus via the vortex veins.
2. No attempt should be made to create a posterior vitreous separation by manual aspiration under air, because of the high risk of globe collapse and retinal injury.

25.4 Processing of Vitreous Specimens

Vitreous specimens should be marked as "urgent" and have to be sent off immediately after surgery to the diagnostic laboratories. Direct communication between the ophthalmic surgeon and the laboratory staff is essential both to ensure that the most suitable tests with regard to the suspected diagnosis will be performed and to avoid delays in processing the specimens. It is recommended that every ophthalmologist who regularly performs diagnostic vitrectomies establish direct contact with the laboratories of the involved specialties.

In Table 25.3, we provide a recommendation on how to portion the intraoperatively harvested vitreous for subsequent laboratory investigations. However, specimen sizes which are needed for investigation as well as the containers for transport (e.g., syringes or tubes) may differ between various laboratories and have to be arranged on site.

Take Home Pearls

- Diagnostic vitrectomy is a helpful tool if conventional diagnostic methods fail to classify a uveitis or if intraocular inflammation does not respond to empirical medical treatment.
- Modern molecular biologic techniques assist analysis of vitreous specimens for infection or masquerade syndromes.

References

1. Adenis JP, Mounier M, Salomon JL, Denis F (1994) Human vitreous penetration of imipenem. Eur J Ophthalmol 4: 115–117
2. Akpek EK, Maca SM, Christen WG, Foster CS (1999) Elevated vitreous interleukin-10 level is not diagnostic of intraocular-central nervous system lymphoma. Ophthalmology 106: 2291–2295
3. Barry P, Behrens-Baumann W, Pleyer U, Seal D (2005) ESCRS guidelines on prevention, investigation and management of post-operative endophthalmitis
4. Becker MD, Bodaghi B, Holz FG, Harsch N, Le Hoang P (2003) Diagnostic vitrectomy in uveitis. Possibilities of molecular biology. Ophthalmologe 100: 796–801
5. Bodaghi B, LeHoang P (2005) Herpes viruses in ocular inflammation. In: Pleyer U, Mondino B (eds.) Uveitis and immunological disorders. Berlin: Springer, pp 141–159
6. Clark WL, Kaiser PK, Flynn HW Jr, Belfort A, Miller D, Meisler DM (1999) Treatment strategies and visual acuity outcomes in chronic *Propionibacterium acnes* endophthalmitis. Ophthalmology 106: 1665–1670
7. Coupland SE, Bechrakis NE, Anastassiou G, Foerster AMH, Heiligenhaus A, Pleyer U, Hummel M, Stein H (2003) Evaluation of vitrectomy specimens and chorioretinal biopsies in the diagnosis of primary intraocular lymphoma in patients with masquerade syndrome. Graefes Arch Clin Exp Ophthalmol 241: 860–870
8. Coupland SE, Heimann H, Bechrakis NE (2004) Primary intraocular lymphoma: a review of the clinical, histopathological and molecular biological features. Graefes Arch Clin Exp Ophthalmol 240: 901–913
9. Coupland SE, Perez-Canto A, Hummel M, Stein H, Heimann H (2005) Assessment of HOPE fixation in vitrectomy specimens in patients with chronic bilateral uveitis (masquerade syndrome). Graefes Arch Clin Exp Ophthalmol 243: 847–852
10. Davis JL, Chan CC, Nussenblatt RB (1992) Diagnostic vitrectomy in intermediate uveitis. In: Boeke WRF, Manthey KF, Nussenblatt RB (eds) Intermediate uveitis. Developments in ophthalmology, vol. 23. Basel: Karger, pp120–132
11. Doft BH, Wisniewski SR, Kelsey SF, Fitzgerald SG, Endophthalmitis Vitrectomy Study Group (2001) Diabetes and postoperative endophthalmitis in the Endophthalmitis Vitrectomy Study. Arch Ophthalmol 119: 650–656
12. Duker JS, Blumenkranz MS (1991) Diagnosis and management of the acute retinal necrosis (ARN) syndrome. Surv Ophthalmol 35: 327–343
13. Endophthalmitis Vitrectomy Study Group (1995) Results of the endophthalmitis vitrectomy study. A randomized trial of immediate vitrectomy and of intravenous antibiotics for the treatment of postoperative bacterial endophthalmitis. Arch Ophthalmol 113: 1479–1496
14. Ferencz JR, Assia EI, Diamantstein L, Rubinstein E (1999) Vancomycin concentration in the vitreous after intravenous and intravitreal administration for postoperative endophthalmitis. Arch Ophthalmol 117: 1023–1027
15. Heiligenhaus A, Helbig H, Fiedler M (2002) Herpesviruses. In: Foster CS, Vitale AT (eds.) Diagnosis and treatment of uveitis. Philadelphia: Saunders, pp 315–332
16. Holland GN and the Executive Committee of the American Uveitis Society (1994) Standard diagnostic criteria for the acute retinal necrosis syndrome. Am J Ophthalmol 117: 663–666
17. Huang ES, Benson JD, Huong SM, Wilson B, van der Horst C (1992) Irreversible inhibition of human cytomegalovirus replication by topoisomerase II inhibitor, etopodide: a new strategy for the treatment of human cytomegalovirus infection. Antiviral Res 17: 17–32
18. Jackson TL, Eykyn SJ, Graham EM, Stanford MR (2003) Endogenous bacterial endophthalmitis: a 17-year prospective series and review of 267 reported cases. Surv Ophthalmol 48: 403–423
19. Kuhn, Ferenc. Personal communication
20. Lueke C, Bartz-Schmidt KU, Baum UE, Heimann K (2000) Treatment of cytomegalovirus retinitis clinically resistant to ganciclovir and foscarnet with intravitreal etoposide. J Toxicol Cutaneous Ocul Toxicol 19: 27–30
21. Luther TT, Bartz-Schmidt KU (1999) Endophthalmitis. Ophthalmologe 96: 758–771
22. Meier P, Wiedemann P (1997) Endophthalmitis—clinical appearance, therapy and prevention. Klin Monatsbl Augenheilkd 210: 175–191
23. Merle-Beral H, Davi F, Cassoux N, Baudet S, Colin C, Gourdet T, Bodaghi B, LeHoang P (2004) Biological diagnosis of primary intraocular lymphoma. Br J Haematol 124: 469–473
24. Ness T, Pelz K (2000) Endophthalmitis: improvement of culture results. Ophthalmologe 97: 33–37
25. Okhravi N, Adamson P, Carroll N, Dunlop A, Matheson MM, Towler HMA, Lightman S (2000) PCR-based evidence of bacterial involvement in eyes with suspected intraocular infection. Invest Ophthalmol Vis Sci 41: 3474–3479
26. Opremcak EM, Foster CS (2002) Diagnostic surgery. In: Foster CS, Vitale AD (eds.) Diagnosis and treatment of uveitis. Philadelphia: Saunders, pp 215–221
27. Park S, Abad S, Tulliez M, Monnet D, Merlat A, Gyan E, Bouscary D, Dreyfus F, Grimaldi D, Dhote R, Rollot F, Kelaïdi C, Nazal EM, Brézin AP, Blanche P (2004) Pseudouveitis. A clue to the diagnosis of primary central nervous system lymphoma in immunocompetent patients. Medicine 83: 223–232
28. Peterson K, Gordon KB, Heinemann MH, DeAngelis LM (1993) The clinical spectrum of ocular lymphoma. Cancer 72: 843–849
29. Read RW, Zamir E, Rao NA (2002) Neoplastic masquerade syndromes. Surv Ophthalmol 47: 81–124

30. Rohrbach JM, Zierhut M (2001) Intraokuläres (okulozerebrales) non-Hodgkin-lymphom. Ophthalmologe 98: 495–507
31. Schiedler V, Scott IU, Flynn HW Jr, Davis JL, Benz MS, Miller D (2004) Culture-proven endogenous endophthalmitis: clinical features and visual acuity outcomes. Am J Ophthalmol 137: 725–731
32. Siepmann K, Rohrbach JM, Duncker G, Zierhut M (2004) Intraocular non-Hodgkin's lymphoma and its therapy—a case series of ten patients. Klin Monatsbl Augenheilkd 221: 266–272
33. Silverstein BE, Conrad D, Margolis TP, Wong IG (1997) Cytomegalovirus-associated acute retinal necrosis syndrome. Am J Ophthalmol 123: 257–258
34. Taban M, Behrens A, Newcomb RL, Nobe MY, Saedi G, Sweet PM, McDonnell PJ (2005) Acute endophthalmitis following cataract surgery. A systematic review of the literature. Arch Ophthalmol 123: 613–620
35. Therese KL, Anand AR, Madhavan HN (1998) Polymerase chain reaction in the diagnosis of bacterial endophthalmitis. Br J Ophthalmol 82: 1078–1082
36. Thurau S (2003) Practical advice for recovery and successful processing of vitrectomy samples. Ophthalmologe 100: 802–807
37. Voros GM, Pandit R, Snow M, Griffiths PG (2006) Unilateral recurrent acute retinal necrosis syndrome caused by cytomegalovirus in an immune-competent adult. Eur J Ophthalmol 16: 484–486
38. Walters G, James TE (2001) Viral causes of the acute retinal necrosis syndrome. Curr Opin Ophthalmol 12: 191–195
39. Whitcup SM (2004) Acute retinal necrosis and progressive outer retinal necrosis. In: Nussenblatt RB, Whitcup SM (eds.) Uveitis. Fundamentals and clinical practice. St. Louis: Mosby, pp 201–209
40. Whitcup SM (2004) Masquerade syndromes. In: Nussenblatt RB, Whitcup SM (eds.) Uveitis. Fundamentals and clinical practice. St. Louis: Mosby, pp 409–419
41. Whitcup SM, de Smet MD, Rubin BI, Palestine AG, Martin DF, Burnier M Jr, Chan CC, Nussenblatt RB (1993) Intraocular lymphoma. Clinical and histopathological diagnosis. Ophthalmology 100: 1399–1406
42. Widder RA, Bartz-Schmidt KU, Geyer H, Brunner R, Kirchhof B, Donike M, Heimann K (1995) *Candida albicans* endophthalmitis after anabolic steroid abuse. Lancet 345: 330–331
43. Zierhut M, Baatz H, Coupland S, Deuter C, Heiligenhaus A, Heinz C (2006) Uveitis and the aging. Ophthalmologe 103: 765–772

Chapter 26

Choroidal Biopsy

Christoph M.E. Deuter, Sabine Biester, Karl Ulrich Bartz-Schmidt

Core Messages

- A decision to perform choroidal biopsy should balance the risk of surgical complications against the value of the information potentially gained.
- Choroidal biopsy can be performed if primary intraocular lymphoma (PIOL) is suspected despite prior negative diagnostic vitrectomy.
- Infectious chorioretinitis may require choroidal biopsy if microbiologic, immunologic, and molecular testing of vitreous or aqueous humor is negative.

Contents

26.1	Introduction	267
26.2	Indications	267
26.3	Surgical Procedure	268
26.4	Processing of Specimens	268
References		269

This chapter contains the following video clips on DVD: Video 42 shows Diagnostic Vitrectomy with air, Video 43 shows Choroidal biopsy (Surgeon: Karl-Ulrich Bartz-Schmidt), Video 44 shows Subretinal aspiration and choroidal biopsy in ocular lymphoma (Surgeon: Matthias Becker) and Video 45 shows Choroidal biopsy (Surgeon: Marc de Smet).

26.1 Introduction

Surgical procedures to perform chorioretinal biopsy while preserving the integrity and function of the eye were described for the first time by Peyman and coworkers in the 1980s [5, 6]. Remarkable progress in vitreoretinal surgery has been made since then, including therapeutic subretinal surgery for resection of choroidal neovascularization membranes and endoresection of choroidal melanomas. Advanced vitreoretinal surgical techniques are rarely used in the diagnosis of posterior uveitis; however, the informative value of diagnostic vitrectomy may be limited in cases where the pathology is primarily located at the level of the choroid and the retina [4]. Thus the decision to perform choroidal biopsy may be warranted in cases in which the risks of surgical complications are outweighed by the potential gain of information that may help in the treatment of either the biopsied eye or the fellow eye [1].

26.2 Indications

In the literature, several cases have been reported in which chorioretinal biopsy was used to diagnose severe posterior uveitis of unknown etiology. Multifocal choroiditis, ocular sarcoidosis and acute retinal necrosis have been investigated in this manner [1, 4]. However, in our opinion, the most important indication to perform choroidal biopsy is the suspicion of primary intraocular lymphoma (PIOL). This sight- and life-threatening diffuse large cell B-cell lymphoma, which belongs to the so-called masquerade syndromes that mimic uveitis, has been described in more detail in the previous chapter on diagnostic vitrectomy. Diagnosing PIOL is often challenging. Lymphoma cells are fragile and may be damaged during diagnostic vitrectomy or during processing. Although diagnostic vitrectomy is the most common technique used in the diagnosis of PIOL, it often fails to confirm or definitively exclude the diagnosis even if repeated [2]. In such cases, and especially if a subretinal

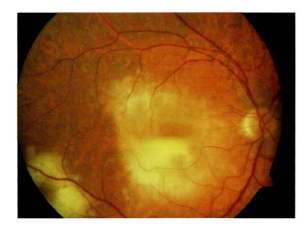

Fig. 26.1 Subretinal masses in PIOL

or choroidal infiltrate is present (Fig. 26.1), choroidal biopsy should be considered to confirm the diagnosis in order to initiate adequate treatment rapidly.

26.3 Surgical Procedure

Prior to choroidal en bloc biopsy, the area for excision is selected based on location of the infiltrated choroid, respecting the visual impact of the biopsy. If possible, the macular area is always avoided, but it is also important to avoid nasal or superior block biopsy if possible because of the importance of the temporal and inferior visual fields. However, the goal of biopsy is to obtain an adequate specimen, and this may require invasion of visually important areas. As is the case for vitreous biopsy, systemic steroids should be discontinued at least 2 weeks before the procedure in eyes with suspected intraocular lymphoma.

A traditional 20-G, three-port approach is preferred because of more secure extraction of the choroidal tissue block through an enlarged sclerotomy and the likelihood of silicone oil exchange.

Phakic patients may benefit from small incision lens surgery with foldable hydrophobic acrylic lens in combination with an implantation of a PMMA capsular tension ring prior to biopsy. The phako tunnel should be placed at the 12 o'clock position, because suturing of the inferotemporal sclerotomy after vitrectomy might lead to opening of a temporal corneal incision. Usually the eyes have already had the vitreous completely removed during a prior diagnostic vitrectomy, with separation of the posterior vitreous. If not, the posterior hyaloid should be removed before biopsy. The procedure is started with a small retinotomy at the peripheral edge of the planned biopsy area. A localized retinal detachment is created by injection of balanced salt solution using a double lumen cannula. Alternatively, a 40-G Teflon cannula can be used for both retinotomy and injection. At least a 180° detachment 1–2 mm posterior to the abnormal area is necessary. After anterior retinotomy using the automated handpiece or scissors, the retina is folded back, exposing the retinal pigment epithelium and choroid. If the BIOM visualization system is used, the retinotomy must be performed with scleral indentation. Indentation is not needed when using a wide-angle contact lens system. To hold the detached retinal flap in place, perfluorocarbon liquid (PFCL) is injected. Endodiathermy is used to coagulate choroidal vessels surrounding the biopsy area before excision with Heimann scissors. Alternatively, continuous frequency doubled green endolaser (continuous mode 500 mW) can be used to cut and coagulate the choroid. The tissue bloc is then detached from the underlying sclera by a spatula and extracted using forceps through an enlarged sclerotomy.

To reattach the retina, PFCL is removed completely and reinjected after unfolding of the retina. Following complete reattachment of the retina, standard laser photocoagulation and PFCL silicone oil exchange is performed. The use of a capsular tension ring will inhibit silicone oil spillover into the anterior chamber. The tissue block is rapidly transferred to the pathology laboratory for processing.

Typically, a first attempt to remove silicone oil can be made at 3 months. The IOL power should be calculated as refraction after silicone oil removal, especially when the macular region is preserved during the biopsy procedure.

26.4 Processing of Specimens

Choroidal biopsies are fixed in 4%-buffered formalin and sent to an experienced pathology laboratory as rapidly as possible. For the diagnosis of PIOL, these tissue specimens allow a larger range of immunohistochemical investigations than vitreous aspirates. Conventional histology of PIOL in the choroidal specimens reveals infiltration of atypical lymphocytes. The neoplastic cells are medium to large-sized with a basophilic cytoplasm, oval-shaped nuclei and conspicuous nucleoli. Mitotic figures sometimes can be seen [3].

Vitreous specimens that were also harvested during the procedure of choroidal biopsy should be processed as described in the previous chapter on diagnostic vitrectomy.

Take Home Pearls

- In the hands of an experienced vitreoretinal surgeon, choroidal biopsy represents an important diagnostic tool for severe inflammatory disorders of unclear origin affecting the retina or choroid.
- Suspected intraocular lymphoma may be an indication for choroidal biopsy if previous diagnostic vitrectomy has failed to confirm or exclude the diagnosis.

References

1. Chan CC, Palestine AG, Davis JL, De Smet MD, McLean IW, Burnier M, Drouilhet JD, Nussenblatt RB (1991) Role of chorioretinal biopsy in inflammatory eye disease. Ophthalmology 98: 1281–1286
2. Coupland SE, Bechrakis NE, Anastassiou G, Foerster AMH, Heiligenhaus A, Pleyer U, Hummel M, Stein H (2003) Evaluation of vitrectomy specimens and chorioretinal biopsies in the diagnosis of primary intraocular lymphoma in patients with masquerade syndrome. Graefes Arch Clin Exp Ophthalmol 241: 860–870
3. Coupland SE, Heimann H, Bechrakis NE (2004) Primary intraocular lymphoma: a review of the clinical, histopathological and molecular biological features. Graefes Arch Clin Exp Ophthalmol 240: 901–913
4. Martin DF, Chan CC, de Smet MD, Palestine AG, Davis JL, Whitcup SM, Burnier MN Jr, Nussenblatt RB (1993) The role of chorioretinal biopsy in the management of posterior uveitis. Ophthalmology 100: 705–714
5. Peyman GA, Juarez CP, Raichand M (1981) Full-thickness eye-wall biopsy: long-term results in 9 patients. Br J Ophthalmol 65: 723–726
6. Peyman GA, Raichand M, Schulman J (1986) Diagnosis and therapeutic surgery of the uvea—part I: surgical technique. Ophthalmic Surg 17: 822–829

Chapter 27

Retinal Biopsy

Janet L. Davis

Core Messages

- The simplest biopsy technique that will provide an answer should be selected.
- More aggressive biopsies can be performed if simpler techniques are inadequate.
- Tissue biopsies are limited in most cases to sight- or life-threatening disorders such as intraocular infections or intraocular lymphoma.
- Various techniques for biopsy have been described, but only a small number of cases are reported in the literature.
- Selection of technique and site should be individualized for each patient.

Contents

27.1	Introduction	271
27.2	Surgical Techniques	272
27.2.1	Subretinal Aspiration	272
27.2.2	Endoretinal Biopsy	273
27.2.3	*Ab Externo* Chorioretinal Biopsy	274
References		274

27.1 Introduction

Gholam Peyman is credited with the technique of ab interno retinal biopsy, initially in experimental animals [1] and then in a small series of 14 patients with disparate diagnoses [2]. Various series and case reports have appeared that correlate histopathologic results of biopsy with clinical diagnoses [3–10]. Rao proposed the strategy of biopsy of the most accessible tissue first [3]. For most cases of viral retinitis, the most accessible tissue is aqueous humor, and excellent results from specimens obtained by paracentesis [11] make diagnostic vitrectomy unnecessary in most cases. Aqueous humor analysis to detect elevated levels of interleukin-10 may provide a minimally invasive way to screen for intraocular lymphoma [12].

When a diagnosis of intraocular lymphoma is suspected, diagnostic vitrectomy is usually performed. In a series of 84 biopsy specimens from 80 patients, 12 cases of intraocular lymphoma were identified based on the vitreous specimen, and an additional 3 were diagnosed after chorioretinal biopsy with an automated cutter and 2 after enucleation [10]. Lymphoma has also been diagnosed by direct biopsy of the retina [13], in which a sample of the retina is removed (endoretinal biopsy), and by chorioretinal biopsy ab externo. Peyman was the first to describe successful diagnosis of lymphoma by this technique [14]. Chapter 25 of this volume describes a method of biopsying subretinal tissues that involves disinsertion of 180° of peripheral retina, followed by retinal detachment repair.

Retinal biopsy and chorioretinal biopsy find applications in diseases other than lymphoma. The preponderance of cases in the literature are from viral retinitis at the time of retinal detachment repair [7] which often is more easily diagnosed by PCR of intraocular fluid. Multifocal choroiditis and subretinal fibrosis, sarcoidosis, tuberculosis, candidal endophthalmitis, HTLV-1-associated leukemia, and viral retinitis have been diagnosed by these techniques [5–8]. They may be applicable to other infections that preferentially affect the subretinal tissues, such as *Nocardia*, and are difficult to culture from the vitreous (Fig. 27.1a,b). Use of these techniques assumes that simpler diagnostic methods such as diagnostic paracentesis or diagnostic vitrectomy have not yielded a diagnosis. Occasionally, they may be combined with diagnostic vitrectomy to reduce the risk of a second procedure if the vitreous specimen is inadequate. Vitrectomy with elevation of the hyaloid is required before any tissue biopsy.

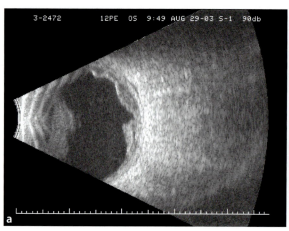 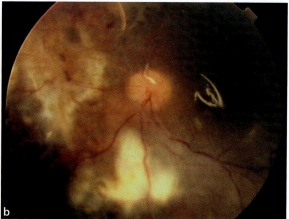

Fig. 27.1 **a** Ultrasound of the left eye at presentation of a 58-year-old woman with systemic lupus erythematosus on oral corticosteroids with complaints of reduced vision. Vision was hand motions, and there was a large white subretinal deposit involving the nasal half of the retina. Vitreous cultures were negative. Subretinal aspiration of the mass grew *Nocardia asteroides*. A systemic focus was eventually identified in a foot ulcer. **b** Fundus, left eye. The eye was imaged after subretinal aspiration and repair of retinal detachment with silicone oil. The majority of the abscess has cleared with high doses of intravenous trimethoprim-sulfamethoxazole and intravitreal amikacin, but persistent deposits are visible below the optic nerve, confined to the subretinal space at the level of the retinal pigment epithelium without retinal invasion. All deposits eventually cleared after further antibiotic treatment. Detachment probably occurred because the aspiration site could not be adequately lasered due to persistent deposits in the subretinal space. Primary infusion of silicone oil may have avoided this complication, but would have created a different set of problems, such as inability to effectively use intravitreal amikacin and compartmentalization of the inflammation

When tissue is acquired, the biopsy specimen is generally divided in the operating room into portions for histology, culture and/or PCR, and immunopathology. Consultation with laboratory personnel is advised prior to biopsy.

27.2 Surgical Techniques

27.2.1 Subretinal Aspiration

Removal of material from the subretinal space by aspiration is the easiest and least traumatic of biopsy methods. Intraocular lymphoma is particularly favorable for subretinal aspiration because it forms yellow retinal pigment epithelial detachments filled with highly concentrated and freely mobile cells (Fig. 27.2a, b).

Subretinal aspiration with fine needles can provide a specimen for cytologic examination [9, 15]. Conventional sharp-pointed needles may be less suitable for aspiration of these shallow collections of cells because the tip impales the choroid before the bevel is well within the cellular deposit. A 20-gauge silicone-tipped extrusion needle, conventionally used in repair of retinal detachment by vitrectomy, has several advantages in subretinal aspiration. The flexible tip can be cut to the desired length, shallowly beveled if desired, and inserted easily through a knife slit in the retina. The tube bends so that it can remain parallel to the retina in the subretinal space and travel a short distance. Even directed vertically, it is atraumatic to the choroid. The other advantage is that the cells can be seen entering the tubing. Aspiration into a 3-cc syringe with no more than 0.5–1 ml infusate from the central vitreous cavity provides a good cytologic specimen. Endolaser photocoagulation can be applied around the biopsy site, but the retinal hole is likely self-healing; short-acting gas tamponade should provide ample time for this to occur if it is desirable to avoid photocoagulation, for example in macular lesions.

In the technique described by Bechrakis et al. [16] and used in the review series of Coupland et al. [10], biopsy of subretinal tissue was performed by penetrating the retina with a knife blade as for subretinal aspiration above and inserting the vitreous cutter in the subretinal space. Using high aspiration pressure and low cutting

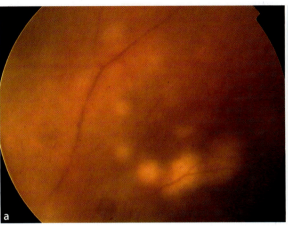
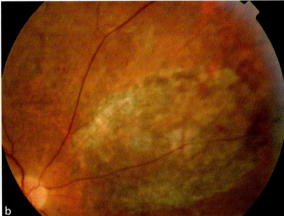

Fig. 27.2 a Fundus of the right eye of an 83-year-old man with complaints of floaters. There are solid detachments of the retinal pigment epithelium characteristic of intraocular lymphoma. Diagnostic vitrectomy was performed. Examination of the vitreous specimen did not confirm the diagnosis of intraocular lymphoma, but material from aspiration from these lesions did. During surgery, the flexible silicone cannula permitted drainage of the three largest lesions from a single retinotomy. b Fundus of the right eye after vitrectomy and external beam radiation. There are laser photocoagulation scars surrounding the involved area, and the media are now clear

rate, the surgeon takes a few bites of the underlying mass. No laser photocoagulation was used, and tamponade with a short-acting gas was sufficient to maintain retinal attachment. In Bechrakis's original series, biopsy of solid tumors was described. Tumors such as intraocular lymphoma that are easily aspirable probably do not require cutting. The vitrectomy probe could be used to aspirate subretinal contents, especially 25-gauge instrumentation in which the port is closer to the tip of the instrument. All aspirations through the vitrector should be done into a syringe connected directly inline without a stopcock, as close to the vitrector handle as possible.

Subretinal aspiration of exudative fluid may be helpful in the diagnosis of metastasis and uveal melanocytic proliferation [7, 17].

27.2.2 Endoretinal Biopsy

Direct biopsy of the retina is conceptually simple. A pathologic area is identified, cut free, and removed from the eye. Selection of the site of biopsy is more critical than with subretinal aspiration as tissue will be removed. Although most authors discuss removal of pieces of 1–2 mm [13, 18], such small biopsies may be inadequate, or lost, or prevent division. In addition, it is considered desirable to include a portion of normal retina at the border zone if possible to assist in orientation of the specimen. Size up to 3–5 mm is not unreasonable. Consideration should be taken of the surgeon's hand position to facilitate cutting and the position of large retinal vessels, which, if they cannot be avoided, can be closed with diathermy. Diathermy use should be minimized to avoid tissue injury.

Square biopsies are easier to cut than round ones. It is not necessary to detach the retina, as has been described [13]. Either the retina can be incised with a sharp knife, or one blade of a vertical or horizontal cutting vitreoretinal scissor is inserted through the retina. Cuts are made on four sides, freeing three corners. The remaining corner remains attached to the retina to prevent loss of the biopsy. The specimen is then aspirated into a 10-cc syringe attached to an 18–19-gauge extrusion needle, using the force of aspiration to break the remaining connection to the retina. Additional fluid 2–3 cc is aspirated from the central vitreous cavity, and the translucent specimen is visualized in the syringe [19].

Transfer to a sterile Petri dish is then made by removing the plunger and pouring the specimen into the dish. The retinal biopsy can be "beached" by tilting the plate and the excess fluid carefully dried. Fixation at this point with formalin or paraformaldehyde may help transfer the specimen atraumatically. Forceps removal or allowing the specimen to float freely out of one of the sclerotomies is unnecessarily damaging and risks loss of the specimen [18].

Endoretinal biopsy probably requires endolaser photocoagulation and gas–fluid exchange. Silicone oil tamponade could be considered if good adhesion could not be obtained in diseased tissue or the patient could not position adequately.

Choroidal biopsy can be easily performed through the retinal biopsy site. The biopsy is more difficult to cut, and more difficult to elevate from the sclera than the endoretinal biopsy. Diathermy is needed to reduce bleeding.

27.2.3 *Ab Externo* Chorioretinal Biopsy

Localization of the biopsy site is a critical preoperative procedure. Ideally, the site should be anterior to the equator, rendering this impractical in many cases. Superior locations are preferred. If retina is to be removed, preoperative demarcation of the biopsy site with laser may help reduce the risk of postoperative retinal detachment.

Published descriptions of biopsy technique can be consulted [6, 14, 18, 20]. Vitrectomy with placement of an infusion line helps stabilize the globe. Care must be taken to position the line so that a full rotation of the eye can be obtained. Muscle sling sutures, as for scleral buckling, are helpful. A Flieringa ring sutured to sclera surrounding the biopsy site will also help stabilize the globe.

Circular flaps are easier to close with sutures than square ones. Partial-thickness trephination can be helpful, leaving a one-clock-hour hinge. Deep dissection leaving only the inner laminae of sclera produces a sturdy hinged flap. Diathermy at the edge of the biopsy site can reduce the risk of hemorrhage. The inner sclera, uvea, and retina are incised with a sharp blade, grasped with forceps, and cut free with scissors or a blade. As for endoretinal biopsy, square or rectangular biopsies are easier to cut. The flap is then sutured in place with multiple interrupted 9-0 nylon sutures, leaving the knots exposed. Fibrin or cyanoacrylate glue can be helpful if the flap is not watertight. Additional vitrectomy, laser, air, or gas–fluid exchange can be performed at this point.

Take Home Pearls

- Subretinal aspiration is a simple, atraumatic, and useful technique suited to cellular deposits such as intraocular lymphoma.
  — Laser demarcation is optional.
  — Short-acting gas tamponade is advised.
- Endoretinal biopsies should be of sufficient size to permit comprehensive testing.
  — Laser demarcation is advised.
  — Gas tamponade is usually adequate.
  — Silicone oil tamponade can be considered.
- Choroidal biopsies can be removed though an endoretinal site.
  — More bleeding is expected.
  — Choroidal biopsies are harder to remove.
- Chorioretinal biopsy *ab externo* is probably best suited to cases in which an entire lesion is being excised, i.e., tumors, as *ab interno* biopsy appears safer and should suffice for most indications.

References

1. Peyman GA, Barrada A. Retinochoroidectomy ab interno. Ophthalmic Surg 1984; 15(9):749–751
2. Peyman GA. Internal retinal biopsy: surgical technique and results. Int Ophthalmol 1990; 14(2):101–104
3. Cote MA, Rao NA. The role of histopathology in the diagnosis and management of uveitis. Int Ophthalmol 1990; 14(5–6):309–316
4. Chan CC, Palestine AG, Davis JL, de Smet MD, McLean IW, Burnier M et al. Role of chorioretinal biopsy in inflammatory eye disease. Ophthalmology 1991; 98(8):1281–1286
5. Barondes MJ, Sponsel WE, Stevens TS, Plotnik RD. Tuberculous choroiditis diagnosed by chorioretinal endobiopsy. Am J Ophthalmol 1991; 112(4):460–461
6. Martin DF, Chan CC, de Smet MD, Palestine AG, Davis JL, Whitcup SM et al. The role of chorioretinal biopsy in the management of posterior uveitis. Ophthalmology 1993; 100(5):705–714
7. Rutzen AR, Ortega-Larrocea G, Dugel PU, Chong LP, Lopez PF, Smith RE et al. Clinicopathologic study of retinal and choroidal biopsies in intraocular inflammation. Am J Ophthalmol 1995; 119(5):597–611
8. Levy-Clarke GA, Buggage RR, Shen D, Vaughn LO, Chan CC, Davis JL. Human T-cell lymphotropic virus type-1 associated T-cell leukemia/lymphoma masquerading as necrotizing retinal vasculitis. Ophthalmology 2002; 109(9):1717–1722

9. Rao M. Primary intraocular lymphoma diagnosed by fine needle aspiration biopsy of a subretinal lesion. Retina 2002; 22(4):512–513
10. Coupland SE, Bechrakis NE, Anastassiou G, Foerster AM, Heiligenhaus A, Pleyer U et al. Evaluation of vitrectomy specimens and chorioretinal biopsies in the diagnosis of primary intraocular lymphoma in patients with masquerade syndrome. Graefes Arch Clin Exp Ophthalmol 2003; 241(10):860–870
11. Tran TH, Rozenberg F, Cassoux N, Rao NA, Lehoang P, Bodaghi B. Polymerase chain reaction analysis of aqueous humour samples in necrotising retinitis. Br J Ophthalmol 2003; 87(1):79–83
12. Cassoux N, Giron A, Bodaghi B, Tran TH, Baudet S, Davy F et al. IL-10 measurement in aqueous humor for screening patients with suspicion of primary intraocular lymphoma. Invest Ophthalmol Vis Sci 2007; 48(7):3253–3259
13. Cassoux N, Charlotte F, Rao NA, Bodaghi B, Merle-Beral H, Lehoang P. Endoretinal biopsy in establishing the diagnosis of uveitis: a clinicopathologic report of three cases. Ocul Immunol Inflamm 2005; 13(1):79–83
14. Peyman GA, Juarez CP, Raichand M. Full-thickness eye-wall biopsy: long-term results in 9 patients. Br J Ophthalmol 1981; 65(10):723–726
15. Levy-Clarke GA, Byrnes GA, Buggage RR, Shen DF, Filie AC, Caruso RC et al. Primary intraocular lymphoma diagnosed by fine needle aspiration biopsy of a subretinal lesion. Retina 2001; 21(3):281–284
16. Bechrakis NE, Foerster MH, Bornfeld N. Biopsy in indeterminate intraocular tumors. Ophthalmology 2002; 109(2):235–242
17. Sternberg P Jr, Tiedeman J, Hickingbotham D, McCuen BW, Proia AD. Controlled aspiration of subretinal fluid in the diagnosis of carcinoma metastatic to the choroid. Arch Ophthalmol 1984; 102(11):1622–1625
18. Gonzales JA, Chan CC. Biopsy techniques and yields in diagnosing primary intraocular lymphoma. Int Ophthalmol 2007; 27(4):241–250
19. Moshfeghi DM, Dodds EM, Couto CA, Santos CI, Nicholson DH, Lowder CY et al. Diagnostic approaches to severe, atypical toxoplasmosis mimicking acute retinal necrosis. Ophthalmology 2004; 111(4):716–725
20. Nussenblatt RB, Davis JL, Palestine AG. Chorioretinal biopsy for diagnostic purposes in cases of intraocular inflammatory disease. Dev Ophthalmol 1992; 23:133–138

Subject Index

5-fluoroudine (5-Furd) 28
5-fluorouracil (5-FU) 27, 28, 89, 169, 174, 224
5-fluorouracil, 5-fluorouridine, Mitomycin, Taxol, Daunorubicin, EDTA and FGF-Saporin 27
5-FU 27, 28
γ-globulin 147

A

ab interno laser sclerostomy 88
ab interno retinal biopsy 271
ablation 232
absorbable sutures (AS) 77
ACE (angiotensin-converting enzyme) 64
acetazolamide 51, 95, 151, 160, 161
acquired immunodeficiency syndrome (AIDS) 226
acrylic IOLs 155
active antiretroviral therapy (HAART) 262
acute retinal hemorrhagic retinal vasculitis 211
acute retinal necrosis (ARN) 103, 225, 267
acute retinal necrosis syndrome (ARNS) 107, 108, 248, 259
acyclovir 117, 247, 261
after cataract 150, 158
Ahmed 170
Ahmed glaucoma valve 170, 175
AIDS 210, 247, 260
air-bubble size 81
air-bubble unfolding 81
air vitrectomy 263
albumin 147
ALK 76
alpha adrenoreceptor agonists 168
amblyopia 90, 146, 148, 150, 153, 161, 162
amniotic membrane 76
amniotic membrane graft 186
amniotic membrane transplantation 64
amniotic membrane transplantation (AMT) 76, 77
Amphotericin B 259, 260
Amsler's sign 116, 141
Amsler tests 161
AMT 76
anesthesia 93
angiographic 205
angiography 42, 112
angiotensin converting enzyme 99

anterior capsule opacification (ACO) 138, 147, 159
anterior capsule tears 115
anterior chamber-associated immune deviation (ACAID) 36
anterior chamber depth 112
anterior chamber paracentesis 9
anterior chamber puncture 240
anterior hyaloid membrane 152
anterior lamellar keratoplasty (LKP) 73
anterior vitrectomy 146, 152, 159
anti-angiogenic factors 204
anti-vascular endothelial growth factor (anti-VEGF) 6
antibiotic 94
antibody 239
anticoagulant therapy 212
antigen-presenting cells (APC) 36
antigens 36
antiproliferative agents 27
antiviral drug resistance 247
ants' eggs 48
APC 36
aphakia 123, 170
aphakic contact lenses 146
apraclonidine 168
arcus senilis 178
argon laser peripheral iridoplasty 134
argon laser photocoagulation 212
arifical anterior chamber (AAC) 76, 79, 81
associated surgery 91
atrophy of the iris 93
autologous conjunctival-limbal transplantation 251
autologous conjunctiva transplantation 186
Avastin (bevacizumab) 178
Azathioprine 51, 212

B

B-Scan ultrasonography 50, 232
BAB 137, 138
BAB breakdown 147
Baerveldt 170
Baerveldt glaucoma drainage device 176
Baerveldt glaucoma drainage implant 175
balanced salt solution (BSS) 64
bandage contact lens 65

band keratopathy 50, 63, 86, 88, 156, 157, 162, 178
Beehler pupil dilator 114
Behçet's disease (BD) 12, 39, 40, 42, 43, 100, 128, 210
– intravitreal TA 12
best corrected visual acuity 41
beta-blocking agents 160
bevacizumab 161
bevacizumab (Avastin®) 142
binocular indirect ophthalmoscopy (BIO) 39
biocompatibility 121, 122, 147
biodegradable dexamethasone implant 21
biopsy 247
birdshot chorioretinopathy 203, 204
birdshot retinochoroidopathy 11, 249
blebitis 175
bleb leaks 89
blood-retinal barrier (BRB) 24, 36, 210
– inner blood–retinal barrier 7
– outer blood–retinal barrier 7
blood–aqueous barrier (BAB) 87, 100, 113, 122, 127, 137, 147, 156
blood–aqueous barrier breakdown 112
borreliosis 247
brimonidine 160, 168
brinzolamide 160
Brown syndrome 181

C

campimetry 91
can-opener technique 151
candida 35
capsular bag 147
capsular bending rings 159
capsular biocompatibility 148
capsular contraction 138
capsular contraction syndrome 140
capsular dislocation 140
capsular fibrosis 159
capsular opacification 86
capsular response 139
capsular retraction 147
capsular rim tears 93
capsular tension ring 116, 268
capsulectomy 89, 106, 156
capsule shrinkage 152
capsulorhexis 93, 111, 124
capsulotomy 106, 139
carcinoma in situ of the conjunctiva and cornea 251
Castroviejo calipers 77
cat-scratch disease 210
cataract 9, 50, 85, 105, 106, 112, 117, 137, 162
cataract surgery 86, 91, 99
ceftazidime 259
cefuroxime 94

central retinal artery occlusion (CRAO) 9
central retinal vein occlusion (CRVO) 8
central serous chorioretinopathy (CSCR) 9
chelation with EDTA 64, 156
chest X-ray 99
childhood uveitis 145
cholinergic drugs 87
chorioretinitis 112
choroidal biopsy 267
choroidal detachment 232
choroidal folds 160
choroidal granuloma 247
choroidal neovascularization (CNV) 6, 12, 203
– intravitreal TA 8
choroidal swelling 100
chronic open-angle glaucoma (COAG) 8
chronic suppurative otitis media. *see* CSOM
cidofovir 232, 261
ciliary body 232
ciliary body ablation 232
ciliary body failure 133, 134, 232
ciliary body traction 232
ciliary body traction detachment 233
ciliary traction membranes 160
Cionni rings 140
ciprofloxacin 28
circumlinear capsulorhexis 117
cis-4-hydroxyproline (CHP) 28
cleansing 138
CME 7, 11, 40, 42, 43, 47, 48, 49, 50, 54, 87, 88, 95, 100, 101, 148, 151, 153, 160, 162
– pseudophakic 11
CMV retinitis 107
coagulation cascade 94
coagulation factors 147
Coats' disease 10
coaxial illumination 54
cocoon 152
collagen 169
collagen fibrils 38
collagen IV 155
color tests 90
combination 186
complement cascade 95, 147, 211
complement system 94
confocal microscopy 246
confocal scanning laser 205
congenital hereditary endothelial dystrophy 63
conjunctival autograft 246
contact lens 108, 150, 153, 162
continuous circular capsulorhexis (CCC) 93
continuous curvilinear capsulorhexis 151
core vitrectomy 204
corneal abscess 246

corneal edema 67
corneal endothelial guttae 88
corneal melt descemetocele formation
– with or without perforation 67
corneal opacities 112
corneal opacity 67
corneal perforation 76
corneal specular microscopy 133
corneal transplantation 67
corneal trephine 79
corticosteroid 5, 40, 51, 101, 113, 160, 174
– intravitreal concentration 6
– intravitreal corticosteroid injection 5
– mechanism 7
cotton wool spots 210
COX-2 inhibitors 27
crescent knife 246
Crohn's disease 211
cryocoagulation 142
cryotherapy 47, 213, 222
crystallins 147
CsA 28, 42
culture 258
culture of vitreous samples 258
cyclitic membrane 48, 50, 87, 89, 104, 133, 134, 152, 156, 221
cyclitic membrane formation 89
cycloablation therapy 88
cyclodestruction 170
cyclodestructive procedures 174, 175, 194
cyclodialysis cleft 232
cyclodialysis spatula 178
cyclophosphamide 249
cyclophotocoagulation 175
cyclosporine A (CsA) 28, 41, 212
cystoid macula edema 162
cystoid macular edema (CME) 10, 86, 99, 111, 115, 122, 141, 148, 161, 203, 204
– "pseudophakic" CME 11
– refractory macular edema 6
cystotome 152
cytokine 36, 37, 39
cytokine assays 241
cytology 241
cytomegalovirus (CMV) retinitis 8, 103, 203, 226, 259

D

DECT or DMECT Descemet's membrane endothelial cell transplantation 74
deep lamellar endothelial keratoplasty (DLEK) 79
deep sclerectomy 169, 246
delayed hypersensitivity 36
Descemet-stripping 73
Descemet's membrane 132

descemetocele 76
descemetorhexis (DX) 73, 79, 80
descemetorhexis with endokeratoplasty (DXEK) 71, 79
descemetorhexis with endokeratoplasty (DXEK or DSEK) 73
– deep anterior lamellar keratoplasty (DALK) 73
– mid-anterior lamellar keratoplasty (MALK) 73
– penetrating keratoplasty (PKP) 73
– superficial anterior lamellar keratoplasty (SALK) 73
– total anterior lamellar keratoplasty (TALK) 73
descemet stripping with endothelial keratoplasty (DSEK) 79
detachment 47
dexamethasone 6, 28, 96, 100, 106, 115, 151
– intravitreal dexamethasone 13
dexamethasone sustained delivery device (DEX-BDD, Posurdex™) 7
diabetic macular edema (DME) 204
diclofenac 65, 96
donor corneal button 76, 78
dorzolamide 160
doxorubicin 28
drainage devices 170

E

Eales disease 12, 43, 210, 212, 221, 227
– intravitreal TA 12
Early Treatment Diabetic Retinopathy Study (ETDRS) 11
ECA endothelial cell activation 74
echothiophate 178
ECT endothelial cell transplantation 74
EDTA (Ethylene diamine tetraacetic acid) chelation 64
either imipenem 258
electrophysiological test 149, 150
electroretinography 42
electrotransfer 26
Elschnig pearl 152
Elschnig pearl formation 139
Elvax disc 27
endocycloablation 175
endodiathermy 268
endolaser 268
endolaser photocoagulation 54
endophotocoagulation 213
endophotocoagulator 175
endophthalmitis 28, 169, 175, 227, 240, 248, 256, 257, 259
– infectious endophthalmitis following intravitreal injection of TA 8

- intravitreal corticosteroids in the treatment of infectious endophthalmitis 13
- sterile inflammatory reaction 6

endoresection of choroidal melanomas 267
endothelial cell activation 73
endothelial cell transplantation 73
endothelial graft rejection 67
endotoxin-induced uveitis (EIU) model 30
enlarged sclerotomy 268
enucleation 246
epikeratophakia 153
epinephrine 156
epiretinal membrane (ERM) 37, 38, 86, 95, 112, 153, 203, 204, 212
episcleral nodules 251
epitheloid 147
epitheloid cells 138
Epstein-Barr virus 248
ERM 39, 42, 43
ERM peeling 40, 212
erythematous systemic lupus (SLE) 211
ethylene vinyl acetate (EVA) 24
etoposide 261
EVS Study 263
excimer laser 64
excimer laser ablation 65
experimental autoimmune uveitis (EAU) 28
experimental PVR models 28
external fistula 232
external leakage 232
external wound leakage 232
extracellular matrix proteinases 211
extracellular matrix proteins 38
exudative retinal detachment 54
eye wall resection 247

F

Fas ligand (CD95L) 36
feeder vessels 212
fibrin formation 100, 122
fibrin membrane 148, 151
fibrinogen 147
fibrinous pupillary membranes 146
fibronectin 147, 148, 155
fibrous vitreous band 221
filtering operation 134
filtering surgery 169, 174
flare 87
flare meter 113
Flieringa ring 274
flow cytometry 249
fluconazol 259
fluconazole 29, 260
fluocinolone acetonide (Retisert™) implant 8

fluocinolone acetonide depot (Retisert™) 14
fluocinolone acetonide intravitreal implant 18, 174
- characteristics 18
- efficacy 18
- patient selection 20
- safety 19
- surgical complications 20
- surgical procedure 20

fluocinolone acetonide intravitreal implants 51
fluorescein angiographic (FA) 210
fluorescein angiography 39, 40, 49, 50, 149, 150, 161, 212
fluorescein leakage 210
fluorophotometry 140
fluoroquinolone 76
fluorouracil 28
flurbiprofen 91
foldable hydrophobic acrylic lens 90
forced hydrodissection 77, 78
foreign body giant cells 127
foreign body inflammatory response 94
foreign body reaction 147, 148
formalin 268
foscarnet 247, 261
Fox eye shield 76
frosted branch angiitis 211
Fuchs cyclitis 112, 113
Fuchs heterochromic cyclitis (FHC) 89, 100, 116
Fuchs heterochromic iridocyclitis (FHC) 85, 86, 88, 132, 133, 138, 146
Fuchs uveitis 161
Fuchs uveitis syndrome 41, 42, 153, 162

G

ganciclovir 29, 261
GDD surgery 174
general anesthesia (GA) 79
giant cell reaction 147
giant cells 138, 147
glaucoma 48, 50, 86, 88, 99, 104, 105, 112, 141, 147, 159, 162, 212
glaucoma drainage devices (GDD) 174, 175
gliosis 37
glistenings 125
glycolide-co-lactide-co-caprolactone copolymer (PGLC) 28
Goldmann–Witmer coefficient (GWc) 242, 261
Goldmann three-mirror lens 48, 54
gonioprism 134
gonioscopy 178, 232
goniosynechiolysis 135, 178
goniotomy 171, 196
gout 63

H

H-factor protein 211
Hanna corneal punch 79
Hanna suction trephine 81
Hanna vacuum trephine 77
haptics 147
Heimann scissors 268
hemorrhage 42, 141, 210
heparin 94, 100, 224
heparin surface-modified (HSM) PMMA IOLs 155
herpes iridocyclitis 161
herpes simplex 132, 133
herpes simplex (HSV-1, HSV-2) 239
herpes simplex virus (HSV) types 1 and 2 259
herpes simplex virus type 1 247
herpes zoster 132, 133
herpetic uveitis 117
heterochromia 248
heterochromic iridocyclitis 242
high-frequency echography 141
high IOP 95
highly active antiretroviral therapy (HAART) 107, 226, 260
high molecular OVD 134
HLA-B27 88
HLA B27-associated uveitis 132
HLA class I 36
HOPE fixative 262, 264
Hoskins or a Ritch nylon suture lens 187
host corneal surgery 76
HSV-2 248
HSV 1 and 2, VZV, CMV, EBV 264
HTLV-1-associated leukemia 271
human amniotic membrane (HAM) 77
human herpes virus, designated HHV-8 248
hyalocytes 36, 38
hyaluronan 38
hyaluronic acid 140
hydrodissection 152
hypercalcemia 63
hypertension 42
hyphema 89, 116, 141, 157, 161
hypopyon 39, 257
hypotension 89
hypotonous 232
hypotonous maculopathy 169
hypotony 13, 42, 48, 86, 88, 89, 90, 100, 105, 133, 134, 141, 146, 152, 160, 178, 231
– hypotony maculopathy 13
– hypotony maculopathy secondary to chronic uveitis associated with juvenile idiopathic arthritis 13
hypotony-maculopathy 231, 233

I

I-vation® 21
idiopathic arthritis-associated uveitis 88
idiopathic recurrent branch retinal arterial occlusion 211
idiopathic retinal vasculitis aneurysms and neuroretinitis (IRVAN) 211
IFN-α2a 248
IFNγ 39
IL-10 36
IL-2 receptor 37
imipenem 259
immune privilege 36, 37
immune recovery 203
immune recovery uveitis 11
immune response 239
immunohistochemistry 246, 247, 249
immunological tolerance 35, 36
immunomodulation 212
immunosuppression 35, 40, 41, 43, 100, 145, 212
immunosuppressive and immunomodulatory drugs 35
immunosuppressive medication 204
immunosuppressives 40
immunosuppressive therapy 37, 106, 113
indirect ophthalmoscopy with scleral depression 220
infectious mononucleosis 248
infliximab 12
in situ hybridization 247
in situ PCR 247
interferometry 149
interleukin-10 271
intermediate uveitis 88, 104, 133, 225, 232
internal limiting membrane (ILM) 204
interstitial keratitis 133
intracapsular implantation 138
intraepithelial dysplasia 251
intraocular inflammation 35
intraocular lens (IOL) 104, 121, 137
intraocular lymphoma 241, 256, 271
intraocular pressure (IOP) 6, 7, 87, 167
intraoperative floppy-iris syndrome (IFIS) 115
intraretinal hemorrhages 210
intravenous pulse therapy 100
intravitreal methotrexate 8
intravitreal TA 12
intravitreal triamcinolone 161, 204
invasive squamous cell carcinoma 251
IOL 147
IOL design 155
IOLMaster 150
IOP 87
iridectomy 88, 133, 134, 135, 140, 160, 168, 169
iridocorneal angle 167

iridocyclectomy 249
iridocyclitis 168
iridotomy 87, 88, 93, 115, 134, 135, 156, 157, 160
iris–lens synechiae 112
iris atrophy 85, 86, 88, 89, 112, 117
iris bombé 152, 160, 168
iris capture 140, 152
iris hook 93, 113, 114, 115, 156
iris neovascularization 85
iris nodule 248
iris nodule or granuloma 252
iris prolapse 115, 117
iris spatula 93
iris tuberculoma 247
ischemia 50, 51

J
JCA 88
jeweler's forceps 183
JIA 153, 162
JIA-associated iridocyclitis 133
JIA-associated uveitis 148
juvenile chronic arthritis 86
juvenile idiopathic arthritis (JIA) 104, 117, 132, 146, 157, 175
juvenile idiopathic arthritis (JIA) associated uveitis 100, 138
juvenile idiopathic arthritis associated iridocyclitis 85
juvenile rheumatoid arthritis 232
juvenile xanthogranuloma (JXG) 248

K
kaposi sarcoma (KS) 248
kaposi sarcoma herpes virus-associated uveitis 248
Kelly punch 191
keratectomy 64
keratitis 247
keratoplasty 11
- ALK 73, 76
- anterior lamellar keratoplasty (ALK) 73, 74
- automated endothelial keratoplasty (DLEK, DSEK, DXEK, DSAEK) 73
- DALK 73
- DALK deep ALK 74
- DLEK 73
- DLEK deep lamellar endothelial keratoplasty 74
- DSAEK descemet stripping with automated endothelial keratoplasty 74
- DSEK, DXEK, DSAEK 73
- DSEK descemet-stripping endothelial keratoplasty 74
- DXEK-A DXEK automated 74
- DXEK-L DXEK laser (femtosecond laser) 74
- DXEK-M DXEK manual 74
- DXEK descemetorhexis with endokeratoplasty 74
- endokeratoplasty 73
- FDLEK flap-associated DLEK 74
- full-thickness 67
- graft rejection 11
- MALK 73
- MALK mid-ALK 74
- optical lamellar keratoplasty 73
- PLK posterior lamellar keratoplasty 74
- posterior lamellar 67
- SALK 73
- SALK superficial ALK 74
- TALK 73
- TALK total ALK 74
Koeppe nodules 88
Koyanagi-Harada (VKH) syndrome 104
Krupin implants 170

L
lamellar corneal dissector 77
lamellar corneal surgery 67
laminin 155
LASEK 64
LASEK alcohol cup 65
laser 212
laser flare meter photometry 113
laser flare photometry 149
laser peripheral iridotomy 168, 174
laser photocoagulation 215
laser retinopexy 222
laser suture lysis 183
LEC 142, 155
lens 101
lens-related uveitis 133
lensectomy 89, 103, 146, 152, 158, 213
lens epithelial cell (LEC) 138, 147
Lens Opacity Classification System (LOCS) 39
lepromatous uveitis 247
leprosy 247
liposomes 26, 29
log minimum angle of resolution (logMAR) 38
Lucentis (ranibizumab) 178
Lyme disease 99, 210, 247
lytic cocktails 160

M
macrophages 37, 138, 147
macular atrophy 112
macular edema (ME) 7, 8, 39, 41, 42, 105, 112, 203, 204, 210, 212
macular holes 42
macular ischemia 112
macular pucker 162
magnetic resonance imaging 50

MALT lymphoma 249
masquerade syndrome 38, 88, 241
Mediterranean spotted fever 210
melt 76
membrane 105
membranectomy 156
metalloproteinase 211
metaplasia 122
methotrexate 51
methylprednisolone 41, 100, 101, 151, 212, 259
methylprednisolone acetate 51
microaneurysms 210
microbial culture 241
microincisional cataract surgery (MICS) 93
microkeratome 76
microkeratome-assisted automated preparation 76
mini spatula 246
miosis 156, 157
miotics 140, 178
mitomycin 232
mitomycin C (MMC) 89, 169, 174
modern phacoemulsification 105
Molteno implant 89, 170
monitored anesthesia care (MAC) 76
monocytes 138
mononuclear 36
mononuclear cells 35
moria anterior lamellar therapeutic keratoplasty
   (ALTK) unit 76
mucosa-associated lymphoid tissue (MALT) 249
Müller glial cells 30
multifocal chorioretinitis 37, 40, 90
multifocal choroiditis 11, 12, 203, 204, 267, 271
multilayered AMT 77
multiple sclerosis 42, 50, 210
MVR blade 106
mycophenolate mofetil (MMF) 41
mydriatics 140
myofibroblasts 139, 159

N
Nd:YAG/argon laser iridotomy 134
Nd:YAG goniosynechiolysis 170
Nd:YAG laser 54, 87
Nd:YAG laser capsulotomy 107
Nd:YAG laser iridotomy 87, 140
Nd:YAG laser vitreolysis 178
necrotizing viral retinopathies 259
neovascularization 10, 39, 47, 49, 50, 51, 86, 88, 159,
   211, 212
– of the iris 10
neovascularization of retinal vessels 148
neuropeptide 36
nitric oxide synthetase 211

non-Hodgkin lymphoma 262
nonabsorbable sutures (NAS) 77
nonpenetrating glaucoma surgery 169
nonsteroidal anti-inflammatory drug 100
Norrie disease 63
NSAID 91, 95, 96
nucleotide sequencing 247

O
occlusion therapy 148, 149, 161
occlusive retinal vasculitis (ORV) 210
OCT 42, 204
ocular hypertension 112
ocular implantable drug delivery system 24
ocular posttransplant lymphoproliferative
   disorder 247
ocular surface squamous neoplasia 251
oculocerebral lymphoma 262
oligo(deoxy)nucleotides 30
ophthalmic viscoelastic devices (OVD) 132
optical coherence tomography (OCT) 39, 50, 112,
   161, 210
optical coherent tomography 149
optic atrophy 90
opticin 38
optic neuropathy 112
oral steroids 42
orbital cellulitis 248
orbital lymphoma 249
outcome of cataract surgery by phacoemulsification
   in Fuchs heterochromic cyclitis 117

P
Paget disease 63
panretinal photocoagulation 178, 212
paracentheses 113
paracetamol 65
pars plana 38
pars plana exudates 47, 48
pars plana vitrectomy (PPV) 39, 203, 223, 258
pars planitis (PP) 42, 48, 49, 85, 88, 95, 210
pars planitis syndrome 88
particulate drug delivery system 26
patch graft 185
patient 90
PCO 142, 148, 155, 159
PCR 241, 242, 245, 247, 264
PDDS 28
pediatric cataract 121
pediatric glaucoma 194, 196
PEGylation 26
penetrating keratoplasty (PKP) 67, 72, 81
perfluorocarbon liquid (PFCL) 268
periocular corticosteroid injection 5

period of quiescence before surgery 113
perioperative immunosuppression 41
peripheral anterior synechiae 168, 178
peripheral iridectomy 174
peripheral iridoplasty 174
peripheral iridotomy 117, 174
peripheral stromal scrubbing 80
PFCL 268
phacoanaphylactic uveitis 138
phacoantigenic uveitis 148, 149
phacoemulsification 103, 104, 111, 146, 158, 213
phacoemulsification machine 114
phimosis 159
phototherapeutic keratectomy (PTK) 64, 65, 156
phthisical eye 133
phthisis 42, 105, 141, 152, 160, 162
phthisis bulbi 48, 50, 86, 90, 104, 170
pigment deposit 88
pilocarpine 178
PLA 28
plasma cell 239
platelet-derived growth factor 38
PLGA 27, 28
pneumatic retinopexy 222
POE 27
poly(lactic-co-glycolic acid) (PLGA) 24
polyanhydrides 25
- 1,3-bis(carboxyphenoxypropane) (PCPP) 25
- sebatic acid (SA) 25
polyarteritis nodosa 210, 211
polycaprolactone (PCL) 25, 28
- porous reservoir 25
polyfluorocarbon (Teflon) 123
polylactic acid (PLA) 24
polymer 24
- Complications associated with the implantation 24
polymerase chain reaction (PCR) 242, 258, 261
polymethylmethacrylate (PMMA) 121, 122
polymethyl methacrylate (PMMA) pupil dilator ring 114
polymorphonuclear leukocyte (PMN) 147
Polyvinyl alcohol (PVA) 24
Posner–Schlossman iridocyclitis 87
Posner–Schlossman syndrome 88
posterior capsular opacification 89
posterior capsular rupture 112
posterior capsule opacification (PCO) 27, 93, 95, 107, 108, 121, 138, 139, 147, 158
posterior capsule opacity 213
posterior capsulorhexis 146
posterior capsulotomy 117
posterior hyaloid 106
posterior hyaloid removal 213
posterior lamellar keratoplasty (PLK) 73

posterior scleritis 168
posterior subcapsular cataract (PSC) 9, 88
posterior synechiae 105, 146, 156, 157
posterior vitreous detachment (PVD) 38, 41, 48, 204, 211
postoperative fibrin formation 176
postoperative hypertension 141
postoperative PVR 224
Posurdex™ 14, 18, 21
potential acuity measurement (PAM) 90
povidone-iodine 8
PPV 40, 161
prednisolone 41, 96, 100, 101, 114
prednisolone acetate 5
prednisolone acetate 1% 91, 100
prednisolone succinate 100
prednisone 91
prephthisical 232
presumed ocular histoplasmosis syndrome (POHS) 12
primary central nervous system lymphoma (PCNSL) 262
primary intraocular lymphoma 250
primary intraocular lymphoma (PIOL) 262, 267
primary posterior capsulorhexis (PPCCC) 140, 159
progressive outer retinal necrosis (PORN) 259
prolene haptics 94
proliferative vitreoretinopathy (PVR) 10, 27, 29, 37, 108
prostaglandin analogs 87
prostaglandins 7
prostaglandin synthesis 122
protein levels in the anterior chamber 113
pseudoendophthalmitis 8
pseudohypopyon 8
psoriatic arthritis 232
pupillary block 134, 160, 168
pupillary membrane 87, 104, 156, 162
pupillary seclusion 87
pupil size 148
pupil stretching 114
PVA–EVA 28
PVR 42, 232

Q
questionnaire 99

R
"Rip Cord" technique 182
recombinant tissue plasminogen activator (rt-PA) 28, 87, 101
Reiter's syndrome 232
renal failure 63
retinal cryotherapy 52

Subject Index

retinal detachment 9, 48, 50, 86, 88, 107, 141, 148, 153, 168, 210, 213, 220, 221
retinal ischemia 210
retinal laser photocoagulation 54
retinal pigment epithelium (ARPE-19) cells 9
retinal pigment epithelium (RPE) 36
retinal vasculitis (RV) 209, 210, 247
retinitis-pigmentosa-like changes 50
retinopathy 256
retinoschisis 54
retinotomy 268
Retisert® 18, 174, 233
retroillumination of the iris 117
Roth spots 257
RPE 36, 37
RPE atrophy 162
rubeosis 141, 161
rubeosis iridis 89, 212
rupture of the posterior capsule 115

S

sarcoidosis 12, 37, 42, 88, 89, 99, 100, 132, 133, 153, 204, 210, 211, 232, 251, 267, 271
Sato knife 159
scanning laser ophthalmoscope 112
scleral buckling procedures 213
scleral buckling surgery 222
scleral buckling versus primary vitrectomy in rhegmatogenous retinal detachment study (SPR study) 223
scleral depression 106
scleral grafting 247
scleral nodule 246
scleral trocar 213
scleritis 246, 250
scleromalacia 246
SCORE (Standard of Care versus Corticosteroids for Retinal Vein Occlusion) 6
SCORE study 8
scotomata 210
secondary glaucoma 150
secondary implant 127
sector iridectomy 246
Seidel test 186
selective tissue corneal transplantation (STCT) 67
serous macular detachment 160
serpiginous choroiditis 12
setons 170
sharp optic edges 125
sheathing 88, 210
shrinkage 159
shunt vessels 212
silicone IOLs 155
silicone oil 231, 268

silicone oil tamponade 107
Sinskey hook 81, 114
sirolimus 28
smooth-tipped irrigating cyclodialysis spatula 134
snowball 42, 48, 88
snowbank 48, 88
snowbanking 42, 48
snowflake-like opacification in the lens optic 125
snowflake degeneration 125
Standardization of Uveitis Nomenclature (SUN) working group 39
steroid 42, 95, 161
steroid responders 8
Stevens muscle hooks 181
Stevens tenotomy scissors 181
Still disease 63
strabismus 162
straight crescent blade 76
streptokinase 87
submacular surgery 204
subretinal space 28, 272
subretinal surgery 267
Super Quad 160 lens 54
surgical peripheral iridectomy 174
sustained-release dexamethasone implant 14
sympathetic ophthalmia 12, 36, 37, 156, 169, 170
– intravitreal TA 12
synechiae 85, 86, 87, 88, 100, 113, 140, 160, 162
synechiolysis 134, 140
syphilis 87, 132, 133
systemic corticosteroid 100
systemic erythematous lupus 210
systemic lupus erythematosis 232

T

T-flux implant 169
T-lymphocytes 35, 36, 37, 38, 39
taco insertion into AC 80
tamoxifen 28
tamsulosin (Flomax) 115
tarsorrhaphy 186
telangiectasia 210
TGFb2 30
TGFβ 36
thrombospondin 1 37
thymidine kinase 247
tissue adhesive 76, 78
tissue plasminogen 140
tissue plasminogen activator (TPA) 160, 191
TNF-α 30, 37
tolerance induction 36
topical corticosteroid 96
topical corticosteroid eyedrops 100
topical steroid 41

topoisomerase II inhibitor 261
Touton giant cell 249
toxoplasmic retinochoroiditis 12
- intravitreal dexamethasone in combination with intravitreal clindamycin 12
toxoplasmosis 52, 99, 117, 210, 232
trabecular meshwork (TM) 134
trabeculectomy 88, 89, 169, 174, 196, 246
trabeculodialysis 88
traction retinal detachment 54
transforming growth factor β (TGFβ) 36
transpupillary 105
trephine 246
triamcinolone 28, 43, 106, 115, 140, 141, 158, 160, 161
triamcinolone acetonide (TA) 6, 41, 51, 100, 114, 115, 151, 158
- preservative-free formulations 8
trypan blue ophthalmic solution 77, 78
trypan blue staining 117
tube extender 185
tube inserter 185
tuberculosis 87, 99, 132, 133, 210, 247, 271
Tutoplast 185
Tyndall phenomenon 122

U

UBM (ultrasonic biomicroscopy) 232
UGH syndrome 133
ultrasonic biomicroscope (UBM) 232
ultrasonography 149
ultrasound 149, 231
ultrasound biomicroscopy (UBM) 133, 168
useful vision 177
uveal biocompatibility 148
uveal effusion 148, 160, 168
uveal response 138
uveitic macular disease 204
uveitic macular edema (UME) 204
uveitis 38, 88, 247
uveitis, glaucoma, and hyphema (UGH) syndrome 155
uveitis-glaucoma-hyphema (UGH) syndrome 132

V

valacyclovir 117
Valganciclovir 261
valves 170
vancomycin 258, 259
- intravitreal vancomycin 13
Vannas 76

Vannas scissors 93, 133, 135, 183, 246
varicella zoster 239
varicella zoster virus (VZV) 259
vascular endothelial growth factor (VEGF-A) 211
vasculitis 39, 42, 88, 161
VEGF 7
viscodissection 135
viscoelastics 93
viscoelastic substance 113
visual acuity (VA) 38, 41, 148, 210
visual deprivation amblyopia 148
visual field 150
visual rehabilitation 146
Vitrasert 29
vitrectomy 35, 56, 103, 106, 156, 212, 213, 215
vitrectomy probe 93
vitreomacular traction (VMT) 204, 205
vitreoretinal adhesion 47
vitreoretinal endoscope 231
vitreoretinal traction 210
vitreous body 38
vitreous haze 39, 88
vitreous hemorrhage 9, 42, 49, 50, 86, 88, 153, 210, 212
vitreous infiltrates 40
vitreous opacity 41, 112, 116, 148, 153
vitreous specimens 264
vitreous tap 258, 263
vitritis 48
VKH syndrome 90
Vogt-Koyanagi-Harada (VKH) syndrome 12, 168
- intravitreal TA 12
Vogt-Koyanagi-Harada disease (VKH) 37, 232

W

warfarin (Coumadin), 178
Wegener's granulomatosis 211
Weiss rings 205
Westcott 76
Westcott scissors 181, 183
white dot syndrome 37

X

Xylocaine 2% jelly 76

Y

YAG laser 160
yttrium aluminum garnet (YAG) laser 135

Z

zonular dialysis 116